Routledge Studies in Health in Africa

Series Editor: Pieter Fourie

1. **The Normalization of the HIV and AIDS Epidemic in South Africa**
   Katinka de Wet

2. **Preventing HIV Among Young People in Southern and Eastern Africa**
   Emerging Evidence and Intervention Strategies
   Edited by Kaymarlin Govender and Nana K. Poku

Preventing HIV Among Young People in Southern and Eastern Africa

This book provides an overview of the current epidemiology of the HIV epidemic among young people in Eastern and Southern Africa (ESA) and examines the efforts to confront and reduce the high level of new HIV infections among young people.

Taking a multi-dimensional approach to prevention, the contributors discuss the many challenges facing these efforts, in view of the slow progress in curbing the incidence of HIV among young people, focusing particularly on the structural and social drivers of HIV. Through an examination of these issues, chapters in this book provide valuable insights on how to mitigate HIV risk among young people and what can be regarded as the catalysts to mounting credible policy and programmatic responses required to achieve epidemic control in the region. The contributors draw on examples from a range of primary and secondary data sources to illustrate promising practices and challenges in HIV prevention, demonstrating links between conceptual approaches to prevention and lessons learnt from implementation projects in the region.

Bringing together social scientists and public health experts who are actively engaged in finding effective solutions, the book discusses which interventions work, why they work and the limitations and gaps in our knowledge to curb the epidemic among young people. As such it is an important read for researchers focusing on HIV/AIDS and public health.

Kaymarlin Govender is the Research Director at the Health Economics and HIV/AIDS Research Division (HEARD), University of KwaZulu-Natal, South Africa.

Nana K. Poku is the Executive Director at the Health Economics and HIV/AIDS Research Division (HEARD), University of KwaZulu-Natal, South Africa.

Preventing HIV Among Young People in Southern and Eastern Africa

Emerging Evidence and Intervention Strategies

Edited by Kaymarlin Govender and Nana K. Poku

Routledge
Taylor & Francis Group
LONDON AND NEW YORK

First published 2021
by Routledge
2 Park Square, Milton Park, Abingdon, Oxon OX14 4RN

and by Routledge
52 Vanderbilt Avenue, New York, NY 10017

Routledge is an imprint of the Taylor & Francis Group, an informa business

British Library Cataloguing-in-Publication Data
A catalogue record for this book is available from the British Library

Library of Congress Cataloging-in-Publication Data
A catalog record for this book has been requested

ISBN: 978-1-138-61584-7 (hbk)
ISBN: 978-0-429-46281-8 (ebk)

Typeset in Baskerville
by Apex CoVantage, LLC

Contents

Foreword

Around the world, young people bear the brunt of new HIV infections. Yet it is this particular population who also face challenges and barriers to accessing the services and programs they need in order to protect themselves. These barriers, real and perceived exist in the form of prejudicial and discriminatory attitudes among health care workers, criminalising laws, constrained policies, inefficient and unwieldy health systems and unfriendly clinics and services. Many would say we have failed young people all over the world and contributed to a sense of poor wellbeing and unsatisfactory health outcomes. We are also beginning to see a change where not only young people have found their voice but also there is increased recognition of the urgent need to intervene. However, there is still much to be done. This book written by a stellar collaboration of authors from a diverse number of research and implementation organisations, agencies and interest groups provides an excellent road map of how to go about this, at least in the Eastern Southern African region where the HIV epidemic has been rampant. It comes at a critical time in the HIV epidemic history- charged with an ambitious set of goals from UNAIDS to be met by 2030 in order to see an end to AIDS. It is also clear that unless we make headway in the groups of young people around the world, those goals will be missed.

The edited volume is structured, in its first section, to bring the reader up to date on where we are with HIV and young people in Eastern and Southern Africa and what some of the proposed and known reasons for this are. In the second part of the volume, the gears shift to possible interventions: we are introduced to what has been shown to work, what may be tried and where the knowledge gaps remain. Whilst the focus is understandably on young women and girls for sound epidemiologic reasons, the book does also cover the very important topics of young men and adolescent boys and those groups of young people who are at particularly high risk of HIV acquisition yet face some of the greatest barriers to tailored services; namely young men and transgender women who have sex with men, young people who sell sex and young people who use and inject drugs. We should also see how we can apply these ideas and lessons to young detainees, migrants and other marginalised young people. In addition, whilst HIV is the main theme, the authors collectively recognise the value of integrated service delivery for youth including other health priorities such as sexual, reproductive and mental health components. The writing is succinct and well referenced with an easily accessed reference section after each chapter.

I highly recommend this book for implementers, researchers, policy makers and all who are concerned about the state and wellbeing of young people. As is pointed out, there are applicable lessons in the era of COVID19 and to other areas of health. Failing to address the plight and needs of young people will certainly mean a prolongation of the HIV epidemic but more importantly, will also mean a missed opportunity to invest in the health of young people today, who after all are the adults of tomorrow and the parents of the world's next generation.

Professor Linda-Gail Bekker
Professor of Medicine and the Director of the Desmond Tutu HIV Centre, University of Cape Town, South Africa
Past president of the International AIDS Society (2016–2018)

Figures

Tables

Boxes

Contributors

Carolien Aantjes

Research Fellow, HEARD, College of Law and Management Sciences, University of KwaZulu-Natal, Durban, South Africa, 7535

Alice Armstrong

HIV/AIDS Specialist, Eastern and Southern Africa Regional Office, United Nations Children's Fund, Nairobi, Kenya

Russell Armstrong

Senior Research Officer, HEARD, College of Law and Management Sciences, University of KwaZulu-Natal, Durban, South Africa, 7535

Anurita Bains

Representative, Lesotho Country Office, United Nations Children's Fund, Maseru, Lesotho

Deborah Baron

STRIVE Research Consortium, Researcher and Technical Head: Good Participatory Practice, Wits Reproductive Health and HIV Institute (Wits RHI), University of Witwatersrand, Johannesburg, South Africa

Tara Beattie

STRIVE Research Consortium, Associate Professor in HIV Epidemiology, Department of Global Health and Development, Faculty of Public Health and Policy, London School of Hygiene and Tropical Medicine (LSHTM), London, UK

Asha Belsan

Senior Program Management Specialist at World Vision, Inc.

Shelby Benson

Director for Health and OVC (Orphans and Vulnerable Children) Technical Lead at World Vision, Inc.

Chris Castle

Chief of Section, Section of Health and Education, Division for Peace and Sustainable Development, UNESCO Paris

Dennis Cherian

Associate Vice President for Health and Nutrition at CORUS international, Baltimore, Maryland, USA

Christopher J. Colvin

Associate Professor, School of Public Health and Family Medicine, Division of Social and Behavioural Sciences, University of Cape Town, Cape Town, South Africa; Associate Professor, Department of Public Health Sciences, University of Virginia

Richard G. Cowden

Research Associate, Human Flourishing Program, Institute for Quantitative Social Science, Harvard University, Cambridge, MA, USA

Tamaryn L. Crankshaw

Senior Research Fellow, HEARD, College of Law and Management Sciences, University of KwaZulu-Natal, Durban, South Africa, 7535

Julie DeSoto

Program Manager and Adolescent Health Technical Lead at World Vision, Inc., The George Washington Milken School of Public Health, Washington, DC, USA

Gloria Ekpo

Former HIV and AIDS Senior Technical Advisor at World Vision, Inc.

Jane Freedman

Cresspa Centre for Sociological and Political Research of Paris, Professor at Paris 8 University

Tamar Gabelnick

Public Policy Advisor, Elizabeth Glaser Pediatric AIDS Foundation

Mitzy Gafos

STRIVE Research Consortium Co-research Director, Associate Professor, London School of Hygiene and Tropical Medicine (LSHTM)London, UK

Gavin George

Senior Research Fellow, HEARD, College of Law and Management Sciences, University of KwaZulu-Natal, Durban, South Africa, 7535

Lesley Gittings

Postdoctoral researcher, Centre for Social Science Research, University of Cape Town, Cape Town, South Africa; Factor-Inwentash Faculty of Social Work, University of Toronto, Toronto, Canada

Kaymarlin Govender

Research Director, HEARD, Professor, College of Law and Management Sciences, University of KwaZulu-Natal, Durban, South Africa, 7535

James Hargreaves

STRIVE Research Consortium. Professor of Epidemiology and Evaluation, London School of Hygiene and Tropical Medicine (LSHTM), London, UK

Lori Heise

STRIVE Research Consortium. Professor, Department of Population, Family and Reproductive Health, Johns Hopkins Bloomberg School of Public Health, Johns Hopkins School of Nursing, Baltimore, Maryland, USA

Joanna Herat

Senior Programme Specialist, Section of Health and Education, Division for Peace and Sustainable Development, UNESCO Paris

Rebecca Hodes

Director, AIDS and Society Research Unit, Centre for Social Science Research, University of Cape Town, Cape Town, South Africa

Susie Hoffman

Associate Professor of Clinical Epidemiology (in Psychiatry), HIV Center for Clinical and Behavioral Studies, Division of Gender, Sexuality and Health, New York State Psychiatric Institute and Columbia University Irving Medical Center, and Department of Epidemiology, Mailman School of Public Health at Columbia University, New York, NY, USA

Priscilla Idele

Deputy Director, UNICEF Office of Research – Innocenti, United Nations Children's Fund, Florence, Italy

Rhoda Igweta

Associate Director, Public Policy and Advocacy, Elizabeth Glaser Pediatric AIDS Foundation

Saidi Kapiga

STRIVE Research Consortium, Co-research Director, Professor of Epidemiology and International Health, London School of Hygiene and Tropical Medicine (LSHTM), Scientific Director of the Mwanza Intervention Trials Unit (MITU) Mwanza, Tanzania

Elizabeth A. Kelvin

Associate Professor, Department of Epidemiology and Biostatistics, CUNY Graduate School of Public Health and Health Policy and Investigator, CUNY, Institute for Implementation Science in Population Health, City University of New York, New York, NY, USA

Philip Kreniske

Assistant Professor of Clinical Medical Psychology in (Psychiatry), HIV Centre for Clinical and Behavioural Studies, Division of Gender, Sexuality and Health, New York State Psychiatric Institute and Columbia University Irving Medical Center, New York, NY, USA

Lebohang Letsela

STRIVE Research Consortium. Monitoring and Evaluation Specialist, Soul City Institute for Social Justice, Johannesburg, South Africa

Andrea Low

HIV Clinical and Scientific Director PHIA Project, ICAP at Columbia University and Assistant Professor of Epidemiology, Mailman School of Public Health at Columbia University, New York, NY, USA

Rita Laura Lulua

Education and Skills Lead, Mastercard Foundation Uganda and Former Project Director, SAGE Project under DREAMS IC, World Vision Uganda

Patricia Machawira

Regional Advisor on HIV and Health Education for Eastern and Southern Africa, UNESCO Harare

Joanne E. Mantell

Professor of Clinical Medical Psychology (in Psychiatry), HIV Center for Clinical and Behavioral Studies, Division of Gender, Sexuality and Health, New York State Psychiatric Institute and Columbia University Irving Medical Center, New York, NY, USA

Gerry Mshana

STRIVE Research Consortium. Principal Research Scientist, National Institute for Medical Research (NIMR), Mwanza, Tanzania

Victor Ochaya

Design, Monitoring and Evaluation Specialist, World Vision Uganda

Maryanne Ombija

Technical Advisor, Adolescent HIV Prevention and Treatment, Elizabeth Glaser Pediatric AIDS Foundation

Renato Pinto

Health Manager, Angola Country Office, United Nations Children's Fund, Luanda, Angola

Nana K. Poku

Executive Director, HEARD, and Vice Chancellor University of KwaZulu-Natal, Durban, South Africa, 7535

Tyler Porth

Statistics Specialist, Data and Analytics Section, New York Headquarters Office, United Nations Children's Fund, New York, NY, USA

Michelle Remme

STRIVE Research Consortium. Research Lead, United Nations University International Institute for Global Health (UNU-IIGH), Kuala Lumpur, Malaysia

Janet Seeley

STRIVE Research Consortium Research Director, Professor of Anthropology and Health at the London School of Hygiene and Tropical Medicine (LSHTM), London, UK; Mtubatuba, South Africa; Entebbe, Uganda

Annamarie Bindenagel Šehović

Honorary Research Fellow, Politics and International Studies (PAIS), University of Warwick, UK; Associate Fellow, Potsdam Center for Policy and Management (PCPM), University of Potsdam, Germany; Senior Analyst, Global Governance Institute (GGI), Brussels; Senior Analyst, In On Africa (IOA), Johannesburg, South Africa; Founder, Bindenagel Consulting, cc, South Africa

Catherine M. Slack

HIV AIDS Vaccines Ethics Group, School of Applied Human Sciences, College of Humanities, University of KwaZulu-Natal, Pietermaritzburg, South Africa

Anne Stangl

STRIVE Research Consortium, Senior Behavioral Scientist, International Center for Research on Women (ICRW) Washington, DC, USA; President, Hera Solutions, LLC, Baltimore, Maryland, USA

Kirsten Stoebenau

STRIVE Research Consortium, Assistant Research Professor Behavioural and Community Health, School of Public Health, University of Maryland, Baltimore, Maryland, USA

Ann E. Strode

School of Law, College of Law and Management Studies, and HIV/AIDS Vaccines Ethics Group, School of Applied Human Sciences, College of Humanities, University of KwaZulu-Natal

Elona Toska

Senior Researcher, Centre for Social Science Research; Associate Lecturer, Department of Sociology, University of Cape Town; Research Associate, Department of Social Policy and Intervention, University of Oxford, UK

Leigh A. Tucker

Lecturer and Clinical Psychologist, Psychology Department, Faculty of Community and Health Sciences, University of the Western Cape, South Africa

Robert Wamala

Deputy Director, Innovations Development and Partnerships, Directorate of Research and Graduate Training, Makerere University

Joyce Wamoyi

STRIVE Research Consortium. Senior Social and Behavioural Social Research Scientist, National Institute For Medical Research (NIMR) in Mwanza, Tanzania

Renay Weiner

STRIVE Research Consortium, Director of Research and Training for Health and Development, Johannesburg, South Africa

Nompumelelo Zungu

Research Director, Health and Wellbeing Research Unit, Human Sciences Research Council, Pretoria, 0001, South Africa; University of Pretoria, Department of Psychology, Pretoria, 0002, South Africa

Abbreviations

AADM	Adolescent Assessment and Decision-Makers
AA HA!	Accelerated Action for the Health of Adolescents
ABYM	Adolescents Boys and Young Men
ACGPR	African Charter on Human and Peoples Rights
ACHPR	African Commission on Human and Peoples Rights
ACT	Accelerated Children's HIV Treatment
AGYW	adolescent girls and young women
AHS	African Health Strategy
AIDS	acquired immune deficiency syndrome
ALHIV	adolescents living with HIV
AMSHeR	African Men for Sexual Health and Rights
ARASA	AIDS and Rights Alliance for Southern Africa
ART	antiretroviral therapy
AU	African Union
AVAC	AIDS Vaccine Advocacy Coalition
AYA	adolescents and young adults
CARMMA	Campaign for the Accelerated Reduction of Maternal Mortality in Africa
CGS	cross-generational sex
CIOMS	Council for International of Medical Sciences
COMESA	Common Market for Eastern and Southern Africa
CRC	Convention on the Rights of the Child
CSE	comprehensive sexuality education
DRC	Democratic Republic of the Congo
DREAMS	Determined, Resilient, Empowered, AIDS-free, Mentored and Safe
EAC	East African Community
EGPAF	Elizabeth Glaser Pediatric AIDS Foundation
EHPSA	Evidence for HIV Prevention in Southern Africa
EID	(re-)emerging infectious diseases
ELA	Empowerment and Livelihood for Adolescents
ESA	Eastern and Southern Africa(n)
EUP	early and unintended pregnancies
FDA	Food and Drug Administration

GABA	gamma-aminobutyric acid
GBV	gender-based violence
GF	Global Fund
GFATM	Global Fund to Fight AIDS, TB and Malaria
HEARD	Health Economics and HIV and AIDS Research Division
HIV	human immunodeficiency virus
HIVST	HIV self-testing
HLM	High Level Meeting on HIV
HPTN	HIV Prevention Trials Network
HTC	HIV testing and counselling
ICESCR	International Covenant on Economic, Social and Cultural Rights
IDU	intravenous drug user
IMF	International Monetary Fund
IPV	intimate partner violence
LGBTI	lesbian, gay, bisexual, transgender and intersex
M&E	monitoring and evaluation
MSM	men who have sex with men
MTG	Moving the Goalposts
MYSA	Mathare Youth Sport Association
NACA	National AIDS Coordinating Agency
NGO	non-governmental organisation
OAFLA	Organization of African First Ladies against HIV/AIDS
OHCHR	Office of the High Commissioner for Human Rights
OVC	orphans and vulnerable children
PEPFAR	President's Emergency Plan for AIDS Relief
PMTCT	prevention of mother-to-child transmission
PrEP	pre-exposure prophylaxis
PSABH	Primary School Action for Better Health Programme
RCT	randomized controlled trial
REC	research ethics committee
RESPECT	Rewarding Sexually Transmitted Infection Prevention and Control in Tanzania
SADC	Southern African Development Community
SA DOH	South African Department of Health
SASA	South African Sugar Association
SDGs	Sustainable Development Goals
SDH	social determinants of health
SGBV	sexual and gender-based violence
SRH	sexual and reproductive health
SRHR	sexual and reproductive health and rights
SSA	sub-Saharan Africa
STI	sexually transmitted infection
TB	tuberculosis
TWG	technical working group

UNAIDS	Joint United Nations Programme on HIV/AIDS
UNDP	United Nations Development Programme
UNESCO	United Nations Educational, Scientific and Cultural Organization
UNFPA	United Nations Population Fund
UNGA	United Nations General Assembly
UNICEF	United Nations Children's Fund
VCT	voluntary counselling and testing
VMMC	voluntary medical male circumcision
WHC	Women's Health CoOp
WHO	World Health Organization
YKP	young key populations
YPWSS	Young people who sell sex

Acknowledgement

We acknowledge with sincere gratitude funding from the South African National Research Foundation (NRF) and the Swedish International Development Cooperation Agency (Sida) that supported the development of this volume. We also acknowledge the support from Routledge Publishing Team for their guidance and advice.

We are also immensely grateful to colleagues who reviewed many versions of chapters that were included in this volume. Their comments were often critical but also helpful and kind. Among those who deserve special mention are Timothy Quinlan, Stuart Keane, Quarraisha Abdool Karim, Ayesha Kharsany, Lyn Horn, Andrew Gibbs, Mark Tomlinson, Patrick Nyamruze and Janet Seeley. We would also like to thank Christopher Jimu, our research assistant, for his meticulous work on this project. At many stages and in sometimes very different ways, we are also thankful to colleagues at UNAIDS-Eastern and Southern African team and Evidence for HIV Prevention in Southern Africa (EHPSA) program for supporting and encouraging our work during the early phases of this volume.

Finally, but not least, we dedicate this volume to our dearly loved colleagues who are no longer with us.

Noreen Huni, whose tireless work in advocating for the plight of children and young people infected and affected by HIV and AIDS was a source of inspiration to us all.

Anil Mohanlal Bhagwanjee, whose inspirational teaching and activism in the arena of public health served as a beacon of light to many in the field.

Introduction

In Eastern and Southern Africa (ESA), the region most affected by HIV, progress on the prevention of HIV transmission still remains far too slow with young people,[1] particularly among adolescent girls and young women who account for the majority of all new HIV infections. The data paints an unmistakable picture. Three in five new infections in 2019 were among women, and the incidence of HIV infections among adolescent girls and young women (aged 15–24 years) is inordinately high: they are 2.5 times more likely than their male peers to be infected and, in some countries in the region, the disparities in this age cohort is even greater (UNAIDS, 2020). Furthermore, the demographic trend of a 'youth bulge' (UNAIDSa, 2018) in the ESA population, which is associated with changing patterns of fertility, mortality and population growth, now threatens to increase the proportion of HIV infections among young people. As the overall number of young people grows, more young people are at risk of contracting HIV. In 2019 alone, 260,000 new HIV infections were recorded among young people aged 15–24 in the ESA region (UNAIDS, 2020). This negative trend is of concern given that progress towards ending AIDS as a public health threat was already off track before the coronavirus disease 2019 (COVID-19) outbreak. There are already reports from some ESA countries that 'lockdown' actions to minimise the spread of the severe acute respiratory syndrome coronavirus 2 (SARS-CoV-2) have disrupted HIV prevention and treatment services (Jewell et al., 2020). It is therefore not surprising that the UNAIDS-prescribed prevention targets for 2020 are likely to be missed (UNAIDS, 2020).

Young people are particularly at risk to HIV infection at two stages of their lives: very early in the first decade of life when HIV can be transmitted from mother to child, and later when they are adolescents and young adults and become sexually active. While programmes to prevent mother-to-child transmission (PMTCT) have been hugely successful in recent years (UNAIDSb, 2018), reducing new infections among adolescents and young adults has been slow and more difficult to achieve. In countries in the ESA region, where we have seen generalised HIV epidemics[2] mainly occurring through sexual transmission, the difficulty in reducing risk for acquisition of HIV has been very pronounced for this population. On the one hand, there are complex physical, psychological and social changes they experience in the transition from childhood to adulthood. On the other hand, they face economic, cultural, social and legal prejudice as they become sexually active; for example, cultural inhibitions against sexuality education, discrimination from nurses when they seek sexual and reproductive health services, material poverty influencing exploitative sexual relationships and, for adolescents of different gender and sexual orientations, social and legal stigma.

Therefore, the psychosocial, cultural, economic, and legal and policy challenges we face in reducing the number of new sexually acquired HIV infections are complex and interacting, and poses substantial barriers in reducing risky behaviour.

This edited volume has assembled an array of contributions from diverse and knowledgeable academics, programme implementers and policy experts in the field to record the current state of efforts to confront and reduce the high level of HIV infections among young people in ESA.

Purpose of this book

The chapters that make up this volume discuss the diverse psychosocial and structural factors that drive the sexual transmission of HIV in the ESA region and assess interventions for preventing HIV among adolescents and young people. The volume draws on a systematic appraisal and analysis of research, programmes and policy interventions in ESA settings, with critical insights on 'what works' in preventing the sexual transmission of HIV, while also acknowledging our gaps in knowledge on the implementation of interventions. The volume also draws on insights from our contributors on potentially innovative developments to inform useful and credible approaches to HIV prevention.

The book brings together mainly social scientists, HIV programmers and policy experts who are actively engaged in finding effective solutions. Collectively, the chapters discuss the complex and dynamic pathways to HIV risk, HIV prevention interventions that work, why they work and the limitations in our knowledge on how to curb the epidemic among young people.

This edited collection of writings, more specifically, provides a critical situational assessment of current psychosocial and structural developments in the field in preventing HIV. In this volume, we view the drivers of HIV transmission as the many and diverse biological, psychological, behavioural, interpersonal and societal factors which increase the risk of sexual transmission of HIV in any particular setting. While many chapters in this volume focus on HIV as primarily a sexually transmitted disease, they do so in ways that link sexual practices and psychosocial driven behaviours to the broader social, economic, legal, political and institutional factors which increase or decrease the risk of HIV infection (Auerbach, Parkhurst, and Cáceres, 2011).

The contributors to this volume are collectively driven by the concern that HIV infections in ESA are not going down fast enough, and that our global commitment to ending AIDS as a public threat by 2030 will not be achieved

(UNAIDS, 2020); the recent COVID-19 pandemic has only further slowed progress. Though this book was compiled prior to the advent of COVID-19, the recent pandemic has pushed the HIV response towards a critical juncture, both in terms of its immediate trajectory and its sustainability, as well as its place in the new global and development agenda. The unprecedented efforts to respond to the global health emergency of COVID-19 has highlighted the benefits on ensuring the continuity of HIV programming because previous disease outbreaks in ESA have demonstrated that when health systems are overwhelmed, deaths from vaccine-preventable diseases (e.g. tuberculosis) and preventable and treatable conditions like HIV tend to increase (Govender et al., 2020).

There are opportunities for tackling both the HIV and COVID-19 pandemics, yet this also occurs alongside already growing global concerns of stagnating HIV funding and other competing health priorities (e.g. the increasing prevalence of non communicable diseases such as cancer, diabetes, chronic respiratory illnesses and cardiovascular diseases), with existing and limited resources meant to cover multiple health concerns. The various contributions of authors to the volume are as pertinent as ever in this context.

Outline of the book

Collectively, the different chapters confront the challenge to reduce new HIV infections in communities, nations and states in ESA amidst the rapid growth in the population of young people. The book divides the contributions into two parts.

Part I opens with a 'setting the scene' chapter on the background to the state of the HIV pandemic among young people in ESA. Subsequent chapters cover theoretical and conceptual approaches for understanding the high risk of HIV infection among young people, the form and extent of HIV policy and programmes, and the ethical-legal complexities of involving adolescents in research to understand and find answers to improve HIV prevention interventions.

Part II considers evidence for, and challenges in, addressing the social and structural drivers of HIV among the young people, the plight of young members of key populations who face stigma and discrimination, social protection interventions and opportunities for engaging adolescent boys and young men in HIV research and prevention programming.

In Chapter 1, Govender and colleagues describe the epidemiology of HIV among young people in the ESA region. Current epidemiological data is used to outline the trajectory of new infections and numbers of people living with HIV and the mortality rates among young people. The chapter describes the heterogeneity of the HIV epidemic in terms of the differences in HIV data by age, gender and country, gaps in the HIV data and current information on the extent of human rights violations in ESA countries. The chapter makes the point that a lack of precise and context-specific data is an obstacle to HIV prevention programming.

Chapter 2 is a largely theoretical chapter, in which Cowden and colleagues consider psychosocial and development perspectives that accompany the transition from childhood to young adulthood. The authors signal the onset of puberty as a key marker for the psychological and social changes that occur during adolescence, as well as mechanisms at an ecological level that influence pathways to sexual health risks and HIV acquisition.

The next three chapters analyse different aspects of HIV-related policies and programmes. These include developments in HIV programming, recent strategies to leverage HIV-specific data to support national-level programming, the complexities inherent in navigating ethical-legal issues in HIV research with adolescents and the notion of adolescent citizenship in determining access to health services across country borders.

In Chapter 3, Gabelnick and colleagues outline the broad range of global and regional actors who have committed political and financial resources, and how they have coalesced around a distinct set of policies to reduce new infections among adolescent girls and young women. Given the nature and scope of policies within which HIV prevention programming occurs, the authors also reflect on the challenges of implementing HIV programmes at the national level and then offer some recommendations for harmonisation of processes and improving local accountability.

In Chapter 4, Armstrong and colleagues discuss a multi-sectoral, country-level approach being adopted in the region to generating adolescent-specific knowledge to guide HIV programming. The authors outline the phased process of the All In assessments and reflect on some of the successes and lessons learnt, including ongoing challenges required to sustain in-country programming. These authors signal the importance of drawing on local resources 'to know your epidemic, know your response'.

In Chapter 5, Strode and Slack base their discussion of ethical and legal complexities of undertaking research regarding HIV interventions with young people on the conventions of the rights of the child; namely, that all children are right bearers and these rights may only be limited in justifiable circumstances. They go on to argue that this principle ought to inform research and public health programming for children and young people. The authors also point out that while HIV research with adolescents requires navigating legal-ethical complexities, it is necessary and indeed possible to conduct ethically sound research among this population.

In Chapter 6, Šehović adopts the analytical lens of human security to focus on the unique challenges of adolescent populations as these relate to HIV prevention and treatment access. The chapter pays special heed to the role of citizenship, adolescent vulnerability and HIV. By invoking the human security paradigm, this chapter questions traditional approaches to HIV programming, which framed HIV as a threat to state security, and explores HIV intervention possibilities, which place the welfare of individuals and their circumstances at the centre of the analysis. Suggestions are put forward on how to protect vulnerable populations beyond country borders.

Chapters in Part II assess the evidence for 'what works', lessons learnt from HIV prevention programming and the gaps in scientific knowledge. Interventions that pay special attention to social and structural drivers of HIV and interventions that are responsive to local contextual dynamics and population profiles are more likely to be effective. However, HIV prevention programmes also have to be cost-effective and draw on local partnerships for sustainability. There is now growing international evidence and a range of local and regional programme experiences which we can draw upon to improve our understanding of what constitutes effective HIV prevention interventions.

Chapter 7 begins the section, with Gafos and colleagues reviewing interventions among young people in ESA which are designed to mitigate social and structural drivers of HIV. These social and structural drivers include factors such as limited livelihood options, low school attendance and educational attainment, poverty and gender inequality. The authors present a synthesis of existing evidence on what works to alter structural drivers of HIV risk for young people and why this works. They conclude by identifying key challenges for scaling up effective interventions.

In Chapter 8, Freedman and colleagues also focus on structural drivers but in relation to members of young key populations. They examine what is known about HIV risk and barriers to sexual and reproductive health (SRH) services among constituents of young key populations. The authors argue that young key populations have particular SRH and HIV risks as a result of experiencing considerable social discrimination and stigma in addition to the psychosocial challenges of transitioning into adulthood. Given the limited body of research with these 'difficult to access' and 'hidden' populations, the authors point to the multiplicity of pathways towards HIV vulnerability and share some insights for future programming.

Chapter 9 addresses the neglect of adolescent boys and young men in HIV prevention interventions. Mantell and colleagues review factors associated with HIV risks among adolescent boys and young men, current interventions and key gaps in research. They assert that while HIV prevalence increases rapidly at a later age among young men (mid-twenties) than among young women (late teens and early twenties), the social norms that contribute to high-risk behaviour among men are formed in the early adolescent years. Therefore, engaging boys and young men in HIV prevention programming during the formative years of young adulthood is a key aspect of effective prevention interventions.

Continuing the same theme, Gittings and colleagues in Chapter 10 adopt an *in situ* approach to working with adolescent boys and young men in HIV research. They draw on theoretical concepts such as hegemonic masculinities, power and identities to unravel the multiple and complex masculinities that influence HIV risk and HIV-related health outcomes. The authors lean on their experience of conducting qualitative research with participants over a prolonged period of time to show the ingrained nature of masculine norms and raise some interestingly conceptual and ethical questions on working with young men, including ways to address them.

In Chapter 11, Zungu and colleagues make the case for expanding social protection programmes to mitigate the vulnerabilities of adolescents living with HIV, particularly the linkages between poor adherence to treatment and sexual risk behaviours in this population. The chapter maps the complex causal pathways of key interconnected variables and provides recommendations for interventions whilst acknowledging gaps in the evidence.

Chapter 12 looks at the case for comprehensive sexuality education (CSE). Machawira and colleagues track the evolution of CSE for young people in the ESA region and examine its effectiveness on HIV and SRH health outcomes for young people. They conclude that CSE programming can contribute to reducing sexual risk behaviours and improving sexual health. However, they also point out the key challenges for effective programming, notably restrictive legal and policy environments in many ESA countries, limited in-country technical capacity and neglect of marginalised populations (e.g. out-of-school youth). Prevailing social and cultural norms are often seen as a central stumbling block to implementing CSE.

In Chapter 13, DeSoto and colleagues discuss the implementation of a School-Community Accountability for Girls Education programme in Uganda to reduce school dropout rates among adolescent girls and young women. This programme sought to reduce dropout rates through implementing a school-community early warning system to identify learners at risk of dropping out through peer-led mentoring and family visits. The authors present the evaluative findings of the intervention and also some lessons learnt during implementation of this community-based project.

The concluding chapter of the book reviews current understandings of what interventions work in mitigating social and structural drivers of HIV risk, where the limitations in current interventions are and how the gaps in our knowledge on HIV programming can be addressed. We also reflect on some key issues in evolving HIV prevention programming for young people in the region.

Notes

1 WHO (2015) defines people between 10 and 19 years of age as 'adolescents' and those between 10 and 24 years of age as 'young people'. It should, however, also be noted that adolescence is more than an age range; it represents a collection of life transitions that include biological and psychological changes, including social role changes. These transition points can occur at different ages for different people and in different contexts.

2 UNAIDS (2011) defines a generalised HIV epidemic as an epidemic that is self-sustaining through heterosexual transmission, and HIV prevalence usually exceeds 1% among pregnant women attending antenatal clinics.

References

Auerbach, J. D., Parkhurst, J. O., & Cáceres, C. F. (2011). Addressing social drivers of HIV/AIDS for the long-term response: Conceptual and methodological considerations. *Global Public Health, 6*(suppl 3), S293–S309.

Govender, K., Cowden, R. G., Nyamaruze, P., Armstrong, R. M., & Hatane, L. (2020) Beyond the disease: Contextualized implications of the COVID-19 pandemic for children and young people living in Eastern and Southern Africa. *Frontiers in Public Health, 8*, 504. doi: 10.3389/fpubh.2020.00504

Jewell, B. L., Mudimu, E., Stover, J., Ten Brink, D., Phillips, A. N., Smith, J. A., . . . Bansi-Matharu, L. (2020). Potential effects of disruption to HIV programmes in sub-Saharan Africa caused by COVID-19: Results from multiple mathematical models. *The Lancet HIV*. doi: 10.1016/ S2352-3018(20)30211-3

UNAIDS (2011). UNAIDS terminology guidelines [cited 2019 May 130]. Available from: https://www.unaids.org/sites/default/files/media_asset/JC2118_terminology-guidelines_en_1.pdf

UNAIDSa (2018). The youth bulge and HIV [cited 2020 August 16]. Available from: https://www.unaids.org/sites/default/files/media_asset/the-youth-bulge-and-hiv_en.pdf

UNAIDSb (2018). Miles to go: Closing gaps breaking barriers righting injustices [cited 2019 May 17]. Available from: https://www.unaids.org/sites/default/files/media_asset/miles-to-go_en.pdf

UNAIDS (2020). AIDSinfo [cited 2019 January 20]. Available from: http://aidsinfo.unaids.org/

WHO (2015). Health for the World's Adolescents. A second chance in the second decade, 2014 [cited 2020 August 11]. Available from: http://apps. who. int/adolescent/second-decade/files/1612_MNCAH_HWA_Executive_Summary. pdf

Part I

1 Epidemiology of HIV among adolescents and young people in the Eastern and Southern African region

What does the data tell us

Kaymarlin Govender, Nana K. Poku, Russell Armstrong and Gavin George

Introduction

Many young people's lives are characterised by rapid changes at the nexus between person and environment. The period of transition into young adulthood is also viewed as a window of positive opportunities to enter early in the biopsychosocial system of the life cycle to promote and improve sexual health. However, doing so requires, among other things, comprehensive data for proactive planning and action before HIV and SRH-related risks and vulnerabilities become entrenched. Regrettably, such data are limited in many settings, which presents a serious impediment to timely action across the spectrum from understanding risks and vulnerabilities, to early intervention, to measuring and monitoring progress. In addition, global targets to reduce new HIV infections, in particular for young people (UNAIDSa, 2016), rarely consider the implications and accountabilities that are specific to this age group. Compared with infants and adults, less is known about the individual and social factors that drive HIV risk behaviours among young people and, consequently, how to address their needs for HIV prevention, care and treatment services.

To address this gap, this opening chapter provides an overview of the epidemiology of HIV among young people in the most heavily affected part of the world, namely Eastern and Southern Africa (ESA). This region remains the most affected by the HIV epidemic, accounting for 43% of the world's HIV infections and 54% of people living with HIV globally (UNAIDS, 2020). The chapter also reviews behavioural and environmental factors that increase HIV risk for young people and highlights the challenges in the availability of reliable relevant data to systematically monitor the HIV response among this critically important population.

New HIV infections among adolescents and young people

In 2019, there were 730,000 new HIV infections in ESA (UNAIDS, 2020). In the same year, about 1.2 million adolescents (10–19 years) and 2.2 million young people (15–24 years) living with HIV were located in ESA (UNAIDS, 2020). Approximately 110,000 new HIV infections occurred among adolescents (10–19) in 2019, and 260,000 in young people (15–24 years) (UNAIDS, 2020). While estimates of new HIV infections are staggering, they mask significant regional and country-level profiles as well as differences in populations (adolescence vs young people, male vs females). These patterns in the epidemic are discussed more fully in this chapter.

In 2019, there were 130,000 new infections globally among adolescent girls (10–19 years) and 280,000 new infections among young women (15–24 years) (UNAIDS, 2020). In the ESA, there were 97,000 new HIV infections among adolescent girls and 110,000 new HIV infections among young women aged 20 to 24 (UNICEF, 2017). Females aged 15-24 accounted for 72% of all new infections. While progressive declines in new HIV infections among adolescents and young people have been noticeable over the past decade and a half (see Figure 1.1a–b), these fall-offs have not been rapid enough. The 'youth bulge' affecting the region has already contributed to these slow declines in new infections placing demands on existing health services. For example, in Mozambique, modelling suggests that there would be 53,000 fewer new infections if population growth had not occurred between 2010–2017 among young people aged 15–24 (18,000 fewer new infections in Uganda and 57,000 fewer in Nigeria) (UNAIDSa, 2018).

The majority of new infections occur among adolescent girls and young women (AGYW) aged 15 and older (58% of new infections in the population of people 15 years and older), which means that reaching the political

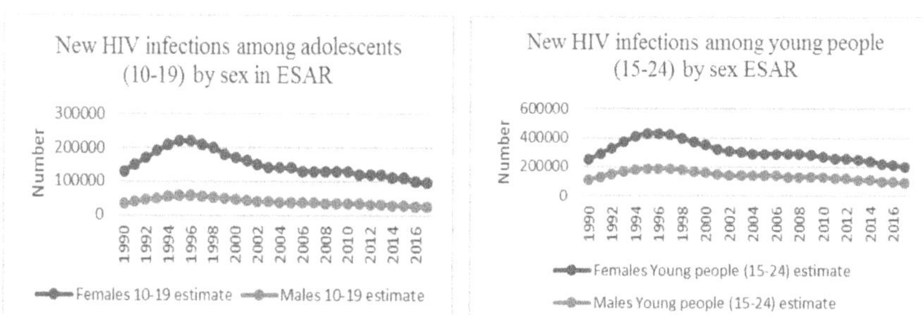

Figure 1.1a–b New HIV infections among adolescents (10–19 years) and young people (15–24 years) in the ESA region

Source: UNAIDS (2020).

declaration target of 2020 (reduce to below 100,000 per year the number of AGYW aged 15–24 newly infected with HIV globally by 2020) will not be achieved (UNAIDSb, 2016). The trend in new infections among young women is worrying in the context of the remarkable progress in the decline in new infections among children (aged 14 years and younger) between 2010 and 2016 in the ESA with more than a 50% reduction in nine countries (UNAIDS, 2020).

Generally, boys and young men in ESA have lower infection rates as compared to AGYW. In 2017, there were 25,000 new infections among 10–19-year-old boys (more than six times lower than girls in the same age range) and 89,000 new infections among 15–24-year-old young men (approximately four times lower than girls in the same age range). Differentiation in country-level profiles is evidenced in recent data which suggests that most new infections occur among adolescent girls (15–19 years) in four countries (South Africa, Kenya, Uganda and Zambia), while the majority of new infections that occur among young women (20–24 years) is present in eight countries of which Tanzania, Mozambique and Zimbabwe rank the highest (UNAIDS, 2020) (Figure 1.2a–b).

South Africa has, by far, the highest estimated number of new infections per week: 1500 among young women (15–24 years) and 640 among young men (15–24 years) (UNAIDS, 2020).

Young people living with HIV

The number of 15–19-year-olds living with HIV in the ESA was as high as 490,000 among adolescent girls and 270,000 among adolescent boys (UNICEF, 2017). When compared to males of the same age group, AGYW represent the largest population of people living with HIV (Figure 1.3a–b). In countries with a generalised epidemic,[1] where data is available, HIV prevalence among adolescent females tends to be considerably higher than among adolescent males, suggesting that context may heighten adolescent girls' sexual risks and vulnerabilities (see Chapter 7 for a detailed discussion on structural drivers of HIV among young people in ESA). Most countries with the highest HIV prevalence rates in the world are in Southern Africa. Age-specific prevalence data show a distinctive sex disparity in HIV prevalence by the age of 15 years.

For example in Eswatini, where adult prevalence is estimated to be the highest globally at over 27% in 2017 (UNAIDSa, 2017), a survey found that HIV prevalence among younger adolescents (10–14 years) is low and more comparative with young children (10 years and younger), but prevalence begins to increase in adolescent girls aged 15–19 and young women 20–24, where it is two and four times as high as boys in the same age ranges (SHIMS2, 2019). HIV prevalence rates can reach nearly 21% in young women aged 20–24, rising to nearly 40% by ages 25–29 (SHIMS2, 2019).

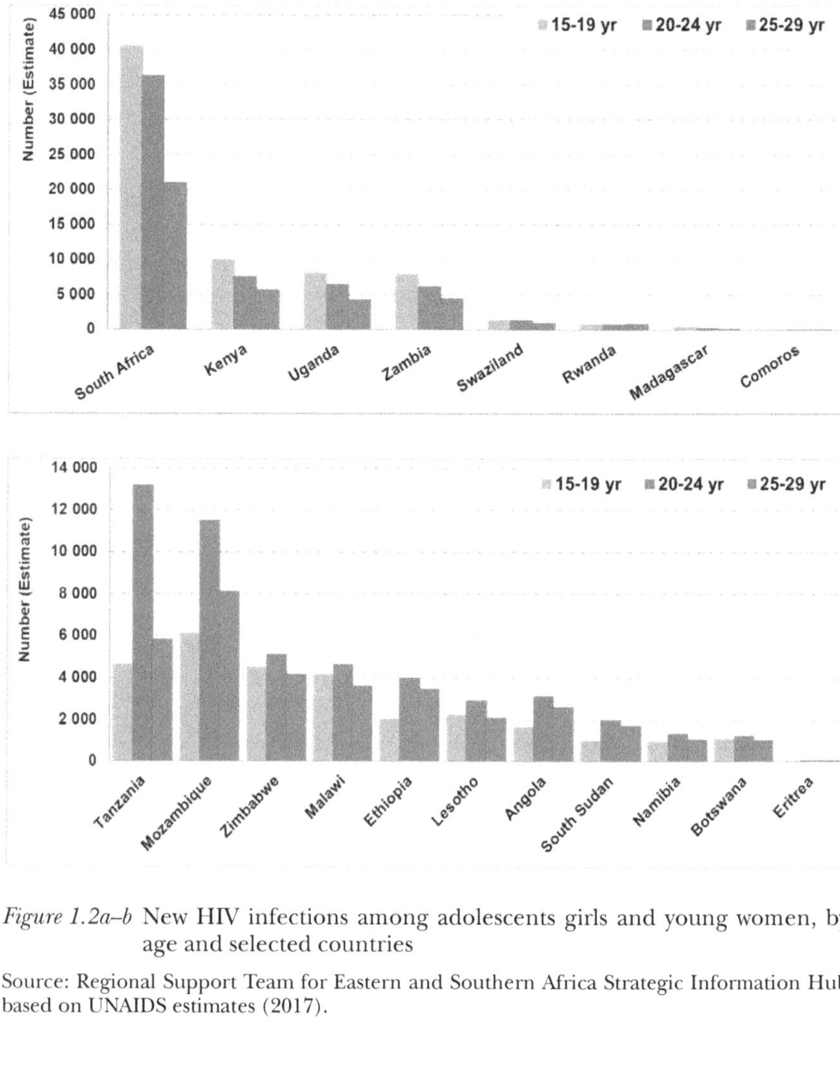

Figure 1.2a–b New HIV infections among adolescents girls and young women, by age and selected countries

Source: Regional Support Team for Eastern and Southern Africa Strategic Information Hub based on UNAIDS estimates (2017).

The high prevalence among this group living with HIV suggests the need to focus on reducing onward transmission through regular testing and early initiation on ART (UNAIDSb, 2016). In fact, the findings of the HPTN052 study have challenged the assumption that HIV treatment and prevention are distinct (Cohen et al., 2011), with a growing body of research demonstrating how HIV treatment and prevention are intrinsically connected (Refer to Chapter 11 for an assessment of the promising approach of social protection which may alleviate the compounded vulnerabilities of young people living with HIV).

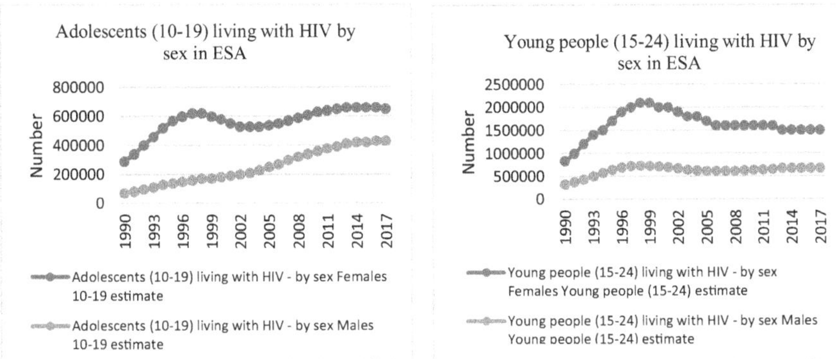

Figure 1.3a–b Adolescents and young people living with HIV in ESA

Source: UNAIDS (2020).

AIDS-related deaths among young people

AIDS-related deaths among adolescents have been steadily declining since 2010 with progressive expansion of ART programmes (see Figure 1.4a–b). However, declines have been more rapid between 2010 and 2019 among young women, from 28,000 to 18,000 (15–24 years), than among young men in the same age range 13,000–12,000 (see Figure 1.4b).

The data on new infections and AIDS-related deaths paints a complex picture of country-level epidemics and differences in patterns by age, gender and location. More generally, AIDS-related deaths are declining among young people, especially among young women, while young men seem to be more at risk of dying from AIDS (refer to Chapter 9, which addresses the issue of boys and young men being left behind in HIV prevention programming).

HIV data among young key populations (YKP)

Certain groups of adolescents and young people may have additional HIV-related vulnerabilities related to one or more characteristics such as sexual orientation, gender identity or gender expression; being sexually exploited[2]; struggling with drug addiction; or being in conflict with the law, including being in a place of detention. The term 'young key populations' (YKP) links these groups together, as they have in common a number of structural barriers and challenges that persist across a wide range of regional and country contexts (Bekker & Hosek, 2015). These

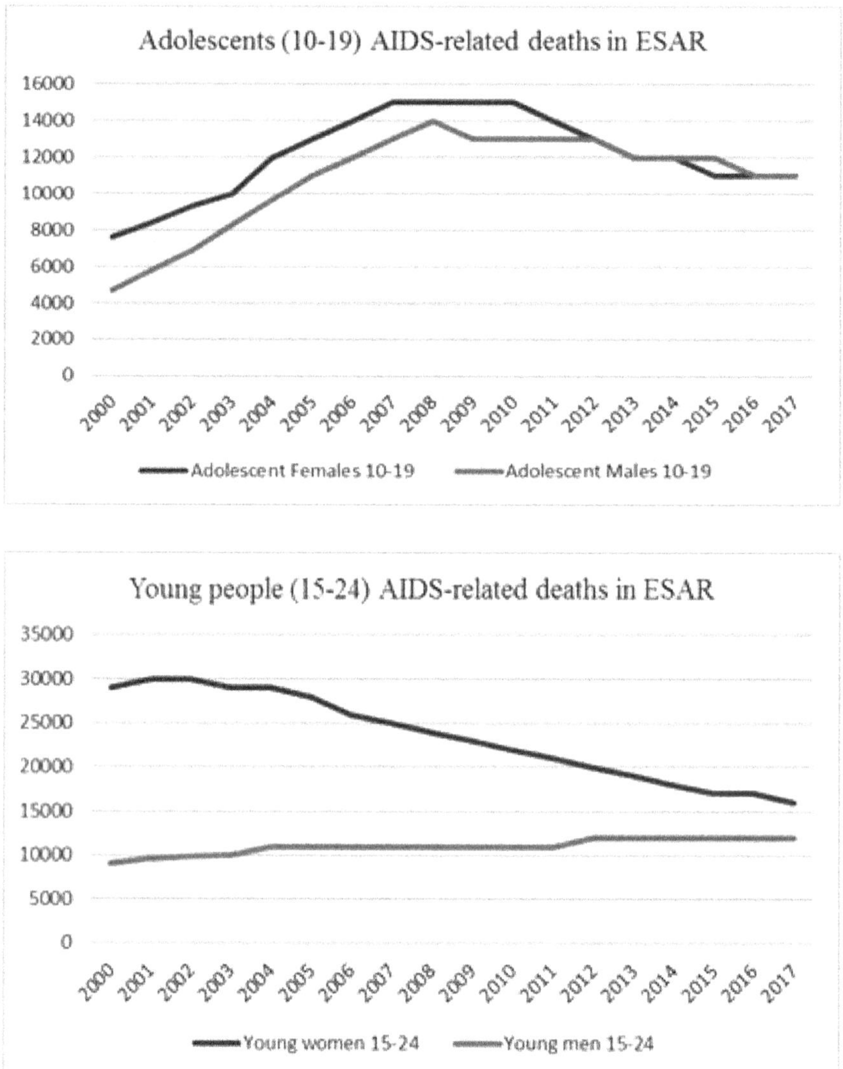

Figure 1.4a–b HIV-related deaths among adolescents (10–19) and young people (15–24) in ESA

Source: UNAIDS (2020).

barriers include a very high incidence of stigma, discrimination and violence, much of which is fuelled by criminalisation and other discriminatory laws and policies, as well as by highly stigmatising and exclusionary social, religious or cultural attitudes, beliefs or practices. As a result, many of these young people face the highest risks of acquiring HIV and the least access to HIV services and related interventions to either prevent HIV infection or to benefit from treatment care and support when they become HIV-positive (Muller, Spencer, Meer, & Daskilewicz, 2018; Cornell & Dovel, 2018).

Although global estimates indicate that more than half of all new adult HIV infections in 2018 occurred among individuals from key population (KP) groups and their sexual partners (UNAIDS, 2020), the situation for ESA is more complex where, in the midst of a generalised epidemic, it was estimated that 25% of all new HIV infections in ESA in 2018 were among KP groups (UNAIDS, 2020). However, the latter statistic masks a significant variation in data according to country, age band and type of KP group. For example, more than a third (39%) of all new HIV infections in Kenya in 2017 occurred among adolescents and young people (aged 15–24 years), an increase from 29% in 2013 (Kenyan Ministry of Health/National AIDS Control Council, 2018). In Madagascar, the only country in ESA where new HIV infections are increasing dramatically (154% since 2010), this figure is estimated to be as high as 50%, primarily among men who have sex with men (UNAIDS**b**, 2018). Comprehensive, disaggregated data is, however, scarce and therefore the detailed regional picture cannot be fully known.

Globally, young people between 15 and 24 years of age who share KP characteristics are at much higher risk of acquiring HIV than their age-matched non-KP peers in the general population (WHOa, 2015). For example, in Mozambique, compared to adult MSM, young MSM reported lower health seeking behaviours, had a low perception of their HIV risk and more reported never having an HIV test (Boothe et al., 2020). The increased risk can be the result of compounding factors which include the many similar vulnerabilities that place all adolescents and young people in the path of HIV infection on the one hand, and the more specific challenges arising from structural/environmental factors on the other hand, such as social stigma and discrimination, physical and sexual violence, lack of community empowerment, violations of human rights, and laws and policies that criminalise drug use, sex work and diverse forms of sexuality, gender identity and gender expression (Bekker & Hosek, 2015; Baggaley, Armstrong, Dodd, Ngoksin, & Krug, 2015; Brook, Morojele, Zhang, & Brook, 2006). There is a growing number of sources demonstrating that the situation is at least similar, if not more complex and serious, for YKP across ESA (Muller et al., 2018).

Data on YKP are limited within contexts of generalised HIV epidemics in the region. Where previous data are available, trends suggest that HIV prevalence (and, by inference, new infections) are disproportionally high among YKP as compared to their age-matched, non-KP peers in the general population. In Zambia, for example, a study carried out in 2013 found that HIV prevalence for young MSM was 8.7% for those under age 20 and 15.7% for those aged 21–25 (Kiefer, Witola, Hansende, Handema, & Siantombo, 2013). By contrast, population-wide HIV prevalence was much lower where it was 4.1% and 7.3% for adolescent (15–19 years) and young (20–24 years) males, respectively (Central Statistical Office, 2015). The situation is similar for young people who use drugs; for example, in a study carried out in 2014 in Mozambique, 19% of male participants aged 18–24 were HIV-positive (Ministério da Saúde (MISAU) and Instituto Nacional de Saúde (INS), 2017). This compared to an HIV prevalence rate of 5.3% among all males aged 20–24 in the country in that same year (MISAU, INE, & ICF, 2019). In 2018, HIV prevalence among women who sell sex in Tanzania was estimated at 15.4% compared to an adult prevalence of 4.6% (UNAIDS, 2019, pp. 68–69). Such differences for young women who sell sex are also pronounced. In Mozambique, among young women who sell sex (15–24 years), this group had almost double (17.2%) HIV prevalence figures compared to women in their same age group (9.8%) (Boothe et al., 2020).

Comparable data for young transgender people or young people in conflict with the law do not exist across ESA. In a recent study across eight African countries, HIV prevalence for adult transgender women was 25% as compared to 14% for cisgendered MSM (Poteat et al., 2017). There was no age-specific disaggregation of the results, although the mean age of the sample was 24 years. ESA has one of the highest rates of HIV prevalence among prisoners globally (Dolan et al., 2016). A number of countries, for complex reasons, incarcerate older adolescents with adults in environments which are characterised by overcrowding, physical and sexual violence and abuse, gang cultures and chronic under-nourishment, among other threats. Young people in these settings face extreme disadvantages to negotiate and secure their personal safety, let alone their sexual and reproductive health (Telisinghe et al., 2016).

While comprehensive data regarding the sexual and reproductive health of young key populations remain elusive across ESA, what can be inferred from data that is available gives a seriously discouraging picture. Among other barriers, discriminatory and exclusionary attitudes and practices pervade the research environment in much of the region, blocking needed attempts to address the significant data gaps. Such efforts are still viewed too often by institutional review boards as either attempts to legitimise or promote criminalised and stigmatised behaviours or identities among adolescents or young people considered to be vulnerable to such negative influences (Delany-Moretlwe et al., 2015). Or they are seen as having little scientific merit or policy-related or programmatic utility, since governments and others express up front their unwillingness to act on research results (Muller et al., 2018). Fortunately, as Chapter 8 in this collection explores, this situation is now beginning to change.

Knowledge and behavioural factors

HIV knowledge

By 2015, 15 out of 21 countries were providing comprehensive sexuality education (CSE) and life skills in at least 40% of primary and secondary schools, and all 21were including sexual and reproductive health (SRH) and CSE training for prospective teachers (UNESCO, 2017). Despite widespread HIV prevention messaging in school and media campaigns, evidence shows low HIV-related knowledge among adolescents: only 26% of the girls and 33% of the boys aged 15–19 in sub-Saharan Africa know how HIV is transmitted and how it can be prevented (UNAIDSa, 2016). Only 36.1% of young people aged 15–24 had correct knowledge about sexual transmission of HIV and rejection of major misconceptions about HIV transmission in South Africa (HSRC, 2019), whilst 44.7% of young women and 42.0% of young men in Zimbabwe (MOHCC, 2019), and 24% of girls and 22% of boys aged 10–14 in Botswana, had comprehensive knowledge about HIV (BAIS, 2013) (see Table 1.1). Lacking the necessary knowledge and skills, younger adolescents are less likely to protect themselves from HIV than older people. Given the importance of sexuality education in the ESA region, Chapter 12 addresses the evolution of CSE programmes in the region and the challenges associated with the scale-up of these programmes. Chapter 13 also discusses the complexities of HIV programming to keep young women in schools. Other studies have established that only 36.1% of young people aged 15–24 had accurate knowledge about the sexual transmission of HIV and rejection of major misconceptions about HIV (HSRC, 2019).

Sexual debut

Sexual debut coincides with adolescence for the majority of people in many countries, where unmarried girls and boys are sexually active before the age of 15 (Doyle, Mavedzenge, Plummer, & Ross, 2012). Among 15–24-year-olds, a higher percentage of young men than young women have had sex before age 15. In South Africa, 19.5% of young men and 7.6% of young women reported having had sex before age 15 (HSRC, 2019), compared to 5.1% of young men and 2.7% of young women in Zimbabwe (MOHCC, 2019) and 4.5% of young men and 2.5% of young women in Eswatini (SHIMS2, 2019). While self report data is unreliable, adolescents who start having sex early are more likely to have sex with high-risk partners or multiple partners, and are less likely to use condoms (Pettifor, O'Brien, MacPhail, Miller, & Rees, 2009; Ningpuanyeh & Sathiya Susuman, 2017). Early sexual debut places young women at risk of tissue injury during intercourse, and the existence of greater proportions of genital mucosa which are present in an immature cervix further increase the risk of HIV infection

Table 1.1 HIV knowledge, testing behaviours, sexual practice and consent laws by age and country

	Know where to get an HIV test		*Ever tested for HIV and received the results*		*Tested for HIV in the last 12 months and received the results*		*Knowledge about HIV prevention among young people*		*Percentage who had 2+ partners in the past 12 months*		*Percentage who reported using a condom during last sexual intercourse*		*Laws requiring parental consent for adolescents to access HIV testing*
	Age 15–19		*Age 15–19*		*Age 15–19*		*Age 15–24*		*Age 15–24*		*Age 15–24*		
	Girls	*Boys*	*Girls*	*Boys*	*Girls*	*Boys*	*Girls*	*Boys*	*Girls*	*Boys*	*Girls*	*Boys*	
Angola	58.0	50.6	21.7	6.9	15.7	4.2	32.5	31.6	1.7	9.4	30.5	39.1	–
Botswana	–	–	–	–	–	–	47.4	47.1	–	–	–	–	Yes (<16 years)
Ethiopia	61.7	73.7	22.4	18.2	12.4	8.9	24.3	39.1	0.3	1.8	21.8	45.5	Yes (<18 years)
Kenya	71.5	90.4	52.7	–	35.3	26.6	56.6	63.7	1.5	9.6	37.5	68.9	Yes (<16 years)
Lesotho	90.2	84.2	56.5	–	40.5	24.9	37.6	30.9	5.1	22.7	67.2	78.2	Yes (<12 years)
Madagascar	34.5	36.3	4.7	–	2.0	0.8	22.9	25.5	2.4	18.2	6.6	8.8	Yes (<18 years)
Malawi	87.1	88.4	47.7	–	31.9	22.0	41.1	44.3	1.3	12.9	49.9	75.3	Yes (<16 years)
Mozambique	75.5	67.2	40.0	–	25.3	10.1	30.8	30.2	2.9	25.3	38.3	40.8	Yes (<12 years)
Namibia	93.2	86.9	41.7	–	28.5	13.9	61.6	51.1	2.8	9.2	–	79.4	Yes (<16 years)
Rwanda	97.9	95.1	52.5	–	27.4	21.9	64.6	64.3	0.7	1.9	61.2	75.0	Yes (<12 years)
South Africa	85.6	87.8	49.1	–	38.4	28.7	46.1	45.6	9.0	25.5	49.8	67.7	Yes (<12 years)
Eswatini	91.5	88.6	52.3	–	40.8	30.4	49.1	50.9	3.8	28.5	58.2	66.7	Yes (<18 years)
Uganda	89.4	89.4	53.6	–	39.4	28.4	45.7	44.8	2.7	14.3	26.4	41.4	Yes (<16 years)
Zambia	89.8	89.1	47.5	–	32.6	19.4	41.5	46.7	1.7	10.6	39.4	40.6	Yes (<16 years)
Zimbabwe	87.0	86.8	46.3	–	29.8	19.4	46.3	46.6	1.3	9.3	44.2	65.7	Yes (<16 years)

Source: UNICEF (2018); UNAIDS (2020); DHS (2014, 2015, 2018); HSRC (2019); SHIMS2 (2019); MOHCC (2019).

(Higgins, Hoffman, & Dworkin, 2010; UNAIDSa, 2016). Early sexual debut is also associated with age-disparate sexual relationships, and these partnerships with older men provide greater exposure to HIV because sex is more frequent, condom use is less consistent, partners are violent and HIV prevalence is higher among men (between 25–30 years) than among adolescent boys (Jewkes, 2002; Evans et al., 2016; De Oliveira et al., 2017). Further, risk of HIV acquisition is higher among young women partly due to the high prevalence of child marriage in Africa (CHR, 2018). Child brides are often unable to effectively negotiate safer sex, leaving themselves vulnerable to sexually transmitted infections, including HIV, along with early pregnancy (UNICEF, 2013).

Condom use and multiple sex partners

Condom use is a critical part of the cascade of interventions for HIV prevention. Unprotected sexual activity and multiple sexual partners increase the risk of HIV infection and other sexually transmitted infections (STIs) among young people. Reported condom use within non-marital partners remains well below 50% in the majority of countries in sub-Saharan Africa (Doyle et al., 2012). In 2017, in South Africa it was estimated that 67.7% of young men aged 15–24 reported using condoms at their last sexual encounter, down from 85.2% in 2008 (HSRC, 2019). Young men aged 15–24 are more likely than their female counterparts to have had more than one sexual partner (25.5% vs 9.0%). However, condom use is more common among young men; 68.1% of young men with more than one partner in the past 12 months reported using a condom with their most recent sexual partner, as compared with 47.3% of young women. Similar trends were noted in Zambia and Kenya, where young men were much more likely than young women to report having multiple sexual partners (11% vs 2%; 9.6% vs 1.5%). Among young women and men who had multiple partners in the past 12 months, 33.7% and 49.1% in Zambia and 37.5% and 68.9% in Kenya, respectively, reported using a condom during their last sexual encounter (DHS, 2018) (see Table 1.1). Interventions with men and boys on HIV prevention often does not acknowledge multiple and complex masculinities, and the experiences and conditions that shape them. Approaches and strategies are needed that dynamically and effectively engage adolescent boys and young men in research, policy and programming (refer to Chapter 10 for a more a critical discussion on HIV research with boys and men and implications for theory and practice).

HIV testing

The World Health Organization recommends regular testing every 6–12 months for people who are engaging in sexual activity and have potential exposure to HIV (WHOb, 2015). Testing for HIV regularly is key to prevent onward HIV transmission and starting antiretroviral treatment early will lead to viral suppression. Despite a high prevalence of HIV infection among adolescents and young adults in ESA, uptake of HIV testing and counselling (HTC) among this population in the region remains sub-optimal. Young women aged 15–24 are more likely than young men in the same age group to know where to get an HIV test, to have been tested for HIV and to have received the test results. In ESA, 71.9% girls (15–19 years) and 77% boys (15–19 years) know where to get an HIV test; 35.2% girls and 26.5% boys have ever been tested for HIV and received the results; and 23.6% girls and 16.1% boys have been tested for HIV in the last 12 months and received the results (UNICEF, 2017) (see Table 1.1). To compound this, most recent data indicate that only 23% of adolescent girls and 17% of adolescent boys aged 15–19 in ESA have been tested for HIV in the past 12 months and received the result of the last test (UNICEF, 2018). However, encouraging data from South African national community surveys reveal an increase in testing rates amongst adolescents and young people from 19.3% in 2005 to 58.8% in 2017 (Jooste et al., 2020).

HIV treatment and care

Access to ART for young people is unknown because data is disaggregated by children under 15 years and adults over 15 years. The majority of young people living with HIV in the region are not receiving care and treatment because they do not know they have HIV as they have not been tested. Among people living with HIV aged 15–24 years in Eswatini and Zimbabwe, 54.1% and 42.4%, respectively, reported awareness of their HIV positive status and ART use (SHIMS2, 2019; MOHCC, 2019). The viral load suppression (VLS) for the same age group in these countries was 50.6% for Eswatini and 45.3% for Zimbabwe. In 2017, in South Africa, an estimated 274,000 young people aged between 15 and 24 were living with HIV and receiving ART (HSRC, 2019). Overall, it is estimated that 47.7% of young people (15–24 years) living with HIV in South Africa in 2017 were virally suppressed (HSRC, 2019). In 2019, suppressed viral loads were highest in Eswatini (92%), Botswana (79%), Zambia (77%), Zimbabwe (73%), Malawi (72%), Kenya (68%) and South Africa (64%) (UNAIDS, 2020). Older adolescents (15–19 years) are the only age group with increasing HIV mortality at a time of massive scale-up of treatment programs and when mortality is declining in all other age groups (UNICEF, 2015). High adolescent HIV mortality reflects critical gaps in the HIV care cascade, including low rates of retention in care and complex challenges with adherence to antiretroviral therapy (ART). Additionally, age-restrictive laws and policies that govern the age of consent for HIV testing and access to sexual and reproductive health services present barriers to young people accessing health services, including ART.

A common concern limiting uptake of HTC among youth is around confidentiality and being judged. This is especially evident among young people who are at risk of HIV infection but may feel as if they would be judged for being sexually active. Many countries have policies and laws restricting adolescent access to testing in clinic settings, with some requiring parental consent for young people to access HTC (UNAIDSa, 2018). In countries where same-sex behaviour and sex work is illegal, YKP face enormous barriers to accessing traditional services due to fear of stigmatisation, discrimination and even criminalisation. Adolescents and young people in ESA face unique legal, policy and environmental challenges in accessing HTC services. Efforts to improve HIV treatment and care requires government to ensure that they provide youth-friendly services where healthcare professionals are non-judgemental and supportive and combat laws and policies that impede access to HCT services.

Surveillance systems, gaps in data and disaggregation

Over the course of the past decade, the global health community have made significant political and financial commitments to reducing HIV infections among young people, particularly adolescent girls and young women (refer to Chapter 3 for an overview of the regional and global responses to prevent HIV among young people). However, measuring the impact of these initiatives in reducing HIV infections is complex given the number of interventions being implemented in various combinations. Actors are also learning while doing, regularly refining solutions as new data becomes available. In the following, we outline current challenges with data to inform effective HIV programming.

HIV science has evolved rapidly, and we now have a number of methods to measure HIV incidence (e.g. cohort estimation, mathematical modelling, inference incidence from antenatal clinic data, laboratory tests, a combination of HIV testing algorithms), each with benefits and limitations (Buthelezi, Davidson, & Kharsany, 2016). More recently, these methods have been complemented by phylogenetic and geospatial epidemiology (Tanser, Bärnighausen, Grapsa, Zaidi, & Newell, 2013). However, some of these methods employ newer technologies, therefore more expertise and resources are required for implementation, especially in low-resourced settings. At present, most national surveillance systems are not fully equipped to implement location-based approaches at sub-national or at health facility levels (Buthelezi, Davidson, & Kharsany, 2016). Lack of specific data means that it becomes difficult to disentangle estimates of adolescent HIV prevalence which currently include both those that have acquired HIV through mother-to-child transmission (vertical transmission) and those who acquired HIV behaviourally through unprotected sex or sharing of non-sterile injecting needles (horizontal transmission). Apart from modelled estimates, we are not clear on what proportions constitute 'vertical' versus 'horizontal' transmissions among all adolescent living with HIV (Prudden et al., 2013). Context-specific data is needed to understand the main modes of transmission in young people. More recently, there has been systematic efforts to gather national data to support the development of more effective programmes and services for adolescents living with and affected by HIV. Chapter 4 discusses progress made in the All In initiative implemented in 14 priority countries in ESA and the impact of the initiative on HIV programming for adolescents across the region.

We have previously noted differences in AIDS-related deaths among adolescents and young people by gender. Apart from UNAIDS estimates, we have little empirical data on adolescent deaths to validate these trends (UNAIDS, 2020). The lack of context-specific data is further compounded by low rates of HIV testing (UNICEF, 2017). Low testing rates among young men could explain the increase in AIDS-related deaths because they are more likely not to know their HIV status, are unlikely to be on ART treatment (UNAIDS**b**, 2017), have a lower cluster of differentiation for when they start treatment, more likely to interrupt treatment or be lost to follow-up. Consequently, men are less likely to achieve viral load suppression, which is associated with higher HIV-related mortality.

The period of adolescence reflects a wide development span, and the characteristics of 10-year-olds are very different to those of 19-year-olds. Currently, there is no standard method for disaggregated data by age band. Even where data exists, disaggregation, sample size and interpretation is often limited. Lack of data on younger adolescents (10–14 years) impedes understanding of sexual practices and nature of sexual risk (e.g. type of sexual partners), which makes it difficult to tailor sexual risk reduction programmes for younger people to reduce HIV acquisition before they get older. For hidden populations, such as young people who are members of key populations, there is a lack of reliable estimates of population sizes which impacts directly on resource allocations for HIV programming (Sawyer et al., 2012). In general, methodological issues including small sample sizes, especially among younger cohorts, and reliance on self-reported behavioural data makes generalisability of behavioural data questionable (see MannionDaniels, 2018). Further, scant data also exists on the broader health and social issues of young populations (e.g. mental health, developmental adjustments to social environments and decision-making skills), with little research looking specifically on the social determinants of health for adolescents and young people as a distinct group from other age groups (also refer to Chapter 2 for an in-depth discussion on social and structural vulnerabilities that are likely to affect the developmental trajectories and health risk behaviour of young people living in ESA).

Many of the data relate to adult samples only or do not disaggregate young people from younger children or adults, yet the contexts and challenges of life as an adolescent and young adult can be markedly different to those of other ages. This is especially so for adolescents, where age of consent policies that are intended to protect minors often have the unintended effect of limiting independent access to health services (e.g. HIV testing, see Table 1.1.) and their ability to participate in HIV related research. Chapter 5 discusses, more critically, some of the complexities of undertaking HIV prevention research with persons who have evolving capacity to make health-related choices and who are accorded special protections in law.

In many countries, adolescents require parental permission to access testing, treatments or procedures. This is a particular problem for minors who do not live with their parents or do not wish to disclose their behaviour to them. For example, young women seeking contraception or safe abortion services are likely to seek care outside of conventional health services (Francome, 2015). While there is substantial evidence for effective interventions to prevent and treat HIV infection in adults, less is known about the delivery of these interventions to adolescents (Mavedzenge, Luecke, & Ross, 2014). Current coverage of services for YKP is generally low (Dhana et al., 2014), and consideration of optimal service delivery models that respond to current barriers to care are now a priority. Further, given the regionality of the HIV epidemic, arguments have been made for HIV interventions as they pertain to and protect vulnerable populations beyond borders (see Chapter 6 for assessing for health security beyond borders of citizenship).

It is acknowledged that multiple types of data (behavioural and sociocultural) are needed to understand social drivers of HIV infections and that specific data-gathering methodologies provide limited understandings on the complexity of HIV epidemics with potentially conflicting accounts. For example, in Botswana condom use is reportedly high and exceeds national targets for both sexes, yet adolescent HIV incidence rates and early pregnancy rates are increasing (UNICEF, 2013). More efforts are needed to interrogate potentially conflicting data reported on adolescents and young people. We can only achieve this through evolving our national data systems to be more comprehensive (biological, behavioural and social data) while improving quality. Further, reliable age-appropriate behavioural questions in surveys that conform to ethically appropriate research with minors are needed. Special consideration should be given to key populations and other situations where illegal behaviour may be involved and where the value of researching these populations needs to be balanced against legal and ethical considerations, and foremost ensuring their safety (Idele et al.,

2014). We need to enhance the abilities of researchers, ethics review committees and funders to undertake sensitive research to support policy and programming.

Conclusion

Intervening early in the life cycle of young people is a priority before they become sexually active and gender roles and associated behaviours become entrenched with potentially negative consequences for later sexual health. To strengthen HIV programming, it is clear that more accurate data on HIV risk is required to enable better programming. Mannion-Daniels (2018) asserts that one solution to the data disaggregation problem is to use five-year age bands (10–14 years; 15–19 years; 20–24 years) (UNICEF, 2016), with further subdivisions also being useful. Good data is essential for informing and shaping effective HIV interventions. Without accurate data gathering, analysis, and reporting systems specific to adolescents and young people, national and international communities can neither measure progress towards reducing new infections nor use the knowledge that comes from such systems to implement efficacious programs that can improve health outcomes for adolescents. Throughout this book, chapter authors make the point for the need to have context-specific HIV data, disaggregated by age, gender and population profile, to improve HIV programming.

Notes

1 The HIV prevalence rate is >1% in the general population.
2 Sex work, in this volume, is used when referring exclusively to adults aged 18 years or older. When referring to those below the age of 18, including 10–17 years olds, reference is made to sexual exploitation of children (in accordance with Article 34 of the Convention on the Rights of the Child, UNGA,1989).

References

Baggaley, R., Armstrong, A., Dodd, Z., Ngoksin, E., & Krug, A. (2015). Young key populations and HIV: A special emphasis and consideration in the new WHO consolidated guidelines on HIV prevention, diagnosis, treatment and care for key populations. *Journal of the International AIDS Society*, 18(1), 85–88.

BAIS (2013). Botswana AIDS impact survey IV. Statistical report [cited 2019 February 23]. Available from: www.statsbots.org.bw/sites/default/files/publications/BOTSWANA%20AIDS%20IMPACT%20SURVEY%20IV%202013.pdf

Bekker, L. G., & Hosek, S. (2015). HIV and adolescents: Focus on young key populations. *Journal of the International AIDS Society*, 18(2 Suppl 1).

Boothe, M., Baltazar, C. S., Sathane, I., Raymond, H. F., Fazito, E., Temmermen, M., & Luchters, S. (2020). Young key populations left behind: The necessity for a targeted response in Mozambique. Available from: https://orcid.org/0000-0002-5362-5106

Brook, D.W., Morojele, N.K., Zhang, C., & Brook, J.S. (2006). South African adolescents: Pathways to risky sexual behavior. *AIDS Education & Prevention*, 18(3), 259–272.

Buthelezi, U.E., Davidson, C.L., & Kharsany, A.B. (2016). Strengthening HIV surveillance: Measurements to track the epidemic in real time. *African Journal of AIDS Research*, 15(2), 89–98.

Central Statistical Office (2015). *Zambia demographic and health survey 2013–2014*. Lusaka: Central Statistical Office [cited 2018 September 18]. Available from: www.dhsprogram.com/pubs/pdf/fr304/fr304.pdf

CHR (2018). A report on child marriage in AFRICA [cited 2019 February 17]. Available from: www.chr.up.ac.za/images/publications/centrepublications/documents/child_marriage_report.pdf

Cohen MS, Chen YQ, McCauley M, Gamble T, Hosseinipour MC, Kumarasamy N, et al. (August 2011). "Prevention of HIV-1 infection with early antiretroviral therapy". *The New England Journal of Medicine*, 365(6): 493–505. doi:10.1056/NEJMoa1105243. PMC 3200068. PMID 21767103

Cornell, M., & Dovel, K. (2018). Reaching key adolescent populations. *Current Opinion in HIV and AIDS*, 13(3), 274–280.

De Oliveira, T., Kharsany, A.B., Gräf, T., Cawood, C., Khanyile, D., Grobler, A., . . . Karim, S. S. A. (2017). Transmission networks and risk of HIV infection in KwaZulu-Natal, South Africa: A community-wide phylogenetic study. *Lancet HIV*, 4(1), e41–e50.

Delany-Moretlwe, S., Cowan, F.M., Busza, J., Bolton-Moore, C., Kelley, K., & Fairlie, L. (2015). Providing comprehensive health services for young key populations: Needs, barriers and gaps. *Journal of the International AIDS Society*, 18, 19833.

Dhana, A., Luchters, S., Moore, L., Lafort, Y., Roy, A., Scorgie, F., & Chersich, M. (2014). Systematic review of facility-based sexual and reproductive health services for female sex workers in Africa. *Globalization and Health*, 10(1), 46.

DHS (2014). Kenya demographic and health survey [cited 2019 February 18]. Available from: www.dhsprogram.com/pubs/pdf/FR308/FR308.pdf

DHS (2015). Zimbabwe demographic and health survey [cited 2019 February 09]. Available from: https://dhsprogram.com/pubs/pdf/FR322/FR322.pdf

DHS (2018). Zambia demographic and health survey 2018 [cited 2020 September 05]. Available from: https://dhsprogram.com/pubs/pdf/FR361/FR361.pdf

Dolan, K., Wirtz, A.L., Moazen, B., Ndeffo-mbah, M., Galvani, A., Kinner, S.A., . . . & Hellard, M. (2016). Global burden of HIV, viral hepatitis, and tuberculosis in prisoners and detainees. *Lancet*, 388(10049), 1089–1102.

Doyle, A.M., Mavedzenge, S.N., Plummer, M.L., & Ross, D.A. (2012). The sexual behaviour of adolescents in Sub-Saharan Africa: Patterns and trends from national surveys. *Tropical Medicine & International Health*, 17(7), 796–807.

Evans, M., Risher, K., Zungu, N., Shisana, O., Moyo, S., Celentano, D.D., . . . & Rehle, T.M. (2016). Age-disparate sex and HIV risk for young women from 2002 to 2012 in South Africa. *Journal of the International AIDS Society*, 19(1), 21310.

Francome, C. (2015). *Unsafe abortion and women's health: Change and liberalization*. Farnham: Ashgate Publishing.

Higgins, J.A., Hoffman, S., & Dworkin, S.L. (2010). Rethinking gender, heterosexual men, and women's vulnerability to HIV/AIDS. *American Journal of Public Health*, 100(3), 435–445.

HSRC (2019). South African national HIV prevalence, incidence, behavior and communication survey [PowerPoint slides]. Available from: https://tbsouth

africa.org.za/sites/default/files/201910%20South%20African%20National%20 HIV%20Prevalence%2C%20Incidence%2C%20Behaviour%20and%20Communication%20Survey%202017.pdf

Idele, P., Gillespie, A., Porth, T., Suzuki, C., Mahy, M., Kasedde, S., & Luo, C. (2014). Epidemiology of HIV and AIDS among adolescents: Current status, inequities, and data gaps. *JAIDS Journal of Acquired Immune Deficiency Syndromes*, 66, S144–S153.

Jewkes, R. (2002). Intimate partner violence: Causes and prevention. *Lancet*, 359(9315), 1423–1429.

Jooste S, Mabaso M, Taylor M, North A, Tadokera R, Simbayi L (2020) Trends and determinants of ever having tested for HIV among youth and adults in South Africa from 2005–2017: Results from four repeated cross-sectional nationally representative household-based HIV prevalence, incidence, and behaviour surveys. PLoS ONE 15(5): e0232883. https://doi.org/10.1371/journal.pone.0232883

Kenyan Ministry of Health/National AIDS Control Council (2018). Kenya AIDS response progress report 2018 [cited 2020 February 13]. Available from: http://www.lvcthealth.org/wp-content/uploads/2018/11/KARPR-Report_2018.pdf

Kiefer, L., Witola, H., Hansende, D., Handema, R., & Siantombo, N. (2013). *Report of the study on HIV prevention for sexual minority groups in Zambia.* Lusaka: Panos Institute for Southern Africa [cited 2019 February 13]. Available from: www.panos.org.zm/wp-content/uploads/2017/04/Panos-Study-on-Sexual-Minorities-in-Zambia-Report.pdf.

MannionDaniels (2018). Adolescents and HIV: Definitions and disaggregation [cited 2019 January 30]. Available from: http://www.ehpsa.org/critical-reviews/age-disaggregation

Mathews, C., Guttmacher, S.J., Flisher, A.J., Mtshizana, Y.Y., Nelson, T., McCarthy, J., & Daries, V. (2009). The quality of HIV testing services for adolescents in Cape Town, South Africa: Do adolescent-friendly services make a difference? *Journal of Adolescent Health*, 44(2), 188–190.

Mavedzenge, S.N., Luecke, E., & Ross, D.A. (2014). Effective approaches for programming to reduce adolescent vulnerability to HIV infection, HIV risk, and HIV-related morbidity and mortality: A systematic review of systematic reviews. *JAIDS Journal of Acquired Immune Deficiency Syndromes*, 66, S154–S169.

Ministério da Saúde (MISAU), Instituto Nacional de Estatística (INE), and ICF (2019). *Survey of indicators on immunization, malaria and HIV/AIDS in Mozambique 2015: Supplemental report incorporating antiretroviral biomarker results.* Maputo, Mozambique, and Rockville, MD: INS, INE, and ICF.

Ministry of Health and Child Care (2019). Zimbabwe population-based HIV impact assessment (ZIMPHIA) 2015–2016: Final report. Available from: https://phia.icap.columbia.edu/wp-content/uploads/2020/02/ZIMPHIA-Final-Report_integrated_Web-1.pdf

Ministry of Health and Social Welfare National AIDS Control Programme (2013). *HIV and STI biological and behavioral survey: A study of female sex workers in seven regions: Dar es Salaam, Iringa, Mbeya, Mwanza, Shinyanga, Tabora and Mara.* India: NACP.

MISAU, INS (2017). *Final report: The Mozambique integrated biological and behavioral survey among people who inject drugs, 2014.* Maputo, Mozambique: MISAU, INS.

Muller, A., Spencer, S., Meer, T., & Daskilewicz, K. (2018). The no-go zone: A qualitative study of access to sexual and reproductive health services for sexual and gender minority adolescents in Southern Africa. *Reproductive Health*, 15(1), 12.

Ningpuanyeh, W.C., & Sathiya Susuman, A. (2017). Correlates of early sexual debut and its associated STI/HIV risk factors among sexually active youths in Malawi. *Journal of Asian and African Studies*, 52(8), 1213–1224.

Pettifor, A., O'Brien, K., MacPhail, C., Miller, W.C., & Rees, H. (2009). Early coital debut and associated HIV risk factors among young women and men in South Africa. *International Perspectives on Sexual and Reproductive Health*, 82–90.

Poteat, T., Ackerman, B., Diouf, D., Ceesay, N., Mothopeng, T., Odette, K.Z., . . . & Mnisi, Z. (2017). HIV prevalence and behavioral and psychosocial factors among transgender women and cisgender men who have sex with men in 8 African countries: A cross-sectional analysis. *PLoS Medicine*, 14(11), e1002422.

Prudden, H.J., Watts, C.H., Vickerman, P., Bobrova, N., Heise, L., Ogungbemi, M.K., . . . & Foss, A.M. (2013). Can the UNAIDS modes of transmission model be improved? A comparison of the original and revised model projections using data from a setting in West Africa. *AIDS (London, England)*, 27(16), 2623.

RST ESA SI Hub based on UNAIDS estimates 2017.

Sawyer, S.M., Afifi, R.A., Bearinger, L.H., Blakemore, S.J., Dick, B., Ezeh, A.C., & Patton, G.C. (2012). Adolescence: A foundation for future health. *Lancet*, 379(9826), 1630–1640.

SHIMS2 (2019). Swaziland HIV Incidence Measurement Survey 2 2016–2017. Final Report [cited 2019 January 30]. Available from: https://phia.icap.columbia.edu/wp-content/uploads/2020/02/SHIMS2_Final-Report_05.03.2019_forWEB.pdf

Tanser, F., Bärnighausen, T., Grapsa, E., Zaidi, J., & Newell, M.L. (2013). High coverage of ART associated with decline in risk of HIV acquisition in rural KwaZulu-Natal, South Africa. *Science*, 339(6122), 966–971.

Tanzania Commission for AIDS (TACAIDS), Zanzibar AIDS Commission (ZAC), National Bureau of Statistics (NBS), Office of the Chief Government Statistician (OCGS), and ICF International (2013). Tanzania HIV/AIDS and malaria indi cator survey 2011–12. Dar es Salaam, Tanzania: TACAIDS, ZAC, NBS, OCGS, and ICF International.

Telisinghe, L., Charalambous, S., Topp, S.M., Herce, M.E., Hoffmann, C.J., Barron, P., . . . & Beyrer, C. (2016). HIV and tuberculosis in prisons in sub-Saharan Africa. *Lancet*, 388(10050), 1215–1227.

UNAIDS (2019). UNAIDS data 2019 [cited 2020 January 20]. Available from: https://www.unaids.org/sites/default/files/media_asset/2019-UNAIDS-data_en.pdf

UNAIDS (2020). AIDSinfo [cited 2019 January 20]. Available from: http://aidsinfo.unaids.org/

UNAIDSa (2016). Ending the AIDS epidemic for adolescents, with adolescents: A practical guide to meaningfully engage adolescents in the AIDS response [cited 2019 January 23]. Available from: www.unaids.org/sites/default/files/media_asset/ending-AIDS-epidemic-adolescents_en.pdf

UNAIDSa (2017). Country fact sheet [cited 2019 February 08]. Available from: file:///C:/Users/210551048/Downloads/Country%20factsheets%20Eswatini%202017.pdf

UNAIDSb (2017). Ending AIDS: Progress towards the 90-90-90 targets [cited 2019 March 16]. Available from: https://www.unaids.org/sites/default/files/media_asset/Global_AIDS_update_2017_en.pdf

UNAIDSa (2018). Miles to go: The response to HIV in Eastern and Southern Africa [cited 2019 January 23]. Available from: www.unaids.org/sites/default/files/media_asset/miles-to-go_eastern-and-southern-africa_en.pdf

UNAIDSb (2016). HIV prevention among adolescent girls and young women [cited 2018 May 23]. Available from: www.unaids.org/sites/default/files/media_asset/UNAIDS_HIV_prevention_among_adolescent_girls_and_young_women.pdf

UNAIDSb (2018). Data. Geneva, Switzerland [cited 2019 March 17]. Available from: www.unaids.org/sites/default/files/media_asset/unaids-data

UNESCO (2017). CSE scale-up in practice: Case studies from Eastern and Southern Africa. [cited 2019 April 18]. Available from: https://hivhealthclearinghouse.unesco.org/sites/default/files/resources/cse_scale_up_in_practice_june_2017_final_.pdf

UNICEF (2013). Ending child marriage. Progress and prospects [cited 2019 February 17]. Available from: https://data.unicef.org/wp-content/uploads/2015/12/Child-Marriage-Brochure-HR_164.pdf

UNICEF (2015). Press release: Adolescent deaths from AIDS tripled since 2000 [cited 2019 January 23]. Available from: www.unicef.org/media/media_86384.html

UNICEF (2016). *Collecting and reporting of sex- and age-disaggregated data on adolescents at the sub-national level.* New York: UNICEF [cited 2019 December 13]. Available from: https://childrenandaids.org/collecting-reporting-sex-age-disaggregated-data

UNICEF (2017). Children and AIDS: Statistical update. UNICEF [cited 2018 May 23]. Available from: https://data.unicef.org/wpcontent/uploads/2017/11/HIVAIDS-Statistical-Update-2017.pdf

UNICEF (2018). Adolescent HIV prevention [cited 2019 February 28]. Available from: https://data.unicef.org/topic/hivaids/adolescents-young-people/

WHOa (2015). HIV and young people who inject drugs. A technical brief [cited 2019 February 13]. Available from: www.unaids.org/sites/default/files/media_asset/2015_young_people_drugs_en.pdf

WHOb (2015). Consolidated guidelines on HIV testing services [cited 2019 February 08]. Available from: https://apps.who.int/iris/bitstream/handle/10665/179870/9789241508926_eng.pdf?sequence=1

2 Conceptual pathways to HIV risk in Eastern and Southern Africa

An integrative perspective on the development of young people in contexts of social-structural vulnerability

Richard G. Cowden, Leigh A. Tucker and Kaymarlin Govender

Introduction

The transition from childhood to adulthood is characterised by substantive biological, psychological, and social changes. A majority of these changes are captured under the umbrella concept of adolescence, a period in which young people undergo biological changes and fulfil key developmental tasks towards independence and self-reliance (Blakemore & Mills, 2014; Linders, 2017). Although legal designations of adulthood (e.g. 18 years of age or older) suggest that fulfilment of this developmental process depends on shared chronological markers, there is extensive interindividual variability in the timing, tempo, and extent to which young people experience developmental changes as they transition from childhood to adulthood. In this chapter, we position adolescence within the broader ambit of the developmental continuum by referring to individuals between 10 and 24 years of age as *young people*.[1]

Compared to their counterparts in more developed parts of the world, young people in Eastern and Southern Africa (ESA) must navigate developmental milestones within environments that often pose significant short- and long-term mental and physical health risks. Understanding developmental changes that accompany the transition to adulthood is key to identifying the challenges that young people experience within the broader sociocultural context in which they live. This chapter provides an overview of theoretical positions that are central to holistically understanding the biopsychosocial development of young people. It also offers a backdrop to subsequent chapters in this book, which focus on delineating mechanisms or processes that may deter health risk behaviours and promote well-being among young people. Drawing on theoretical perspectives rooted in biology, psychology, and

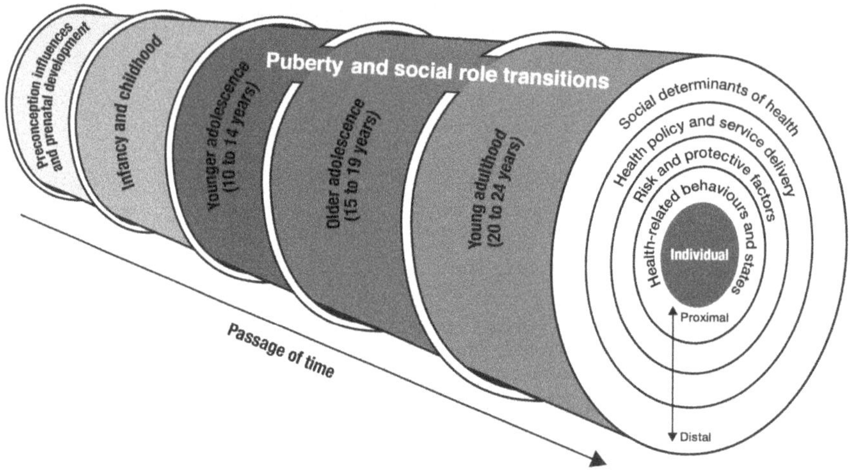

Figure 2.1 Conceptual framework for contextualised development of adolescents and young people

sociology, we outline fundamental processes that independently and conjunctively contribute to the contextualised development of young people (see Figure 2.1 for an overview of the interactive biopsychosocial systems involved in shaping the development of young people). Because HIV continues to have disproportionately devastating effects on young people living in ESA (see UNAIDS, 2017a, 2017b), understanding pathways of risk that have the potential to undermine the health and well-being of young people is integral to guiding the design and implementation of HIV prevention programming for this population.

A life-course perspective on the development of young people

Developmental psychology has traditionally dominated the way in which the experiences of young people have been constructed and understood (Burman, 2008). Traditional developmental discourse tends to assume that healthy and adaptive development is achieved through successful completion of developmental stages and attainment of age-related competencies (Burman, 2008; Hogan, 2005). This narrow perspective features several contentious assumptions, including framing development as a relatively homogenous and universal experience that is progressive, linear, and unidirectional. Emerging evidence suggests that developmental differences among young people are at least partly attributable to distinctions in both the inter- and intraindividual courses of progression, the sociocultural norms and expectations of adolescence, and the environmental context in which development occurs (Foulkes & Blakemore, 2018). Understanding qualitative (e.g. type) and quantitative (e.g. magnitude) differences in developmental experiences is critical to generating well-informed conceptualisations of development that are relevant to the contexts in which young people live.

A life-course perspective acknowledges developmental change in relation to social and structural determinants of health (Brook, Morojele, Zhang, & Brook, 2006; Sawyer et al., 2012). The development of young people unfolds as a transactional process that is the product of bidirectional and synergistic effects of the individual and their experiences within the social environment (Sameroff, 2009). Capacity for adaptive functioning is distributed across interacting systems and reflects evolutionary shifts in biology and culture, with maladaptive patterns representing decreases in functioning within and across multiple systems (Masten, 2014). Importantly, maladjustment can be attributed to or exacerbated by factors at cultural and contextual levels (i.e. social-structural vulnerabilities) that extend beyond the individual (Ungar, 2011). Social-structural vulnerabilities (e.g. lack of education, poverty, gender inequality, discriminatory policies or legal frameworks) tend to heighten exposure of young people to dysfunctional systems, which can disrupt typical trajectories of development and create barriers to successfully navigating pathways of risk. While risky behaviours are a part of the normative dialogue around the development of young people, environments that lack protective processes at social and structural levels may predispose this population to a variety of health risks (e.g. substance abuse, violence), including HIV. In the sections that follow, we consider salient development and role transition processes of young people and contextualise these in relation to some of the social-structural vulnerabilities that exist in ESA.

Developmental processes in contexts of social-structural vulnerability

Pubertal changes

Puberty (mean age of onset is 12 years in males and 11 years in females) is associated with progressive development of sexual and reproductive organs and physical changes indicative of sexual maturity (Blakemore, Burnett, & Dahl, 2010; Byrne et al., 2017). Although the pubertal development process is typical of all adolescents, there are individual differences in the timing and tempo of maturation (Beltz, Corley, Bricker, Wadsworth, & Berenbaum, 2014).

Adolescents who physically mature earlier have been found to be at higher risk of psychological problems because of mismatches between physical growth and their developmental readiness for the biopsychosocial changes that occur (Ge, Brody, Conger, Simons, & Murry, 2002; Ge et al., 2003). For girls, who generally enter puberty earlier than boys (Abreu &

Kaiser, 2016), the risks of maladjustment are sometimes higher (Graber, 2013) because early maturing girls are more likely to stand out from their age-matched peers and affiliate with older peers (Mrug et al., 2014).

Marked economic and gender inequalities in ESA are involved in creating pressure among girls to engage in age-disparate relations or intergenerational sex (i.e. partnerships in which one partner is five or more years younger than the other partner) as a means of fulfilling needs (e.g. socioeconomic freedom and security) that extend beyond interpersonal intimacy and belonging (Mampane, 2018). Age-disparate relationships are sustained by the physical and emotional needs of young people, which are emerging in contexts of deprivation where youth are searching for a gateway to a middle-class lifestyle. The seemingly transactional nature of these relationships continues to activate debate about whether young women are exercising agency or being coerced into such relationships (Wamoyi et al., 2019). Notwithstanding potential rewards or immediate gratification, intergenerational sex has been associated with risky sexual practices and elevated risk of HIV infection (Leclerc-Madlala, 2008; Ritchwood et al., 2016).

High rates of gender-based violence against women within ESA is another social vulnerability that impedes the ability of young women to negotiate safe sex (MacPherson, Richards, Namakhoma, & Theobald, 2014), as they may have concerns over the potential repercussions of not complying with their partner's sexual demands or expectations (O'Sullivan, Harrison, Morrell, Monroe-Wise, & Kubeka, 2006). Gender inequality remains a broader sociocultural issue in many countries within ESA. Legislative policies often lack holistic frameworks to be able to offer sufficient protection and support to young women who experience sexual and gender-based violence (van Eerdewijk et al., 2018). Consequently, the challenges associated with navigating biopsychosocial changes that occur during adolescence may be amplified in high-risk environments where structural mechanisms to combat risk and promote well-being are underdeveloped.

Neurological changes

Adolescence is one of the most sensitive periods for brain development (Steinberg, 2014). During this developmental phase, neuronal networks throughout the brain are optimised and fine-tuned (Arain et al., 2013). Structural changes to the prefrontal cortex, in particular, are linked to important advances in executive functions (Anderson, 2002), including planning, decision-making, and regulation of thought and action (Casey, Jones, & Hare, 2008). Over time, improvements in cognitive control lead to better decision-making processes and inhibition of impulsive behaviour (Blakemore & Choudhury, 2006). Developments in frontal-parietal lobe circuitry contribute to increasingly sophisticated social-cognitive processes that promote interpersonal functioning, including advances in adolescents' proclivity to experience empathy and perspective-taking abilities (Blakemore & Mills, 2014; Dumontheil, Apperly, & Blakemore, 2010).

Key neurochemical processes have been linked to the relative immaturity of the prefrontal cortex during adolescence, including the gamma-aminobutyric acid (GABA) and dopamine systems of neurotransmission (Arain et al., 2013). In the prefrontal cortex, delayed maturation of the GABA system, coupled with elevated levels of dopamine (Wahlstrom, Collins, White, & Luciana, 2010), contribute to adolescents' appetite for novel experiences, exploratory behaviour, and sensation-seeking tendencies (Spear, 2000).

Although the likelihood of risk-taking behaviour increases as young people pursue novel and stimulating experiences (Blakemore et al., 2010), behavioural choices are also affected by the broader environmental context. In ESA, where the prevalence of infectious disease is high (Murray et al., 2012) and access to quality healthcare is limited (Fullman et al., 2018), young people are particularly vulnerable to health consequences associated with risky behaviours. For example, the age at which adolescents are able to independently access medical care varies across countries in ESA, including specific regulations on parental consent for HIV testing (Govender, Nyamaruze, Cowden, & Armstrong, in press). Sometimes, the legal age of consenting to sex (typically 15 or 16 years of age) is lower than the age young people are legally permitted to access sexual and reproductive health services independent of their parents (typically when young people are granted legal status as adults at 18 years of age). Furthermore, social norms and legislative environments in ESA tend to be repressive against young key populations (e.g. those who self-identify as part of the LGBTQ+ community). Many ESA countries maintain policies and legal frameworks that criminalise the identities and sexual activities of key populations (Govender et al., 2018). These kinds of sociopolitical discrepancies and barriers not only conflict with young people's progressive sense of autonomy and capacity to self-regulate, but they may also reduce health-seeking behaviours and obstruct access to HIV care and treatment services (Baggaley, Armstrong, Dodd, Ngoksin, & Krug, 2015).

Psychological changes

With maturation, adolescents' cognitive abilities shift away from concrete operational thought processes (Piaget, 1964) towards higher-order cognitive capabilities (e.g. hypothetical-deductive reasoning, abstract thought, improvements in speed of information processing) that enable young people to weigh risks into decision-making and exert better control over behavioural choices (Steinberg, 2005). Alongside acquisition of general higher-order cognitive abilities, adolescence is accompanied by developments in moral reasoning. Early perspectives (see Kohlberg & Hersh, 1977) conceptualise moral judgement in young people as a progressive socialisation process towards the internalisation of universal moral principles. More recent models (see Rest Narvaez, Thoma, & Bebeau, 2000) emphasise the role of contextually specific influences (e.g. common morality) on the development of moral judgement. Young people make value judgements around sexual practice that are usually dependent on social and structural factors such as poverty, family structure, educational background, gender inequality, and conceptions of romantic relationships. For example, women may fear violence in response to requesting condom use with their sexual partners. Heightened egocentrism (e.g. unrealistic, biased, and self-serving judgements) associated with dominant constructs of masculinity may also undermine adolescents' ability to make independent judgements. Studies have found that expectations of sexual behaviour among men that reflect hypermasculine norms, including sexual appetite, prowess, and conquest (Brown, Sorrell, & Raffaelli, 2005; Shefer, Kruger, & Schepers, 2015), are linked to HIV risk (Fleming, DiClemente, & Barrington, 2016).

Similarly, macro-level environmental factors can influence identity formation processes that are central to development. Young people living in socially repressive contexts have more constraints on their agency to explore, expand, and diversify their social selves. Identity formation processes may be foreclosed or restricted by prevailing norms and policies. For example, many socially conservative countries in ESA have legislative restrictions (e.g. criminalisation of same-sex relations) that reinforce stigma and prejudice against members of key populations. Due to the constraints and prejudices that relevant regulations and policies impose on members of key populations, narrowly defined codes of conduct can have negative effects on the psychological adjustment (e.g. diminished sense of self-worth, feelings of social isolation) of members of young key populations as they transition to adulthood (Govender et al., in press). Young people may also be reluctant to seek sexual and reproductive healthcare services due to concerns about discrimination and potential legal ramifications that may be linked to the behaviours they participate in (Baggaley et al., 2015), which could ultimately lead to unfavourable health outcomes.

Social changes

During adolescence, young people expand their social landscapes beyond familial boundaries to extrafamilial attachment figures (e.g. peers, romantic relationships). They begin to spend more time in the company of their peers (Lam, McHale, & Crouter, 2014) and ascribe greater value to peer opinions and expectations (van Hoorn, van Dijk, Meuwese, Rieffe, & Crone, 2014). Peers serve as role models, provide age- and sex-appropriate standards of acceptable behaviour, and shape behaviour through interactions that reinforce or extinguish behaviour (Crosnoe & McNeely, 2008; Smetana, 2010). Acquired norms may be incorporated into existing standards of behaviour and form part of an individual's subsequent behaviours and decision-making (Berger, 2008). Although the implications of peer influences are heterogenous and can facilitate healthy adjustment (van Hoorn et al., 2014), in vulnerable contexts there are greater risks and consequences of negative peer influences. Adolescents' need to belong and feel accepted may be exploited by peer pressure to conform to deviant or otherwise risky behaviours, particularly those involving substance use (e.g. tobacco, alcohol) and sexual activity (Govender, Cowden, Oppong Asante, George, & Reardon, 2019). These kinds of health-risk behaviours often do not occur in isolation and can synergistically increase risk. For example, adolescents who consume alcohol are more likely to initiate sex at an earlier age and engage in risky sexual practices (e.g. multiple sexual partners) compared to alcohol abstaining peers (Morojele, Nkosi, Kekwaletswe, Saban, & Parry, 2013).

There are also broader contextual dynamics that can affect adolescents' access to recreational substances and ease of engagement in health-risk behaviours. Recent evidence (see Gray-Phillip et al., 2018) indicates that alcohol is readily available for purchase among underage persons in countries within ESA (e.g. South Africa). General accessibility of recreational substances is mediated by environments that enable adolescents to participate in substance use. Studies have found that substance use on school premises tends to be higher when young people believe that repercussions of such activities are unlikely (Evans-Whipp, Plenty, Catalano, Herrenkohl, & Toumbourou, 2013). When sociocontextual consequences of deviant behaviour are outweighed by the perceived benefits, anticipation of generally positive outcomes may affect the decisions of young people to engage in health-risk behaviour (Piontek et al., 2008).

By mid to late adolescence, many young people begin to form intimate romantic relationships (Tanti, Stukas, Halloran, & Foddy, 2011). Dating relationships represent a novel and distinctive type of social engagement for adolescents, which are influenced by prior experiences in attachment relationships (e.g. parents, peers) and further shape a young person's identity, perspectives on relationships, and behaviour (Giordano, Manning, & Longmore, 2006). Perceived pressure to conform to peer norms about romantic relationships influences when young people decide to begin dating relationships, who they enter into relationship with, and the norms they internalise about sexual intimacy within romantic relationships (van Zantvliet, Ivanova, & Verbakel, 2020).

In ESA, social-structural features of the environment (e.g. poverty) are involved in motivating young people to pursue romantic relationships as a means of fulfilling material needs. Young women may engage in transactional sexual relationships to meet basic needs (e.g. food security), gain access to financial support and material gifts, and acquire social status (UNAIDS, 2018). Transactional characteristics of relationships reinforce traditional norms of hegemonic masculinity (e.g. male dominance) and can lead to tolerance of coercion and compliance with male demands about sexual practices (Wamoyi, Fenwick, Urassa, Zaba, & Stones, 2011; Wamoyi et al., 2019). Masculine ideologies (e.g. virility) encourage and endorse risky sexual practices (e.g. multiple, concurrent sexual partners) among young men, which serve as signals of sexual prowess, control over women, and power over other men (Fleming et al., 2016). Together, these kinds of social-structural dynamics conjunctively contribute to fluid partnership patterns (e.g. casual partnering, frequent partner changes) that heighten young people's risk of contracting HIV (Bongaarts, 2007).

Role transitions in contexts of social-structural vulnerability

In contexts of social-structural vulnerability where disruptions in parental or caregiver attachment (e.g. orphanhood, parental absence) are pervasive (Newlin, Reynold, & Nombutho, 2016), young people are at increased risk of prematurely assuming adult roles and responsibilities (e.g. heads of households) for which they are unprepared (Meintjes, Hall, Marera, & Boulle, 2010; Mturi, 2012). Minors who assume positions as head of household are concentrated in ESA (Collins et al., 2016), and the burden of being responsible for the needs of other family members can be emotionally, psychologically, and physically taxing (see Boris et al., 2008; Hartell & Chabilall, 2005; Satzinger, Kipp, & Rubaale, 2012). Furthermore, the challenges of prematurely navigating adult responsibilities in vulnerable social contexts are often compounded by structural constraints that impact employment opportunities, food security, educational attainment, and access to supportive social programming (Collins et al., 2016; Mkhatshwa, 2017).

A similarly abrupt transition to adulthood occurs among young women who are involuntarily married as children. Early child marriages are prevalent in countries within ESA (Koski, Clark, & Nandi, 2017) and may be motivated by intersecting cultural dynamics (e.g. symbolism of social status for men, parents' needs for young women to become 'productive') and the structural vulnerabilities (e.g. prospect of family inheriting bride wealth to alleviate poverty) that exist in the region (Schaffnit, Urassa, & Lawson, 2019). Child marriages not only infringe on rights to self-determination and thwart personal growth opportunities for young women, but they are also linked to highly inequitable, exploitive relationships characterised by gender-based violence and unsafe sexual practices (Kidman, 2017; Raj, Jackson, & Dunham, 2018).

Another prominent early role transition in ESA is motherhood at a young age, where rates of pregnancy and childbearing among adolescent girls remain persistently high (Yakubu & Salisu, 2018). Although it is not uncommon for young women in ESA to have a child as a form of celebrating womanhood (Sennott & Mojola, 2017), unplanned teenage pregnancies and childbirths are driven by broader social (e.g. unequal gender power dynamics, coercive sexual relations) and structural (e.g. poverty, unavailable or inaccessible educational opportunities, barriers to contraception) vulnerabilities in this region (Yakubu & Salisu, 2018). Psychosocial consequences of unplanned and unmarried childbirth may include social stigma and family rejection, which can provoke unsafe abortions and exacerbate the challenges of navigating adult responsibilities of parenthood as an adolescent (see Izugbara, Ochako, & Izugbara 2011; Levandowski et al., 2012). As young girls who bear children are more likely to permanently discontinue their educational pursuits (Wodon et al., 2017), teenage pregnancy and parenthood in vulnerable contexts may have long-term implications for maintaining or perpetuating intergenerational cycles of poverty and gender inequality (Swartz, Colvin, & Harrison, 2018; Wood & Hendricks, 2017).

Vertically infected HIV-positive young people who grow up in ESA are uniquely affected by compounded vulnerabilities as they transition to adulthood. Social stigmatisation may lead to discrimination, social disintegration, and barriers to appropriate support mechanisms (Boushab, Fall-Malick, Ould Cheikh Melaïnine, & Basco, 2017). These consequences aggravate pre-existing psychological distress (e.g. low self-worth, self-stigmatisation, internalising symptoms) during a period when young people are increasingly interested in broadening their social landscapes and their need to belong and feel accepted intensifies (Bennett, Hersh, Herres, & Foster, 2016). Interpersonal and self-imposed HIV-related stigma may reduce help-seeking behaviours and restrict access to healthcare services (Rueda et al., 2016), which are necessary for treating HIV effectively, receiving guidance on safe sexual practices, and obtaining professional support for mental health issues.

Overcoming social-structural vulnerabilities: building resilience in context

Even though structural challenges can create overwhelming obstacles that have the potential to interfere with development, young people living in contexts of social-structural vulnerability frequently emerge well-adjusted (Masten, 2014). Young people are able to adapt successfully in economically disadvantaged and high-risk social environments by drawing upon culturally embedded networks of functionally interrelated resources available to them (Ungar, 2011). Recent reviews of resilience research involving samples of children and youth from countries in ESA (e.g. Betancourt, Meyers-Ohki, Charrow, & Hansen, 2013; van Breda & Theron, 2018) have identified a range of protective processes (e.g. individual, family, community, cultural) that enable resilience, highlighting the diversity of internal and external resources that may be accessible to young people in this region. Mobilisation of community-level resources is a particularly useful means of developing health-enabling environments for overcoming social-structural vulnerabilities (Thomas-Slayter & Fisher, 2011). AIDS-competent communities create health-enabling environments for young people by encouraging engagement and providing avenues for participating in collective dialogue, collectively agreeing on a shared purpose and taking responsibility for the HIV epidemic, and being involved in educating people about HIV prevention and supporting access to healthcare needs (Campbell, Nair, Maimane, & Gibbs, 2009).

Multilevel resilience-enabling resources may be shared among young people across contexts, yet there is heterogeneity in manifestations of resilience among different populations (Ungar, 2008). Interpretations of resilience in contexts of social-structural vulnerability ought to consider self-constructed definitions of successful adaptation among young people (Ungar, 2004). An inclusive perspective that recognises multiple pathways and manifestations of resilience is likely to improve our understanding of how unorthodox pathways may be involved in young people's achievement of non-standard expressions of resilience (Theron, 2016; Ungar, 2008), which can be integrated into the development of contextually relevant HIV prevention programmes for young people living in ESA.

Conclusion

This chapter offered an integrative overview of the contextualised biopsychosocial development of young people in ESA. Although biological change is an inevitable part of adolescent development, there remain maturational disparities and idiosyncratic differences in the way these changes occur. By opening boundaries of childhood and adulthood beyond the typical notion of chronological age, young people may be placed at different points along a developmental trajectory depending on their unique personal circumstances and the social contexts in which they live.

Acquisition of HIV cannot be explained simply at the level of individual behaviour and biology. Rather, HIV risk among young people needs to be interpreted in relation to the broader context of the epidemic. Contextual realities play a key role in how young people negotiate their identities, including their sexual and relational selves. It is important to consider the broader cultural milieu and immediate community influences on societal perceptions of young people and the way in which they perceive themselves. A more holistic view of sexuality may provide a gateway to understanding the role of sociocultural influences on decisions related to sexual activity. Comprehensive frameworks for conceptualising sexual risk behaviour are likely to encourage prevention efforts that take a contextualised, multifaceted approach to targeting risk factors at multiple levels of proximity to the individual.

Note

1 Young people is an inclusive term (see World Health Organization, 2018) that captures phases of younger adolescence (10 to 14 years), older adolescence (15 to 19 years), and young adulthood (20 to 24 years).

References

Abreu, A.P., & Kaiser, U.B. (2016). Pubertal development and regulation. *Lancet Diabetes & Endocrinology, 4,* 254–264. doi:10.1016/S2213-8587(15)00418-0

Anderson, P. (2002). Assessment and development of executive function (EF) during childhood. *Child Neuropsychology, 8,* 71–82. doi:10.1076/chin.8.2.71.8724

Arain, M., Haque, M., Johal, L., Mathur, P., Nel, W., Rais, A., . . . Sharma, S. (2013). Maturation of the adolescent brain. *Neuropsychiatric Disease and Treatment, 9,* 449–461. doi:10.2147/NDT.S39776

Baggaley, R., Armstrong, A., Dodd, Z., Ngoksin, E., & Krug, A. (2015). Young key populations and HIV: A special emphasis and consideration in the new WHO consolidated guidelines on HIV prevention, diagnosis, treatment and care for key populations. *Journal of the International AIDS Society, 18*(Suppl. 1), 19438. doi:10.7448/IAS.18.2.19438

Beltz, A.M., Corley, R.P., Bricker, J.B., Wadsworth, S.J., & Berenbaum, S.A. (2014). Modeling pubertal timing and tempo and examining links to behavior problems. *Developmental Psychology, 50,* 2715–2726. doi:10.1037/a0038096

Bennett, D.S., Hersh, J., Herres, J., & Foster, J. (2016). HIV-related stigma, shame, and avoidant coping: Risk factors for internalizing symptoms among youth living with HIV? *Child Psychiatry & Human Development, 47,* 657–664. doi:10.1007/s10578-015-0599-y

Berger, J. (2008). Identity signaling, social influence, and social contagion. In M.J. Prinstein & K.A. Dodge (Eds.), *Understanding peer influence in children and adolescents* (pp. 181–199). New York, NY: Guilford Press.

Betancourt, T.S., Meyers-Ohki, S.E., Charrow, A., & Hansen, N. (2013). Annual research review: Mental health and resilience in HIV/AIDS-affected children – A review of the literature and recommendations for future research. *Journal of Child Psychology and Psychiatry, 54,* 423–444. doi:10.1111/j.1469-7610.2012.02613.x

Blakemore, S.-J., Burnett, S., & Dahl, R.E. (2010). The role of puberty in the developing adolescent brain. *Human Brain Mapping, 31,* 926–933. doi:10.1002/hbm.21052

Blakemore, S.-J., & Choudhury, S. (2006). Development of the adolescent brain: Implications for executive function and social cognition. *Journal of Child Psychology and Psychiatry, 47,* 296–312. doi:10.1111/j.1469-7610.2006.01611.x

Blakemore, S.-J., & Mills, K.L. (2014). Is adolescence a sensitive period for sociocultural processing? *Annual Review of Psychology, 65,* 187–207. doi:10.1146/annurev-psych-010213-115202

Bongaarts, J. (2007). Late marriage and the HIV epidemic in sub-Saharan Africa. *Population Studies, 61,* 73–83. doi:10.1080/00324720601048343

Boris, N.W., Brown, L.A., Thurman, T.R., Rice, J.C., Snider, L.M., Ntaganira, J., & Nyirazinyoye, L.N. (2008). Depressive symptoms in youth heads of household in Rwanda: Correlates and implications for intervention. *Archives of Pediatrics & Adolescent Medicine, 162,* 836–843. doi:10.1001/archpedi.162.9.836

Boushab, B. M., Fall-Malick, F.-Z., Ould Cheikh Melaïnine, M. L., & Basco, L. K. (2017). Forms of stigma and discrimination in the daily lives of HIV-positive individuals in Mauritania. *Open AIDS Journal, 11*, 12–17. doi:10.2174/1874613601711010012

Brook, D. W., Morojele, N. K., Zhang, C., & Brook, J. S. (2006). South African adolescents: Pathways to risky sexual behaviour. *AIDS Education and Prevention, 18*, 259–272. doi:10.1521/aeap.2006.18.3.259

Brown, J., Sorrell, J., & Raffaelli, M. (2005). An exploratory study of constructions of masculinity, sexuality and HIV/AIDS in Namibia, Southern Africa. *Culture, Health & Sexuality, 7*, 585–598. doi:10.1080/13691050500250198

Burman, E. (2008). *Deconstructing developmental psychology* (2nd ed.). New York, NY: Routledge.

Byrne, M. L., Whittle, S., Vijayakumar, N., Dennison, M., Simmons, J. G., & Allen, N. B. (2017). A systematic review of adrenarche as a sensitive period in neurobiological development and mental health. *Developmental Cognitive Neuroscience, 25*, 12–28. doi:10.1016/j.dcn.2016.12.004

Campbell, C., Nair, Y., Maimane, S., & Gibbs, A. (2009). Strengthening community responses to AIDS: Possibilities and challenges. In P. Rohleder, L. Swartz, & S. Kalichman (Eds.), *HIV/AIDS in South Africa 25 years on* (pp. 221–235). London, UK: Springer.

Casey, B. J., Jones, R. M., & Hare, T. A. (2008). The adolescent brain. *Annals of the New York Academy of Sciences, 1124*, 111–126. doi:10.1196/annals.1440.010

Collins, L., Ellis, M., Pritchard, E. W. J., Jenkins, C., Hoeritzauer, I., Farquhar, A., . . . Nelson, B. D. (2016). Child-headed households in Rakai District, Uganda: A mixed-methods study. *Paediatrics and International Child Health, 36*, 58–63. doi:10.1179/2046905514Y.0000000152

Crosnoe, R., & McNeely, C. (2008). Peer relations, adolescent behavior, and public health research and practice. *Family & Community Health, 31*(Suppl. 1), S71–S80. doi:10.1097/01.FCH.0000304020.05632.e8

Dumontheil, I., Apperly, I. A., & Blakemore, S.-J. (2010). Online usage of theory of mind continues to develop in late adolescence. *Developmental Science, 13*, 331–338. doi:10.1111/j.1467-7687.2009.00888.x

Evans-Whipp, T. J., Plenty, S. M., Catalano, R. F., Herrenkohl, T. I., & Toumbourou, J. W. (2013). The impact of school alcohol policy on student drinking. *Health Education Research, 28*, 651–662. doi:10.1093/her/cyt068

Fleming, P. J., DiClemente, R. J., & Barrington, C. (2016). Masculinity and HIV: Dimensions of masculine norms that contribute to men's HIV-related sexual behaviors. *AIDS and Behavior, 20*, 788–798. doi:10.1007/s10461-015-1264-y

Foulkes, L., & Blakemore, S.-J. (2018). Studying individual differences in human adolescent brain development. *Nature Neuroscience, 21*, 315–323. doi:10.1038/s41593-018-0078-4

Fullman, N., Yearwood, J., Abay, S. M., Abbafati, C., Abd-Allah, F., Abdela, J., . . . Lozano, R. (2018). Measuring performance on the Healthcare Access and Quality Index for 195 countries and territories and selected subnational locations: A systematic analysis from the Global Burden of Disease Study 2016. *Lancet, 391*, 2236–2271. doi:10.1016/S0140-6736(18)30994-2

Ge, X., Brody, G. H., Conger, R. D., Simons, R. L., & Murry, V. M. (2002). Contextual amplification of pubertal transition effects on deviant peer affiliation and externalizing behavior among African American children. *Developmental Psychology, 38*, 42–54. doi:10.1037/0012-1649.38.1.42

Ge, X., Kim, I.J., Brody, G.H., Conger, R.D., Simons, R.L., Gibbons, F.X., & Cutrona, C.E. (2003). It's about timing and change: Pubertal transition effects on symptoms of major depression among African American youths. *Developmental Psychology, 39,* 430–439. doi:10.1037/0012-1649.39.3.430

Giordano, P.C., Manning, W.D., & Longmore, M.A. (2006). Adolescent romantic relationships: An emerging portrait of their nature and developmental significance. In A.C. Crouter & A. Booth (Eds.), *Romance and sex in adolescence and emerging adulthood: Risks and opportunities* (pp. 127–150). Mahwah, NJ: Lawrence Erlbaum Associates.

Govender, K., Cowden, R.G., Oppong Asante, K., George, G., & Reardon, C. (2019). Sexual risk behavior: A multi-system model of risk and protective factors in South African adolescents. *Prevention Science, 20,* 1054–1065. doi:10.1007/s11121-019-01015-3

Govender, K., Masebo, W., Nyamaruze, P., Cowden, R.G., Schunter, B., & Bains, A. (2018). HIV prevention in adolescents and young people in the Eastern and Southern African region: A review of key challenges impeding actions for an effective response. *Open AIDS Journal, 12,* 53–67. doi:10.2174/1874613601812010038

Govender, K., Nyamaruze, P., Cowden, R.G., & Armstrong, R. (in press). *Legal, policy and social barriers to accessing HIV and sexual and reproductive health services among young key populations in Eastern and Southern Africa.* Johannesburg, South Africa: Eastern and Southern Africa Regional Inter-Agency Task Team on Children Affected by AIDS.

Graber, J.A. (2013). Pubertal timing and the development of psychopathology in adolescence and beyond. *Hormones and Behavior, 64,* 262–269. doi:10.1016/j.yhbeh.2013.04.003

Gray-Phillip, G., Huckle, T., Callinan, S., Parry, C. D. H., Chaiyasong, S., Cuong, P.V., . . . Casswell, S. (2018). Availability of alcohol: Location, time and ease of purchase in high- and middle-income countries: Data from the international alcohol control study. *Drug and Alcohol Review, 37*(Suppl. 2), S36–S44. doi:10.1111/dar.12693

Hartell, C.G., & Chabilall, J.A. (2005). HIV/AIDS in South Africa: A study of the socio-educational development of adolescents orphaned by AIDS in child-headed households. *International Journal of Adolescence and Youth, 12,* 213–229. doi:10.1080/02673843.2005.9747953

Hogan, D. (2005). Researching "the child" in developmental psychology. In S. Greene & D. Hogan (Eds.), *Researching children's experience: Approaches and methods* (pp. 22–41). London, UK: Sage.

Izugbara, C.O., Ochako, R., & Izugbara, C. (2011). Gender scripts and unwanted pregnancy among urban Kenyan women. *Culture, Health & Sexuality, 13,* 1031–1045. doi:10.1080/13691058.2011.598947

Kidman, R. (2017). Child marriage and intimate partner violence: A comparative study of 34 countries. *International Journal of Epidemiology, 46,* 662–675. doi:10.1093/ije/dyw225

Kohlberg, L., & Hersh, R.H. (1977). Moral development: A review of the theory. *Theory Into Practice, 16,* 53–59. doi:10.1080/00405847709542675

Koski, A., Clark, S., & Nandi, A. (2017). Has child marriage declined in sub-Saharan Africa? An analysis of trends in 31 countries. *Population and Development Review, 43,* 7–29. doi:10.1111/padr.12035

Lam, C.B., McHale, S.M., & Crouter, A.C. (2014). Time with peers from middle childhood to late adolescence: Developmental course and adjustment correlates. *Child Development, 85*, 1677–1693. doi:10.1111/cdev.12235

Leclerc-Madlala, S. (2008). Age-disparate and inter-generational sex in Southern Africa: The dynamics of hypervulnerability. *AIDS, 22*(Suppl. 4), S17–S25. doi:10.1097/01.aids.0000341774.86500.53

Levandowski, B.A., Kalilani-Phiri, L., Kachale, F., Awah, P., Kangaude, G., & Mhango, C. (2012). Investigating social consequences of unwanted pregnancy and unsafe abortion in Malawi: The role of stigma. *International Journal of Gynecology & Obstetrics, 118*(Suppl. 2), S167–S171. doi:10.1016/S0020-7292(12)60017-4

Linders, A. (2017). Deconstructing adolescence. In A.L. Cherry, V. Baltag, & M.E. Dillon (Eds.), *International handbook on adolescent health and development: The public health response* (pp. 15–28). Cham, Switzerland: Springer.

MacPherson, E.E., Richards, E., Namakhoma, I., & Theobald, S. (2014). Gender equity and sexual and reproductive health in Eastern and Southern Africa: A critical overview of the literature. *Global Health Action, 7*, 23717. doi:10.3402/gha.v7.23717

Mampane, J.N. (2018). Exploring the "blesser and blessee" phenomenon: Young women, transactional sex, and HIV in rural South Africa. *SAGE Open, 8*, 1–9. doi:10.1177/2158244018806343

Masten, A.S. (2014). Global perspectives on resilience in children and youth. *Child Development, 85*, 6–20. doi:10.1111/cdev.12205

Meintjes, H., Hall, K., Marera, D.-H., & Boulle, A. (2010). Orphans of the AIDS epidemic? The extent, nature and circumstances of child-headed households in South Africa. *AIDS Care, 22*, 40–49. doi:10.1080/09540120903033029

Mkhatshwa, N. (2017). The gendered experiences of children in child-headed households in Swaziland. *African Journal of AIDS Research, 16*, 365–372. doi:10.2989/16085906.2017.1389756

Morojele, N.K., Nkosi, S., Kekwaletswe, C.T., Saban, A., & Parry, C. D. H. (2013). *Review of research on alcohol and HIV in sub-Saharan Africa.* Tygerberg, South Africa: South African Medical Research Council. Retrieved from https://www.samrc.ac.za/sites/default/files/attachments/2016-06-27/AlcoholSubSaharan.pdf

Mrug, S., Elliott, M.N., Davies, S., Tortolero, S.R., Cuccaro, P., & Schuster, M.A. (2014). Early puberty, negative peer influence, and problem behaviors in adolescent girls. *Pediatrics, 133*, 7–14. doi:10.1542/peds.2013-0628

Mturi, A.J. (2012). Child-headed households in South Africa: What we know and what we don't. *Development Southern Africa, 29*, 506–516. doi:10.1080/0376835X.2012.706043

Murray, C.J. L., Vos, T., Lozano, R., Naghavi, M., Flaxman, A.D., Michaud, C., . . . Lopez, A.D. (2012). Disability-adjusted life years (DALYs) for 291 diseases and injuries in 21 regions, 1990–2010: A systematic analysis for the Global Burden of Disease Study 2010. *Lancet, 380*, 2197–2223. doi:10.1016/S0140-6736(12)61689-4

Newlin, M., Reynold, S., & Nombutho, M. (2016). Children from child-headed households: Understanding challenges that affect in their academic pursuits. *Journal of Human Ecology, 54*, 158–173. doi:10.1080/09709274.2016.11906998

O'Sullivan, L.F., Harrison, A., Morrell, R., Monroe-Wise, A., & Kubeka, M. (2006). Gender dynamics in the primary sexual relationships of young rural South African women and men. *Culture, Health & Sexuality, 8*, 99–113. doi:10.1080/13691050600665048

Piaget, J. (1964). Part I: Cognitive development in children: Piaget development and learning. *Journal of Research in Science Teaching, 2*, 176–186. doi:10.1002/tea.3660020306

Piontek, D., Buehler, A., Rudolph, U., Metz, K., Kroeger, C., Gradl, S., . . . Donath, C. (2008). Social contexts in adolescent smoking: Does school policy matter? *Health Education Research, 23*, 1029–1038. doi:10.1093/her/cym063

Raj, A., Jackson, E., & Dunham, S. (2018). Girl child marriage: A persistent global women's health and human rights violation. In S. Choudhury, J. T. Erausquin, & M. Withers (Eds.), *Global perspectives on women's sexual and reproductive health across the lifecourse* (pp. 3–19). Cham, Switzerland: Springer.

Rest, J.R., Narvaez, D., Thoma, S.J., Bebeau, M.J. (2000). A neo-Kohlbergian approach to morality research. *Journal of Moral Education, 29*, 381–395. doi:10.1080/03057240020015001

Ritchwood, T.D., Hughes, J.P., Jennings, L., MacPhail, C., Williamson, B., Selin, A., . . . Pettifor, A. (2016). Characteristics of age-discordant partnerships associated with HIV risk among young South African women (HPTN 068). *Journal of Acquired Immune Deficiency Syndromes, 72*, 423–429. doi:10.1097/QAI.0000000000000988

Rueda, S., Mitra, S., Chen, S., Gogolishvili, D., Globerman, J., Chambers, L., . . . Rourke, S.B. (2016). Examining the associations between HIV-related stigma and health outcomes in people living with HIV/AIDS: A series of meta-analyses. *BMJ Open, 6*, e011453. doi:10.1136/bmjopen-2016-011453

Sameroff, A. (2009). The transactional model. In A. Sameroff (Ed.), *The transactional model of development: How children and contexts shape each other* (pp. 3–21). Washington, DC: American Psychological Association.

Satzinger, F., Kipp, W., & Rubaale, T. (2012). Ugandan HIV/AIDS orphans in charge of their households speak out: A study of their health-related worries. *Global Public Health, 7*, 420–431. doi:10.1080/17441690903339652

Sawyer, S.M., Afifi, R.A., Bearinger, L.H., Blakemore, S.-J., Dick, B., Ezeh, A.C., & Patton, G.C. (2012). Adolescence: A foundation for future health. *Lancet, 379*, 1630–1640. doi:10.1016/S0140-6736(12)60072-5

Schaffnit, S.B., Urassa, M., & Lawson, D.W. (2019). "Child marriage" in context: Exploring local attitudes towards early marriage in rural Tanzania. *Sexual and Reproductive Health Matters, 27*, 1571304. doi:10.1080/09688080.2019.1571304

Sennott, C., & Mojola, S.A. (2017). 'Behaving well': The transition to respectable womanhood in rural South Africa. *Culture, Health & Sexuality, 19*, 781–795. doi:10.1080/13691058.2016.1262062

Shefer, T., Kruger, L.-M., & Schepers, Y. (2015). Masculinity, sexuality and vulnerability in 'working' with young men in South African contexts: 'You feel like a fool and an idiot . . . a loser'. *Culture, Health & Sexuality, 17*(Suppl. 2), S96–S111. doi:10.1080/13691058.2015.1075253

Smetana, J.G. (2010). *Adolescents, families, and social development: How teens construct their worlds.* Chichester, UK: John Wiley & Sons.

Spear, L.P. (2000). The adolescent brain and age-related behavioral manifestations. *Neuroscience & Biobehavioral Reviews, 24*, 417–463. doi:10.1016/S0149-7634(00)00014-2

Steinberg, L. (2005). Cognitive and affective development in adolescence. *Trends in Cognitive Sciences, 9*, 69–74. doi:10.1016/j.tics.2004.12.005

Steinberg, L. (2014). *Age of opportunity: Lessons from the new science of adolescence.* New York, NY: Houghton Mifflin Harcourt.

Swartz, A., Colvin, C., & Harrison, A. (2018). The problem or the solution? Early fertility and parenthood in the transition to adulthood in Khayelitsha, South Africa. *Reproductive Health Matters, 26*, 145–154. doi:10.1080/09688080.2018.1537417

Tanti, C., Stukas, A.A., Halloran, M.J., & Foddy, M. (2011). Social identity change: Shifts in social identity during adolescence. *Journal of Adolescence, 34*, 555–567. doi:10.1016/j.adolescence.2010.05.012

Theron, L.C. (2016). Toward a culturally and contextually sensitive understanding of resilience: Privileging the voices of black, South African young people. *Journal of Adolescent Research, 31*, 635–670. doi:10.1177/0743558415600072

Thomas-Slayter, B.P., & Fisher, W.F. (2011). Social capital and AIDS-resilient communities: Strengthening the AIDS response. *Global Public Health, 6*(Suppl. 3), S323–S343. doi:10.1080/17441692.2011.617380

UNAIDS. (2017a). *Ending AIDS: Progress towards the 90–90–90 targets*. Geneva, Switzerland: UNAIDS. Retrieved from https://www.unaids.org/sites/default/files/media_asset/Global_AIDS_update_2017_en.pdf

UNAIDS. (2017b). *UNAIDS data 2017*. Geneva, Switzerland: UNAIDS. Retrieved from https://www.unaids.org/sites/default/files/media_asset/20170720_Data_book_2017_en.pdf

UNAIDS. (2018). *Transactional sex and HIV risk: From analysis to action*. Geneva, Switzerland: Joint United Nations Programme on HIV/AIDS and STRIVE. Retrieved from https://www.unaids.org/sites/default/files/media_asset/transactional-sex-and-hiv-risk_en.pdf

Ungar, M. (2004). A constructionist discourse on resilience: Multiple contexts, multiple realities among at-risk children and youth. *Youth & Society, 35*, 341–365. doi:10.1177/0044118X03257030

Ungar, M. (2008). Putting resilience theory into action: Five principles for intervention. In L. Liebenberg & M. Ungar (Eds.), *Resilience in action* (pp. 17–38). Toronto, Canada: University of Toronto Press.

Ungar, M. (2011). The social ecology of resilience: Addressing contextual and cultural ambiguity of a nascent construct. *American Journal of Orthopsychiatry, 81*, 1–17. doi:10.1111/j.1939-0025.2010.01067.x

van Breda, A.D., & Theron, L.C. (2018). A critical review of South African child and youth resilience studies, 2009–2017. *Children and Youth Services Review, 91*, 237–247. doi:10.1016/j.childyouth.2018.06.022

van Eerdewijk, A., Kamunyu, M., Nyirinkindi, L., Sow, R., Visser, M., & Lodenstein, E. (2018). *The state of African women*. Nairobi, Kenya: International Planned Parenthood Federation Africa Region. Retrieved from https://www.ippfar.org/sites/ippfar/files/2018-09/SOAW-Report-FULL%20VERSION.pdf

van Hoorn, J., van Dijk, E., Meuwese, R., Rieffe, C., & Crone, E.A. (2014). Peer influence on prosocial behavior in adolescence. *Journal of Research on Adolescence, 26*, 90–100. doi:10.1111/jora.12173

van Zantvliet, P.I., Ivanova, K., & Verbakel, E. (2020). Adolescents' involvement in romantic relationships and problem behavior: The moderating effect of peer norms. *Youth & Society, 52*, 574–591. doi:10.1177/0044118X17753643

Wahlstrom, D., Collins, P., White, T., & Luciana, M. (2010). Developmental changes in dopamine neurotransmission in adolescence: Behavioral implications and issues in assessment. *Brain and Cognition, 72*, 146–159. doi:10.1016/j.bandc.2009.10.013

Wamoyi, J., Fenwick, A., Urassa, M., Zaba, B., & Stones, W. (2011). "Women's bodies are shops": Beliefs about transactional sex and implications for understanding gender power and HIV prevention in Tanzania. *Archives of Sexual Behavior, 40,* 5–15. doi:10.1007/s10508-010-9646-8

Wamoyi, J., Heise, L., Meiksin, R., Kyegombe, N., Nyato, D., & Buller, A.M. (2019). Is transactional sex exploitative? A social norms perspective, with implications for interventions with adolescent girls and young women in Tanzania. *PLoS One, 14,* e0214366. doi:10.1371/journal.pone.0214366

Wodon, Q., Male, C., Nayihouba, A., Onagoruwa, A., Savadogo, A., Yedan, A., . . . Petroni, S. (2017). *Economic impacts of child marriage: Global synthesis brief.* Washington, DC: The World Bank and International Center for Research on Women.

Wood, L., & Hendricks, F. (2017). A participatory action research approach to developing youth-friendly strategies for the prevention of teenage pregnancy. *Educational Action Research, 25,* 103–118. doi:10.1080/09650792.2016.1169198

World Health Organization. (2018). *Guidance on ethical considerations in planning and reviewing research studies on sexual and reproductive health in adolescents.* Geneva, Switzerland: World Health Organization. Retrieved from https://apps.who.int/iris/bitstream/handle/10665/273792/9789241508414-eng.pdf?ua=1

Yakubu, I., & Salisu, W.J. (2018). Determinants of adolescent pregnancy in sub-Saharan Africa: A systematic review. *Reproductive Health, 15,* 15. doi:10.1186/s12978-018-0460-4

3 Global and regional initiatives to prevent HIV among adolescents and youth

Fulfilling the promise in Eastern and Southern Africa

Tamar Gabelnick, Rhoda Igweta and Maryanne Ombija

Introduction

Over the course of the past decade, the global health community has shown an increasing interest in reducing HIV infections among youth, with a particular focus on adolescent girls and young women (AGYW) living in sub-Saharan Africa (SSA). Among the many reasons for their heightened concern is emerging data showing stagnating progress in curbing youth HIV infection and mortality rates, much higher infection rates among females than males in this age group, a set of root causes requiring greater attention, and a conducive political environment. As global health institutions seek to end the AIDS epidemic by 2030, more intensive strategies are needed to reduce new infections in this population, going beyond biomedical interventions to tackle the variety of societal, cultural, economic, and political drivers of HIV infection within this group.

Attention to HIV prevention among AGYW has been visible among a broad range of global health actors with significant political and financial resources at their disposal. Global health partners have created several new initiatives, frameworks, and funding streams, complemented by highly ambitious global prevention targets for AGYW. Continental and regional bodies in Eastern and Southern Africa (ESA) have also increased both their public discourse and initiatives on HIV prevention.

Such support is noteworthy: it has been maintained over a sustained period of time, backed by new funding streams, and coalesced around a distinct set of policy issues and recommendations. This chapter will provide an overview of these funding streams on adolescent HIV prevention and the common policy themes they have evoked. The chapter will also briefly examine national-level developments in ESA and provide recommendations on how to ensure the theoretical benefits of these initiatives actually change the reality on the ground.

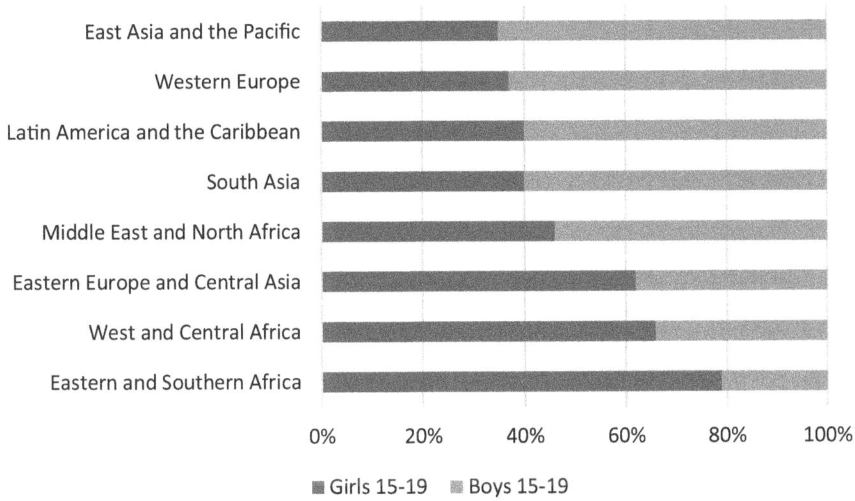

Figure 3.1 Estimated distribution of new HIV infections among adolescents aged 15–19, by gender, 2017

Source: UNAIDS, 2018 estimates (UNICEF, 2018c).

HIV and adolescent girls and young women – re-stating the major issues

Global interest specifically on HIV prevention among AGYW materialized largely after 2010, when reports began to highlight significant age and gender disparities in progress against the HIV epidemic on both prevention and treatment. Data from 2012 to 2015 indicates that AIDS-related diseases were the leading cause of death among adolescents in SSA and the second-most leading cause worldwide (UNAIDS and UNICEF, 2015; UNICEF, 2018a) (see Chapter 1 for more recent data).

While the rates of new HIV infections have decreased among all age groups since the late 1990s, progress among adolescents has stagnated since around 2013 (UNAIDS, 2013; UNICEF, 2017a). The absolute number of new infections is expected to rise steadily over the next decade, with projections of both growing numbers of youth in SSA (referred to as a "youth bulge") (UN DSA, 2015) and steady infection rates. Unless major changes in programs and policies occur, the number of new HIV infections among adolescents in SSA will rise 13% annually until 2030 (UNICEF, 2017a, 2017b).

Earlier chapters in this book have noted that in ESA, HIV prevalence is over twice as high among girls and young women as compared to men, and the countries with the highest levels of prevalence and highest absolute numbers of new infections among young women (15–24 years) are almost all found in ESA (Table 3.1) (Dehne et al., 2016). At the same time,

Table 3.1 HIV among adolescents and youth – global and ESA

	Adolescents living with HIV (10–19) global	*Adolescents living with HIV (10–19) ESA*	*New infections (15–19) Global*	*New infections (15–19) ESA*	*Young women (15–24) preva-lence global*	*Young men (15–24) preva-lence Global*	*Young women (15–24) preva-lence ESA*	*Young men (15–24) preva-lence ESA*
2011	1,600,000	1,200,000	320,000	155,757	0.4	0.3	4.1	1.8
2012	2,100,000	1,300,000	300,000	160,000	0.4	0.3	3.9	1.8
2013	2,100,000	1,400,000	250,000	130,000	0.4	0.3	3.8	1.7
2014	2,000,000	1,200,000	220,000	100,000	0.4	0.3	3.7	1.7
2015	1,800,000	1,100,000	250,000	130,000	0.4	0.3	3.5	1.7
2016	2,100,000	1,300,000	260,000	130,000	0.4	0.3	3.4	1.6
2017	1,800,000	1,100,000	250,000	122,000	–	–	–	–

Source: UNICEF stocktaking reports and statistical updates.

several countries in ESA have made progress in lowering new infections between 2010 and 2017 (UNICEF, 2018c), perhaps due to new programs implemented in this time period.

This marked gender disparity is linked to many socio-economic factors, including legal and societal inequalities and harmful gender norms. AGYW still experience "alarmingly high" levels of intimate partner violence (IPV) (UNAIDS and UNICEF, 2015) and child marriage, both of which raise the risk of HIV infection (Jewkes et al., 2010). Reported rates of IPV among ever-married women in SSA range between 20% and 50% in 18 high-prevalence states (UNAIDS and UNICEF, 2015). Child marriage rates in ESA were 35% in 2016, including around 9% who married before age 15 (UNICEF, 2018b) (refer to Chapter 7).

High rates of school dropout after primary or lower secondary school; discriminatory attitudes, practices, and laws; and other factors limiting girls' economic independence can also drive them to age-disparate sexual relationships and transactional sex. In such cases, the relationships are usually between young girls and older men who have already had several sexual partners and, in many contexts, a relatively high risk of HIV infection. These relationships are also associated with higher levels of IPV and an unequal power balance that can prevent girls from exercising decisions about using protection as well as seeking HIV testing or treatment (Piot et al., 2015, p. 7). An early end to girls' education is associated with a higher risk of HIV and a lower likelihood of seeking help in cases of gender violence (UNICEF, n.d.).

There also remain persistently low levels of access to sexual and reproductive health (SRH) education and HIV services among both genders in this age group (UNAIDS and UNICEF, 2016). For example, in 2016, only 15% of adolescent girls (15–19 years) in SSA had been tested for HIV in

Table 3.2 Drivers of HIV infection among AGYW and common proposed responses

Driver	*Policy/program responses*
Relationships with older partners or transactional sex	Social protection, such as cash transfers; empowerment and engagement of AGYW; PrEP for AGYW in high-incidence areas; voluntary male circumcision
High rates of school dropout (after primary or lower secondary school)	Cash plus care; free primary and secondary school; reintegration of teen mothers in schools; separate sanitary facilities and commodities for girls
IPV	Community mobilization and sensitization; post-violence care; economic empowerment and education
Child marriage	Raise legal and customary age for marriage; provide economic empowerment and education
Stigma and discrimination	Social engagement, political mobilization of youth
Lack of access to comprehensive sexuality education, including on HIV	Comprehensive sexuality education, inside and out of schools
Low levels of testing	Demand creation for adolescents; legal barriers to HIV services, such as age of consent laws; youth-friendly services; HIV self-testing
Low use of condoms	Condom promotion and provision

the past 12 months, and only 27% had comprehensive knowledge of HIV/AIDS (UNICEF, 2018c). Certain laws, policies, and societal stigma and discrimination, especially among healthcare workers, also create barriers to access to prevention services among AGYW (Eba, and Lim, 2017). Table 3.1 provides a summary of these factors, as well as the most common policy and programmatic responses put forward by global and regional policy-makers.

In global and regional fora, these data fueled a belief that the HIV epidemic could not be ended without a sharp decline in infections among AGYW. In new global HIV strategies, policies, and funding streams, AGYW began to receive greater attention than in the past, and a plethora of initiatives was developed to create an "AIDS-free generation," most of them centering around the policy initiatives (see Table 3.2).

Global policy and funding initiatives

As the central HIV advocacy platform with global, regional, and national convening power, UNAIDS has played a leading role in calling attention to the situation of adolescents and youth. Its 2016–2021 strategy seeks to ensure that "young people, particularly young women and adolescent girls, access combination prevention services and are empowered to protect themselves from HIV" through raising levels of secondary schooling, providing social protection to avoid transactional sex, reducing sexual and intimate partner violence, and ending harmful gender norms and practices (UNAIDS, 2010). These themes have been subsequently addressed in many UNAIDS progress reports, biannual governance meetings, guidance documents, HIV-focused panels with the Human Rights Council, and prevention reports and initiatives (UNAIDS, 2015). For example, the UNAIDS and UNFPA-led Global HIV Prevention Coalition endorsed a HIV Prevention 2020 Roadmap in October 2017 with a strong focus on AGYW combination prevention, and the UNAIDS-based secretariat is working with countries to set country-level targets and 100-day action plans (UNAIDS, 2018).

UNAIDS, supported by civil society and many governments, helped develop a strong AGYW orientation for the United Nations General Assembly's 2016 High Level Meeting on HIV (HLM). The HLM Political Declaration adopted by UN member states included a target of reducing new HIV infections among AGYW (15–24 years) to under 100,000 by 2020 (an ambitious 75% reduction from 2010 levels). The Declaration also contains an entire section of political commitments related to eliminating gender-based violence and empowering women and girls.

In 2016, with the end of the largely successful Global Plan (UNAIDS, 2011) to end vertical HIV transmission, UNAIDS and PEPFAR created a successor framework called Start Free, Stay Free, AIDS Free, which emphasized the Plan's less visible prongs,[1] including primary prevention among young women. The framework, led by PEPFAR, UNAIDS, UNICEF, the World Health Organization (WHO) and the Elizabeth Glaser Pediatric AIDS Foundation (EGPAF), created "super fast track" targets including the HLM's target of sharply reducing new infections among AGYW. These "Three Frees" have suffered, however, from a lack of enabling institutional support at the global, regional, and national levels.

UNICEF and UNAIDS launched the All In Fast Track for Adolescents framework in February 2015, a "collaboration platform" intended to drive national awareness and responsiveness to youth in 25 countries that contribute to 86% of all new infections in adolescents. It promotes leadership and advocacy skills among youth and strengthens national programming through better data collection and use and the adoption of innovative services. It set forth ambitious targets, including a 75% reduction in new HIV infections among adolescents by 2020 (UNAIDS and UNICEF, 2015). Together, the PEPFAR Determined, Resilient, Empowered, AIDS-free, Mentored, and Safe program (DREAMS), discussed in more detail later, and All In have been credited with sharply increasing the attention given to HIV prevention among AGYW and prompting others to follow suit, with All In raising the profile of the issue and DREAMS providing the funding for effective interventions (Dehne et al., 2016).

With its role co-leading All In, as co-chair of the Start Free, Stay Free, AIDS Free Framework working group, and through the promotion of other policies and initiatives, UNICEF has played a central role in calling attention to AGYW HIV prevention. Since 2005 it has also issued regular stocktaking reports on the state of the HIV epidemic among children, which pointed to the need for better data disaggregation and other policy changes (Idele et al., 2014). The reports have increasingly focused on the lack of progress for adolescent HIV prevention, with its 2016 report saying the matter was "dire," particularly for adolescent girls ((UNICEF, 2016). UNICEF's 2018–2021 HIV strategy decried the slow progress on HIV prevention among adolescents and designated "scaling up targeted HIV prevention for adolescents" as one of three core objectives.[2]

As the principal international health institution, WHO's increasing attention to adolescent health carries much weight, and it has used its role in setting the global health agenda, issuing normative guidelines and creating developing implementation tools to promote change at the national level.[3] For example, its Global Accelerated Action for the Health of Adolescents (AA-HA!) and guidance on country implementation emphasized the need for better data disaggregation by sex and five-year age bands for the first 25 years of life (WHO, 2017a). WHO HIV self-testing (HIVST) guidance included adolescents and young people among those high-risk groups particularly suited for self-testing, noting age of consent policies may need to specifically address HIVST to be accessible to adolescents (WHO, 2016). The 2016 HIV treatment guidelines recommended PrEP for people considered at substantial risk of acquiring HIV, noting that in ESA such populations include AGYW (WHO, 2017b). WHO guidelines can have a significant impact at the national level, as many countries eventually adopt them and are reluctant to make policy changes before WHO recommends them.

PEPFAR (U.S. President's Emergency Plan for AIDS Relief (PEPFAR), 2017) was among the original stakeholders to raise the issue of empowering adolescent girls and young women backed by a dedicated funding stream. In December 2014, PEPFAR created the DREAMS partnership, spending $761 million over four years to support packages of core prevention interventions in ten ESA countries,[4] with a focus on community-based, innovative activities in high-incidence districts (PEPFAR, 2018). In addition to keeping girls free of HIV, DREAMS aimed to keep girls in school, prevent early pregnancies, prevent sexual violence, and provide post-violence care (see Table 3.2). DREAMS investments were determined in coordination with national authorities based on the country context and priorities, epidemiological data, partners' capacity, and local leadership (see Table 3.3).

DREAMS also set out ambitious prevention targets, which sent a strong political message about the urgency of taking action, and guided implementing partners' activities over that period (PEPFAR, 2015). By the end of the DREAMS partnership (December 2017), PEPFAR reported it had reached over 1 million AGYW and contributed to a reduction of 25%–40%

Table 3.3 DREAMS interventions and countries

Interventions	*Kenya*	*Lesotho*	*Malawi*	*Mozambique*	*South Africa*	*Eswatini*	*Tanzania*	*Uganda*	*Zambia*	*Zimbabwe*
Cash transfers	X				X		X		X	X
Characterization of male partners		X			X					
Combination socio-economic approaches	X	X	X	X	X	X	X	X	X	X
Community mobilization and norms change	X	X	X	X	X	X	X	X	X	X
Condom promotion and provision	X	X	X	X	X	X	X	X	X	
Educational subsidies	X		X	X	X	X	X		X	X
HIV testing and counselling	X	X	X	X	X	X	X	X	X	X
Increase contraceptive method mix	X	X	X	X	X	X	X	X		X
Parenting/caregiver programs	X	X	X	X	X	X	X	X	X	X
Post-violence care	X	X	X	X	X	X	X	X	X	X
PrEP	X				X			X		X
School-based HIV and violence prevention	X	X	X	X	X	X	X		X	X
Social asset building	X	X	X	X	X	X	X		X	

Source: www.pepfar.gov/partnerships/ppp/dreams/c69041.htm (PEPFAR, 2017a).

in new HIV infections among AGYW (15–24 years) in 65% of high-burden communities and lower new infections across almost all DREAMS program districts (PEPFAR, 2017b). PEPFAR planned to continue support for DREAMS-related activities on a bilateral basis after 2017, adding five more countries in 2018.

In collaboration with PEPFAR to ensure complementarity, the Global Fund has also promoted greater support for AGYW programming through its technical briefs, 3-year grants, and special catalytic funds, which it allocates according to national priorities (Table 3.4). In its 2017–2022 global strategy and funding cycle, the Fund demonstrated marked commitment to supporting AGYW HIV prevention programs (GF, 2016). For example, it issued a technical brief on AGYW in high HIV burden settings to support programs strengthened through greater engagement with adolescents themselves (GF, 2017). The GF also created a special $55 million catalytic fund for AGYW in its 2017–2019 funding cycle for 13 countries in ESA, as part of its funding for key and vulnerable populations (see Table 3.3). The fund supports a range of biological, behavioral, and structural interventions with potential to target the key drivers of HIV infection among AGYW (GF, 2018a).

Building on these efforts, the GF launched the HER Campaign in Davos in January 2018. The HER Campaign is a platform for a variety of public and private financial, in-kind, and technical contributions for programs that address AGYW HIV prevention in 13 ESA countries. Citing the risk of a "catastrophic resurgence of the epidemic" among AGYW, the campaign seeks to reduce new infections by 58% over five years in this population (GF, 2018b).

Table 3.4 GF and PEPFAR AGYW funding overview (in millions of US dollars)

Country	*PEPFAR DREAMS (F16–FY17 implementation)*	*GF Targeted AGYW Prevention Activities (2014–2016 Funding Cycle)*	*GF Matching Funds Targeted AGYW Activities (2017–2019 Funding Cycle)*
Botswana	–	6.0	1.0
Cameroon	–	1.8	1.9
Kenya	39.5 (4 districts)	3.5	5.0
Lesotho	14 (2 districts)	2.6	1.5
Malawi	14 (2 districts)	12.0	7.0
Mozambique	20.4 (5 districts)	4.5	6.0
Namibia	–	3.0	1.0
South Africa	66.7 (5 districts)	67.0	5.0
Eswatini	10 (19 districts)	5.0	1.5
Tanzania	16.3 (5 districts)	–	8.0
Uganda	31.4 (10 districts)	–	5.0
Zambia	16.3 (3 districts)	–	4.0
Zimbabwe	20.6 (6 districts)	–	8.0

These initiatives address all the key drivers of the HIV epidemic among AGYW in a variety of mutually reinforcing approaches. They are complemented by a set of regional policy frameworks described below, which also touch on the same themes. While the impact on national activities and new infection rates is not yet certain, it is clear that high levels of political will for this subgroup of the HIV epidemic have been created across all major stakeholders in the HIV community and are standing the test of time in a field of competing and fleeting priorities.

African continental and regional policy frameworks

Since around 2005, African intergovernmental bodies at the continental and sub-regional levels have elaborated a wide array of policy documents that address the health and well-being of adolescents and young people, many of them connected to HIV prevention (African Union, 2011). At the highest level, the African Union (AU) Agenda 2063 (African Union, 2015) lays out Africa's aspirational development goals, including creating an enabling, people-driven environment to empower women, children, and youth to reach their full potential. Implementation of the Agenda would contribute to reducing the risk of HIV infection in adolescents and young people. In addition, the Africa Health Strategy (AHS) (AU DSA, 2016), the 2006 AU Continental Policy Framework on Sexual Reproductive Health and Rights, the 2013 Addis Ababa Declaration on Population and Development in Africa beyond 2014 (UNECA, AUC, and UNFPA, 2013), the Catalytic Framework to end AIDS, TB, and Malaria in Africa (African Union, 2016), and the revised AU Maputo Plan of Action 2016–2030 that operationalizes the SRHR framework all address issues at the core of HIV prevention among adolescents and young people.

The 2001 AU Abuja Declaration on HIV/AIDS, TB, and Other Related Infectious Diseases (African Union, 2001), renewed in 2006 and 2013, urges countries to invest 15% of their annual budgets in health. The 2013 Abuja Declaration encouraged countries to especially focus on increasing access to prevention programmes targeting youth, especially young women, to ensure an AIDS-free generation (African Union, 2013). These AU commitments demonstrate that there is continental endorsement of strategic approaches to addressing HIV and other health challenges for youth, and they are reinforced by AIDS Watch Africa's[5] Strategic Framework (2017–2030), which highlights the disproportionate impact of HIV on young people.

Regionally, the East African Community (EAC), Southern African Development Community (SADC), and the Common Market for Eastern and Southern Africa (COMESA) have promoted collaboration and accountability on ending AIDS among AGYW through various frameworks, policy documents, and model legislation. For example, the 2012 EAC HIV and AIDS Prevention and Management Act promotes a framework to address common priorities in the region and minimize gaps and discrepancies in national HIV laws. An assessment of the application of this legislation cannot yet be conducted, however, since Uganda is the only member state that has reviewed its HIV legislation since its passage. Moreover, the Uganda legislation has been criticized (Hanibal, 2017) as it criminalizes transmission of HIV and requires pregnant women to undergo mandatory HIV testing.

The 2008 SADC model HIV/AIDS legislation was developed to inspire countries to undertake legislative reforms in line with international human rights law and to promote the implementation of effective prevention, treatment, care, and research strategies and programmes on HIV. According to AIDS and Rights Alliance for Southern Africa (ARASA, 2016, p. 26), between 2009 and 2016, several countries in EAS (Angola, DRC, Kenya, Madagascar, Tanzania, and Uganda) disregarded the model law by introducing specific legislation or continuing to use existing legal provisions to criminalize HIV transmission, exposure and/or non-disclosure. In the same period, only Malawi, DRC, and Mozambique had made some progress in reviewing criminalization provisions in their laws. Only two countries in SSA (Comoros and Mauritius) have HIV-specific laws that do not criminalize HIV transmission.

The 2013 Ministerial Commitment on Comprehensive Sexuality Education and SRH Services for Adolescents and Young People in ESA (ESA Commitment) (Young People Today, 2013) was developed in response to the continuing lack of access to such information and services among young people in the region. Twenty-one ESA countries committed to taking bold actions to ensure quality comprehensive sexuality education and youth-friendly SRH services. To date, however, the implementation of the ESA Commitment has been mixed, with several countries not having taken any steps to develop a coordination mechanism or work plan or mobilize any resources, which are critical to driving its implementation (UNESCO, UNFPA and UNAIDS, 2016, p. 26).

Several other continental and regional initiatives have been created over the years to promote progress for AGYW. For instance, the theme of the Organization of African First Ladies against HIV/AIDS (OAFLA) for 2018 is “Transforming Africa through Prioritizing Children, Adolescents and Mothers in the Fights against HIV and AIDS,” focusing political attention on children and adolescents living with and at risk for HIV (African Union, 2018). Other initiatives such as the joint AU/OAFLA Free to Shine Campaign (2018) and the AU Campaign for the Accelerated Reduction of Maternal Mortality in Africa (CARMMA) all add to the continental push to ensure that AGYW have access to comprehensive SRH and HIV prevention services. When resources are available to drive the initiatives at the country level, there has been significant traction and greater likelihood of national impact. In the case of CARMMA, continental political support, a system for integrating the initiative at the country level, and an accountability mechanism are associated with progress on the ground (CARMMA, 2012).

National impact in ESA countries

Global and regional mobilization on AGYW appears to have prompted rising national political awareness and commitment to the issue in ESA, steering policy, guideline, and program development and orienting government and civil society activities towards evidence-based solutions. This connection is most visible when initiatives have been accompanied by funding, which strengthens the hand of the institution seeking national changes while enabling the country to pay for new or expanded programs. National buy-in to global goals and regular interaction between the global/regional bodies and the national authorities also stimulates greater national-level activities. Civil society involvement, both at the community and national levels, supports stronger connections between the aspirations of the initiative and the needs of affected populations.

For example, under the All In framework, UNICEF supported country-by-country assessments and investment cases in 25 countries in a process that included ministries, UN agencies, and young people (UNAIDS and UNICEF, 2016). It also led countries like Kenya, where a national high-profile meeting was held on All In, to give visibility and political attention to the AGYW issue. The Global HIV Prevention Coalition's push for national targets and action plans, backed by a global secretariat and national prevention coalitions, has also prompted several policy revisions and programmatic innovations (UNAIDS, 2018). The establishment of an accountability mechanism, including progress reports with individual country scorecards and community-based monitoring tools, has already appeared to encourage national activities, though civil society shadow reports decry insufficient community involvement in program planning and implementation (International HIV/AIDS Alliance, 2018).

Arguably, the clearest connection between global and local efforts has been due to DREAMS, where PEPFAR partnered with ministries of health (MoH) at the national level and emphasized the generation of evidence to steer programming. PEPFAR-backed largely community-driven intervention packages in a limited number of regions, closely monitoring implementation and data produced by the initiative. As of mid-2018, PEPFAR was still assessing why more progress was made in some districts than others, an analysis that will help shape its planned continuing support for DREAMS in a broader set of countries. It also began a process of consultation with adolescent girls on their priorities, with early feedback centering on enhancing financial opportunities.

As a public-private partnership, DREAMS acted as a catalyst to engage private sector partners and to work in coordination with the development community. DREAMS also created a ripple effect, such as South Africa's creation of She Conquers, a national campaign to take DREAMS beyond the four PEPFAR-supported districts. The Global Fund's 2017–2019 allocations and catalytic investment for AGYW will also build upon DREAMS, with dedicated funding set to arrive in 13 ESA countries in 2018. For example, Eswatini is joining forces with the Global Fund and the National Emergency Response Council on HIV/AIDS, resulting in close to national coverage for adolescent girls and young women (UNAIDS and UNICEF, 2016, p. 18).

Reflecting initiatives at the global and regional levels, most countries in ESA are in the process of reviewing or revising their HIV prevention policies and guidelines for adolescents, and some countries' policies include foci such as gender-based violence and HIV that had not been prioritized in the past (see Box 3.1). In Lesotho, in line with global and regional support for such activities, more policies and guidelines were updated or generated in 2017 than in the past decade combined. In June 2017, Uganda, with HIV prevalence almost four times higher among females aged 15–24 than males, launched the Presidential Fast-Track Initiative for Ending HIV/AIDS as a public health threat in Uganda by 2030, with a focus on girls and young women and their male partners.

Box 3.1 Examples of recent guideline and policy adoption/amendments in ESA

Kenya

- Building a situation room platform to better monitor prevention progress, including on AGYW
- Indicators for cash transfers for adolescents and retention in secondary school to be included in district health management system.

Lesotho

- Adolescent and Young People's Health and Development Strategy revised in 2015
- Comprehensive Sexuality Education Guidelines for Secondary Schools created in 2017, supported by UNESCO and PEPFAR
- 2002 Gender-Based Violence (GBV) Guidelines updated in 2017
- Guidelines for the roll out of pre-exposure prophylaxis (PrEP) developed in 2017; determines eligibility by risk rather than age alone, and includes PrEP for priority populations with high HIV incidence, such as AGYW
- National policy on testing and treatment, including HIV self-testing, revised in 2017; age of consent to increase from 12 to 16 years for testing at facilities

- Essential service packages for AGYW to be reviewed in 2018 and included in 2018–2023 national strategic plan.

Malawi

- National prevention strategy was being developed in 2018, including results framework and targets for AGYW
- A national strategy on condom programming was launched
- An AGYW empowerment/HIV prevention strategy was being developed in 2017–2018.

Mozambique

- Establishment of a national prevention coalition with high-level MoH leadership for the prevention agenda
- High-priority locations for AGYW HIV prevention were defined in 2017.

South Africa

- South African National AIDS Council has re-established a prevention technical task team and technical working groups, including one for AGYW
- National prevention targets are being revised in line with the 2016 HLM targets.

Eswatini

- A national HIV Prevention Road Map was launched, backed by a high-level oversight committee
- The 2017–2019 Global Fund request included increased funding for prevention.

Uganda

- Adolescent Health Policy Guidelines and Service Standards (2011)
- Presidential Initiative for AIDS Strategy on Communication to the Youth
- Investment Case for Reproductive, Maternal, Newborn, Child, and Adolescent Health Sharpened Plan for Uganda, 2016
- National HIV Testing Services (HTS) Policy and Implementation Guidelines – revised 2016; streamlines testing for minors, lowers

the age of consent for HTC to 12 years, and increases the number of young testing providers
- National sexuality education framework approved in 2018.

Tanzania

- A national condom strategy was launched in 2018 with focus on young people's access to condoms
- Plans in 2018 to establish program targets related to AGYW HIV prevention.

Zambia

- Legal and policy barriers to HIV prevention among adolescent girls identified; work ongoing with parliament on age of consent for HIV services
- National technical guidelines on HIV prevention among adolescents developed.

Zimbabwe

- Strengthened coordination on prevention among AGYW
- In 2018 public health bill review, proposals to address policy and legal barriers for adolescents to access health services.

Sources: EGPAF programs; UNAIDS (2018).

On the other hand, where global targets such as those in the Three Frees and the HLM have received less national or global advocacy, it is harder to observe a direct impact of the initiative. Since the creation of the Three Frees, progress has been made, including a 19% decline in the number of adolescent girls and young women acquiring HIV and 85% ART coverage for pregnant women globally. Despite these advances, however, most of the Start Free Stay Free AIDS Free targets will not be met (UNAIDS, 2020). In addition, ESA countries have been slow to implement global guidelines, such as those on PrEP and HIVST for older adolescents, and improving data collection techniques and age disaggregation. Many regional initiatives provide states with suggested packages of services, standards, and legal changes that may have inspired national revisions to laws and policies, but a separate analysis would be needed to review their country-by-country implementation. An analysis of adoption of the 2008 SADC model legislation, for example, shows no significant impact to date (UNAIDS and UNICEF,

2016), nor does the 2012 ESA model legislation appear to have had an impact. And despite the ESA Commitment referred to earlier, a large proportion of schools in SSA still promote abstinence only and teach "life skills" rather than meaningful HIV education or comprehensive sexuality education (CSE) (UNFPA, 2015).

Finally, global and regional initiatives do not appear to have promoted the development of much-needed inter-ministerial collaboration in such areas as education, social protection, and IPV. For example, most schools do not facilitate HIV testing or treatment access, which could be addressed through better coordination between ministries of health and education. Better integration has been seen, however, when global and regional actors underscore the importance of such integration, such as PEPFAR's push for an inter-ministerial strategy in Malawi and its support for sexual violence strategies in Mozambique and Tanzania. But such collaboration, as with all systematic change, requires national commitment for real effectiveness and sustainability.

Conclusion and recommendations

This overview of policy and funding initiatives does not represent the totality of global and regional efforts to cut new HIV infections among AGYW, but it does clearly demonstrate the degree to which global, regional, and national stakeholders have embraced the need to reduce infections among this group as key to ending the HIV epidemic. In boardrooms, conference halls, policy decisions, guidelines, and donor budgets related to HIV, there is firm and consistent support for tackling the root causes of HIV infection among adolescents and young women. Amassing such a level of political will is particularly notable in the face of historically weak backing for the broader prevention agenda (Dehne et al., 2016). The consensus around which policies and programmatic initiatives should be prioritized is also remarkable, with more options on what could work for different cultural contexts and epidemics than ever before.

As policy commitments have been matched with significant donor funds, ambitious global targets, new guidelines, and a consistent set of policy and programmatic recommendations, there would seem to be an extraordinary opportunity for real change for young people in ESA. But while supra-national support appears to be impacting policies and programs at the national and sub-national levels, at this relatively early stage the causative effect is unclear. Measuring the impact of each initiative in reducing HIV infections is also complex given the number of interventions being implemented in various combinations (Krishnaratne et al., 2016). Actors are also learning while doing, regularly refining solutions as new data becomes available.

At this point, some shortcomings related to the development and implementation of top-down initiatives are already apparent. For example, there seems to be insufficient emphasis on building national ownership of global and regional targets, as well as consultation with community-based groups and the affected youth. In addition, global and regional initiatives often lack mechanisms to assign responsibilities, monitor implementation, and hold actors accountable. The following recommendations would support better national-level outcomes:

- Global and regional organizations should work more closely with national authorities to ensure greater national ownership and alignment of national plans with global targets, initiatives, and policies.
- Global and regional organizations should work with civil society, including community-based organizations and young people, to ensure their initiatives respond to the true needs of the people they seek to support.
- Global and regional organizations should establish in-country focal points for their initiatives to maximize communication and promote comprehensive implementation.
- Global and regional initiatives should be backed by funding streams (from donors and/or national budgets) to promote maximum impact and sustainability.
- Global and regional initiatives should include accountability mechanisms with clear assignment of roles and responsibilities, establishment of SMART milestones, and a system of monitoring and evaluation.
- Countries should improve multi-sectoral collaboration between the ministries of health and education and ministries concerned with gender, social protection, and related areas to address multi-layered prevention needs in a coordinated way.
- National authorities should expand youth involvement in advocacy and program design, implementation, and evaluation.
- All stakeholders should support better capacity for disaggregated data collection so progress can be measured separately for younger adolescents, older adolescents, and young men and women.
- All stakeholders should continuously assess programs and policies against evidence and revise them accordingly when necessary.

The types of economic, societal, cultural, and policy changes needed to reduce significantly HIV infection among AGYW will require long-term political commitment and financial support for the types of programmatic interventions described throughout this book. Global and regional efforts are an essential first step to raise the profile and available resources for such activities. But global and regional actors must continue their support over the long term while working with national authorities to build political and financial support. The greatest changes will come only when national governments take full ownership of the issue, leading calls for change, providing adequate financial and human resources, and working closely with communities and youth to ensure effective laws, policies, and programs are implemented.

Notes

1 The four prongs of the Global Plan were primary HIV prevention, family planning for women living with HIV, HIV testing and treatment for women living with HIV, and HIV care and treatment for children and their families.
2 Available at: <www.unicef.org/aids/files/Unicef-HIV_Vision_Summary_Final_May2017.pdf [Accessed 15 February 2018].
3 One visible signal of WHO's interest in adolescent health was in the addition of "adolescents" to its 15-year maternal, newborn, and child health strategy: the Global Strategy for Women's, Children's, and Adolescents' Health 2016–2030, which emphasizes a number of socio-economic issues for HIV prevention among AGYW.
4 The ten focus countries are Kenya, Lesotho, Malawi, Mozambique, South Africa, Eswatini, Tanzania, Uganda, Zambia, and Zimbabwe.
5 AIDS Watch Africa is an advocacy platform of African heads of state and government within the AU.

References

African Union, 2001. *AU Abuja Declaration on HIV/AIDS, TB, and Other Related Infectious Diseases.* [pdf] Available at: <www.aidswatchafrica.net/index.php/commitments/declarations/document/29-2001-abuja-declaration/14> [Accessed 2 February 2018].

African Union, 2011. *African Youth Decade 2009–2018 Plan of Action: Accelerating Youth Empowerment for Sustainable Development.* [pdf] Available at: <www.un.org/en/africa/osaa/pdf/au/african_youth_decade_2009-2018.pdf> [Accessed 2 February 2018].

African Union, 2013. *Declaration of the Special Summit of the African Union on HIV/AIDS, Tuberculosis and Malaria: Abuja Actions Toward the Elimination of HIV and AIDS, Tuberculosis and Malaria in Africa by 2030.* [pdf] Available at: <http://alma2030.org/sites/default/files/head_of_state_meeting/abuja_declaration.pdf> [Accessed 2 February 2018].

African Union, 2015. *Agenda 2063 Framework Document: The Africa We Want.* [pdf] Available at: <https://au.int/sites/default/files/documents/33126-doc-03_popular_version.pdf> [Accessed 2 February 2018].

African Union, 2016. *Catalytic Framework to end AIDS, TB and Malaria in Africa by 2030.* [pdf] Available at: <https://au.int/sites/default/files/newsevents/workingdocuments/27513-wd-sa16949_e_catalytic_framework.pdf> [Accessed 2 February 2018].

African Union, 2018. *Twentieth (20th) Ordinary General Assembly of Organization of African First Ladies Against HIV/AIDS (OAFLA).* [online] Available at: <https://au.int/en/newsevents/20180129/twentieth-20th-ordinary-general-assembly-organization-african-first-ladies> [Accessed 15 February 2018].

African Union Department of Social Affairs (AU DSA), 2016. *Africa Health Strategy 2016–2030.* [pdf] Available at:<https://au.int/sites/default/files/documents/24098-au_ahs_strategy_clean.pdf> [Accessed 2 February 2018].

ARASA, 2016. *ARASA TB HIV and Human Rights 2016 Report*, p. 26. [pdf] Available at: <www.arasa.info/files/3314/8119/1044/ARASA_2016_Human_Rights_report.pdf> [Accessed 14 May 2018].

CARMMA, 2012. *CARMMA Country Scorecards.* [Online] Available at: <www.carmma.org/node/299> [Accessed 16 May 2018].

Dehne, K. et al., 2016. HIV prevention 2020: A framework for delivery and a call for action. *Lancet HIV*, 3:323–332. [online] Available at: <www.thelancet.com/pdfs/journals/lanhiv/PIIS2352-3018(16)30035-2.pdf> [Accessed 15 February 2018].

Eba, P. M. and Lim, H., 2017. Reviewing independent access to HIV testing, counselling and treatment for adolescents in HIV-specific laws in sub-Saharan Africa: Implications for the HIV response. *Journal of the International AIDS Society*, 20(1): 21456. [online] Available at: <https://onlinelibrary.wiley.com/doi/epdf/10.7448/IAS.20.1.21456> [Accessed 15 February 2018].

Free to Shine, 2018. *About Free to Shine*. [online] Available at: <http://freetoshineafrica.org/about/> [Accessed 16 May 2018].

Hanibal, G., 2017. *Uganda: New Law Criminalizes HIV/AIDS Transmission, Requires Pregnant Women to Undergo HIV Testing*. [online] Available at: < www.loc.gov/law/foreign-news/article/uganda-new-law-criminalizes-hivaids-transmission-requires-pregnant-women-to-undergo-hiv-testing/> [Accessed 14 May 2018].

Idele, P. et al., 2014. Epidemiology of HIV and AIDS among adolescents: Current status, inequities, and data gaps. *Journal of Acquired Immune Deficiency Syndrome*, 1(66):144–153. [online] Available at: <www.ncbi.nlm.nih.gov/pubmed/24918590> [Accessed 15 February 2018].

International HIV/AIDS Alliance, 2018. *Shadow Prevention Reports Highlight Significant Gaps*. [online] Available at: < www.aidsalliance.org/news/1136-shadow-prevention-reports-highlight-significant-gaps> [Accessed 1 August 2018].

Jewkes, R. K. et al., 2010. Intimate partner violence, relationship power inequity and incidence of HIV infection in young women in South Africa: A cohort study. *Lancet*, 376(9734):41–48. [online] Available at: <www.thelancet.com/pdfs/journals/lancet/PIIS0140-6736(10)60548-X.pdf> [Accessed 15 February 2018].

Krishnaratne, S. et al., 2016. Interventions to strengthen the HIV prevention cascade: A systematic review of reviews. *Lancet HIV*, 3(7):307–317. [online] Available at: <www.thelancet.com/pdfs/journals/lanhiv/PIIS2352-3018(16)30038-8.pdf> [Accessed 15 February 2018].

PEPFAR, 2015. *Fact Sheet: 2015 United Nations General Assembly Sustainable Development Summit*. [online] Available at: <https://2009-2017.pepfar.gov/documents/organization/247548.pdf> [Accessed 15 February 2018].

PEPFAR, 2017a. *Working Together for an AIDS-Free Future for Girls and Women*. [online] Available at: <www.pepfar.gov/partnerships/ppp/dreams/index.htm> [Accessed 15 February 2018].

PEPFAR, 2017b. *New PEPFAR Results Reach Historic Highs in HIV Prevention and Treatment*. [online] Available at: <www.pepfar.gov/press/releases/2017/276082.htm> [Accessed 15 February 2018].

PEPFAR, 2018. *PEPFAR's Focus on Girls, Adolescent Girls and Young Women*. [online] Available at: <www.wilsoncenter.org/sites/default/files/ambassador_deborah_birx_pepfars_focus_on_girls_adolescent_girls_and_young_women.pdf> [Accessed 3 August 2018].

Piot, P. et al., 2015. Defeating AIDS – advancing global health. *Lancet*, 386(9989):171–218. [online] Available at: <www.thelancet.com/action/showCitFormats?pii=S0140-6736%2815%2960658-4&doi=10.1016%2FS0140-6736%2815%2960658-4> [Accessed 15 February 2018].

The Global Fund, 2016. *Global Fund Strategy 2017–2022, Investing to End Epidemics*. [pdf] Available at: <www.theglobalfund.org/media/1176/bm35_02-theglobalfundstrategy2017-2022investingtoendepidemics_report_en.pdf> [Accessed 15 February 2018].

The Global Fund, 2017. *Technical Brief: Adolescent Girls and Young Women in High-HIV Burden Settings.* [pdf] Available at: <www.theglobalfund.org/media/4576/core_adolescentgirlsandyoungwomen_technicalbrief_en.pdf> [Accessed 15 February 2018].

The Global Fund, 2018a. *Presentation to Stay Free Working Group.*

The Global Fund, 2018b. *HER: HIV Epidemic Response.* [online] Available at: <www.theglobalfund.org/en/her/> [Accessed 15 February 2018].

UN Department of Economic and Social Affairs (UN DSA), 2015. *Youth Population Trends and Sustainable Development.* POPFACTS, No. 2015/1. [pdf] Available at: <www.un.org/en/development/desa/population/publications/pdf/popfacts/PopFacts_2015-1.pdf. [Accessed 15 February 2018].

UNAIDS, 2010. *Getting to Zero: 2011–2015 Strategy Joint United Nations Programme on HIV/AIDS (UNAIDS).* [pdf] Available at: <http://files.unaids.org/en/media/unaids/contentassets/documents/unaidspublication/2010/20101221_JC2034E_UNAIDS-Strategy_en.pdf> [Accessed 15 February 2018].

UNAIDS, 2011. *Global Plan towards the Elimination of New HIV Infections among Children by 2015 and Keeping their Mothers Alive.* [pdf] Available at: <www.unaids.org/en/resources/documents/2011/20110609_JC2137_Global-Plan-Elimination-HIV-Children_en.pdf> [Accessed 15 February 2018].

UNAIDS, 2013. *Global Report: UNAIDS Report on the Global AIDS Epidemic 2013.* UNAIDS. [pdf] Available at: <www.unaids.org/sites/default/files/media_asset/UNAIDS_Global_Report_2013_en_1.pdf> p. 17 [Accessed 15 February 2018].

UNAIDS, 2015. *Invest in HIV Prevention.* [pdf] Available at: <www.unaids.org/sites/default/files/media_asset/JC2791_invest-in-HIV-prevention_en.pdf> [Accessed 15 February 2018].

UNAIDS, 2018. *Implementation of the HIV Prevention 2020 Road Map.* UNAIDS. [pdf] Available at: <www.unaids.org/sites/default/files/media_asset/jc2927_hiv-prevention-2020-road-map-first-progress-report_en.pdf> [Accessed 15 February 2018].

UNAIDS, 2020. *Progress towards the Start Free, Stay Free, AIDS Free targets.* UNAIDS. [pdf] Available at: https://www.unaids.org/sites/default/files/media_asset/start-free-stay-free-aids-free-2020-progress-report_en.pdf > [Accessed 3 September 2020].

UNAIDS and UNICEF, 2015. *All In #EndAdolescentAIDS.* UNAIDS. [pdf] Available at: <www.unaids.org/sites/default/files/media_asset/20150217_ALL_IN_brochure.pdf> [Accessed 15 February 2018].

UNAIDS and UNICEF, 2016. *All In to End the Adolescent AIDS Epidemic a Progress Report.* UNAIDS. [pdf] Available at: <www.unaids.org/sites/default/files/media_asset/ALLIN2016ProgressReport_en.pdf> [Accessed 1 May 2018].

UNECA, AUC, and UNFAP, 2013. *Addis Ababa Declaration on Population and Development in Africa beyond 2014.* [pdf] Available at: <www.unfpa.org/sites/default/files/resource-pdf/addis_declaration_english_final_e1351225_1.pdf> [Accessed 2 February 2018.]

UNESCO, UNFPA and UNAIDS, 2016. *Fulfilling Our Promise to Young People Today 2013–2015 Progress Review The Eastern and Southern African Ministerial Commitment on Comprehensive Sexuality Education and Sexual and Reproductive Health Services for Adolescents and Young People.* [pdf] Available at: <http://youngpeopletoday.net/wp-content/uploads/2016/07/ESA-Commitment-Report-Digital.pdf> [Accessed 15 February 2018].

UNFPA, 2015. *The Evaluation of Comprehensive Sexuality Education Programmes: A Focus on the Gender and Empowerment Outcomes.* [pdf] Available at: <www.unfpa.

org/sites/default/files/pub-pdf/UNFPAEvaluationWEB4.pdf> [Accessed 15 February 2018].

UNICEF, 2016. *For Every Child, End AIDS, Seventh Stocktaking Report, 2016.* UNICEF [pdf] Available at:<www.unicef.org/publications/files/Children_and_AIDS_Seventh_Stocktaking_Report_2016_EN.pdf.pdf> [Accessed 15 February 2018].

UNICEF, 2017a. *Children and AIDS: Statistical Update.* UNICEF. [pdf] Available at: <https://data.unicef.org/wp-content/uploads/2017/11/HIVAIDS-Statistical-Update-2017.pdf> [Accessed 15 February 2018].

UNICEF, 2017b. *Key Global Charts and Figures.* UNICEF. [excel] Available at: <https://data.unicef.org/topic/hivaids/adolescents-young-people/> [Accessed 15 February 2018].

UNICEF, 2018a. *Patterns of Mortality Change as Children Enter Adolescence.* [online] Available at: <https://data.unicef.org/topic/adolescents/mortality/#_ftn3> [Accessed 3 May 2018].

UNICEF, 2018b. *Child Marriage is a Violation of Human Rights, but is All Too Common.* [online] Available at: <https://data.unicef.org/topic/child-protection/child-marriage/> [Accessed 14 May 2018.].

UNICEF, 2018c. *Turning the Tide against AIDS will Require More Concentrated Focus on Adolescents and Young People.* [online] Available at: <https://data.unicef.org/topic/adolescents/hiv-aids/> [Accessed 14 May 2018].

UNICEF, n.d. *Goal: Promote Gender Equality and Empower Women.* [online] Available at: <www.unicef.org/mdg/index_genderequality.htm> [Accessed 15 February 2018].

U.S. President's Emergency Plan for AIDS Relief (PEPFAR), 2017. *Adolescent Girls & Women: Creating Gender Equity.* [online] Available at <www.pepfar.gov/priorities/girlswomen/index.htm> [Accessed 15 February 2018].

World Health Organization (WHO), 2016. *Guidelines on HIV Self-Testing and Partner Notification Supplement to Consolidated Guidelines on HIV Testing Services.* [online] Available at: <http://apps.who.int/iris/bitstream/10665/251655/1/9789241549868-eng.pdf?ua=1> [Accessed 15 February 2018].

WHO, 2017a. *Global Accelerated Action for the Health of Adolescents (AA-HA!) Guidance to Support Country Implementation.* [pdf] Available at: <Global Accelerated Action for the Health of Adolescents (AA-HA!). guidance to support country implementation> [Accessed 15 February 2018].

WHO, 2017b. *WHO Implementation Tool for Pre-Exposure Prophylaxis (PrEP) of HIV Infection.* [pdf] Available at: <http://apps.who.int/iris/bitstream/10665/258515/1/WHO-HIV-2017.29-eng.pdf?ua=1> [Accessed 15 February 2018].

Young People Today, 2013. *Ministerial Commitment on Comprehensive Sexuality Education and Sexual and Reproductive Health Services for Adolescents and Young People in Eastern and Southern African (ESA).* [pdf] Available at: <www.unesco.org/new/fileadmin/MULTIMEDIA/HQ/HIV-AIDS/pdf/ESACommitmentFINALAffirmedon7thDecember.pdf> [Accessed 14 May 2018].

4 The All In assessments

Leveraging data to achieve results for adolescents in Eastern and Southern Africa

Alice Armstrong, Anurita Bains, Renato Pinto, Tyler Porth and Priscilla Idele

Introduction

As Eastern and Southern Africa (ESA) hosts 62% of the world's adolescents living with HIV, and with adolescent girls and young women continuing to be disproportionately affected by HIV, adolescents and young people contribute significantly to shaping the future course of the HIV epidemic in ESA (UNICEF, 2017a). In 2015, girls accounted for three out of four new infections among adolescents aged 15–19 in ESA (UNICEF, 2017a). There is, therefore, an urgent need to address the health and well-being of adolescents affected by and living with HIV. Yet until recently, little was known about the impact of HIV on their lives.

It is against this backdrop that we have seen a growing call for global advocacy and policy attention to adolescents and young people, which culminated in the launch of the All In to End Adolescent AIDS (All In) initiative in February 2015 (Joint United Nations Programme on HIV/AIDS, 2015a; UNICEF, 2015). All In sought to address the critical gaps in data on HIV response for adolescents, defined by the UN as the population 10–19 years of age. Through a structured systematic approach, the All In country assessments gathered national data to support the development of more effective strategies, policies, programmes and services for adolescents living with and affected by HIV (Joint United Nations Programme on HIV/AIDS and United Nations Children's Fund, 2015; United Nations Children's Fund, 2015).

Since early 2013, governments and the international community have become aware that adolescents and young people were being left behind in the HIV response and that urgent action was required. However, due to the lack of disaggregated data by age and/or sex in many countries, we have an incomplete picture of the HIV, health and social support needs of adolescents. Decision-makers do not know the extent of HIV infection and associated drivers and inequalities, making it difficult to design and implement population-specific interventions that are responsive to the particular needs of adolescents living with, at risk of and affected by HIV (UNICEF, 2016a).

Three years after All In's launch, countries in ESA have experienced far-reaching progress across multiple areas of adolescent HIV programming, laying the groundwork for improved adolescent HIV outcomes. This chapter outlines the progress made in the All In initiative and the critical insights of its impact on HIV programming for adolescents across the ESA region. These findings have been collated through a desk review of All In country assessment reports, observations during site visits and interviews with 43 individuals including government officials, national and sub-national implementing partners, UN representatives and funding partners.

HIV evidence and programme gaps for adolescents and young people

Adolescence is a period of rapid physical, neurodevelopmental and psychosocial changes, with cognitive development and social transitions continuing into the early twenties (WHO, 2014a). These changes affect adolescents' health, decision-making, vulnerability, risk behaviour and access to services. Accordingly, age is a highly important factor in the case of adolescents because it marks differences with regard to their relative risk of HIV infection, rates of infection, and opportunities for access to counselling, diagnosis, care and treatment (WHO, 2014a). Therefore, understanding age-specific needs in adolescents is critical for generating relevant evidence to inform national health and HIV programming.

A challenge is that there are different and sometimes overlapping age bands used in collecting data on adolescents, thus masking the age-specific differences within this age group (Idele et al., 2014). Global and national data systems have historically grouped adolescents into broad age brackets, either with those age 14 and younger or with those age 15 and older (Slogrove et al., 2017) or as part of young people (15–24 years). The lack of disaggregated data by age or sex, in particular at the sub-national level, means that sub-populations of adolescents and young people have been invisible in data-driven and evidence-informed programming efforts (UNICEF, 2016a).

Indicators across the HIV prevention and treatment cascade are missing, especially for measuring access, the use of community-based interventions and linkage between services (Idele et al., 2014). Further, important indicators are not harmonized for these adolescents. For example, national indicators related to violence utilize age bands of 13–17, whereas HIV data reporting utilizes age bands of 10–14 and 15–19. Additionally, the level of vulnerability and risk are not well understood, as definitions vary and measurements are not well established (Govender et al., 2018). Without these data, there is an incomplete picture of the health and social support needs of adolescents and young people. In turn, national responses are unable to monitor the progress of the HIV epidemic or HIV-related outcomes and, therefore, without adequate information to assess the resource needs, often the resources allocated to address HIV in adolescents and young people are inadequate.

The challenge in generating data, especially among younger adolescents, is often due to real and perceived complexities of conducting research on adolescents (Idele et al., 2014). For example, institutional ethics review board requirements deter researchers and sometimes programmes from including individuals younger than 18 years of age. This deterrent is often exacerbated in the cases of those who are particularly vulnerable (i.e. key populations) or whose behaviour is stigmatized and criminalized (Joint United Nations Programme on HIV/AIDS, 2015a). For adolescents, health data from administrative and programme sources is often limited to adolescent girls who attend family planning or antenatal care, as most adolescents are healthy and infrequently use health services (Idele et al., 2014). Additionally, in many countries, data collection systems remain weak and thus require considerable investment (Idele et al., 2014).

Road to All In – enabling change for and with adolescents

A number of factors led to the demand for an initiative that would recognize adolescents as a distinct population group, address the lack of disaggregated metrics and estimates and support effective interventions for them. Previous understanding of HIV among adolescents and young people has relied heavily on estimates and research studies often extrapolated from child or adult populations (Idele et al., 2014). UNICEF's secondary analysis of 2012 UNAIDS estimates indicated that adolescent girls and young women were disproportionately affected by new HIV infections, there was an increase in adolescents HIV-related deaths, and that sub-Saharan Africa carried the most significant HIV burden in this age group (UNICEF, 2013). Similarly, the World Health Organization's (WHO) 2013 Global Health Estimates for adolescents identified HIV as the leading cause of death for adolescents in Africa (WHO 2006, 2014a). At the same time, both qualitative and quantitative research began to highlight significant challenges for these populations compared to other age groups. Studies indicated low uptake of prevention interventions, challenges to access, low coverage (Ferrand et al., 2009) and poor quality of services (WHO and KIT, 2012; Li et al., 2010), in addition to higher rates of loss to follow-up (Lamb et al., 2014; Grimsrud et al., 2014), adherence challenges (Nachega et al., 2009), poor virological outcomes and an increased need for psychosocial support for those living with HIV (Lowenthal et al., 2014; Hodgson et al., 2012; Mellins and Malee, 2013).

As the magnitude of these challenges was being understood, it became more apparent that contextual evidence was needed on how HIV programmes targeted these age groups. Further, many programmes and interventions that were being implemented were not evaluated. It was clear that evidence of effective interventions was lacking for adolescents and young people. For example, a systematic review of the evidence to prevent HIV/AIDS in young people in 2010 found only four interventions showing sufficient evidence to enable implementation to scale (Napierala Mavedzenge, Doyle and Ross, 2011). Of the available evidence, this was often found too weak and of poor quality, as outcomes measured did not include biological markers, studies did not review multiple interventions and the data analysis lacked rigour (Napierala Mavedzenge, Doyle and Ross, 2011; MacPherson et al., 2015).

Given the increased understanding of the needs of adolescents and the gaps in quality data, governments and partners in countries began to request technical support in programming for adolescents and young people living with HIV, including those from key populations. This led to an increased policy focus and advocacy efforts at the global level. UNICEF conducted a comprehensive global review of HIV infections among adolescents and young people in 2011 and in 2012 (UNICEF, 2011, 2013), together with WHO, that paved the way for the development of the first adolescent-specific global recommendations on HIV testing (WHO, 2013). WHO's (2014b) guidelines for key populations included specific consideration for young key populations and, in parallel, the Inter-agency Technical Working Group developed a series of technical briefs (Joint United Nations Programme on HIV/AIDS, 2015a). Increased attention to broader adolescent health issues was observed, with the publication of the first WHO Health for the World's Adolescents report in 2014 (WHO, 2014a). On the basis of this work, UNICEF further advocated for age disaggregation of all core HIV indicators to include children and adolescents in the WHO (2015a) Consolidated Strategic Information Guidelines for HIV in the Health Sector. In all these efforts there was a clear call for better evidence, including the disaggregation of programmatic data and targeted interventional research.

To accelerate national-level change, it was acknowledged that a focused agenda and movement was needed, with a key focus on improved data availability and quality, leading to the conceptualizing of the All In initiative in 2014 and an official launch in 2015.

All In: a global platform for country-level change

Launched in February 2015 in Kenya, All In is a collaborative initiative aimed at accelerating gains towards ending the AIDS epidemic by 2030, by ensuring that no adolescents are 'left behind' in the HIV response. All In builds on the global goals set at the June 2016 United Nations General Assembly Special Meeting on HIV/AIDS by uniting governments, youth organizations, civil society groups and researchers around three measurable targets by 2020: (1) reduce new HIV infections among adolescents by at least 75%; (2) reduce AIDS-related deaths among adolescents by at least 65%; and (3) end stigma and discrimination (Joint United Nations Programme on HIV/AIDS and United Nations Children's Fund, 2015; UNICEF, 2015). Co-convened by UNICEF and UNAIDS, the platform focused on four action areas in 25 priority countries (see Box 4.1).

Box 4.1 All In action areas

- Engage, mobilize and support adolescents as leaders and agents of social change.
- Sharpen adolescent-specific elements of national AIDS programmes by improving data collection and analysis, and use to drive programming and results.
- Foster innovation in approaches that improve the reach of services for adolescents and increase the impact of prevention, treatment and care programmes.
- Advocate and communicate at the global, regional and country levels to generate political will to invest in adolescent HIV and mobilize resources.

Priority countries for All In were identified on the basis of the level of HIV incidence in adolescents and high HIV prevalence among adults; thereafter, they were selected on the basis of ensuring global geographic representation and in which tangible results could be achieved and demonstrated over a five-year period. Of the initial 25 priority countries, 14 were in ESA, reflecting the large adolescent populations and significant HIV burden in this region (Joint United Nations Programme on HIV/AIDS and United Nations Children's Fund, 2015; UNICEF, 2015). The 14 countries are Botswana, Ethiopia, Kenya, Lesotho, Malawi, Mozambique, Namibia, Rwanda, South Africa, Eswatini, Uganda, United Republic of Tanzania, Zambia and Zimbabwe.

All In country assessments: from national to sub-national level

Central to All In is the promotion and use of evidence to support the development of effective strategies, policies, programmes and services for adolescents living with and affected by HIV. Country assessments were designed to address the critical gap of adolescent-specific HIV-related data to strengthen planning and implementation for improved outcomes for adolescents (UNICEF, 2016b). The assessments were guided by a systematic process to identify equity and performance gaps impacting on adolescent HIV programming. These gaps served to inform priority actions to improve the effectiveness of national adolescent HIV responses.

Assessments were primarily centred around HIV outcomes but included a broad and multi-sectoral range of data and analyses to assist with contextualizing the HIV-related gaps for adolescents within the broader perspective of their holistic health, protection, education and general well-being.

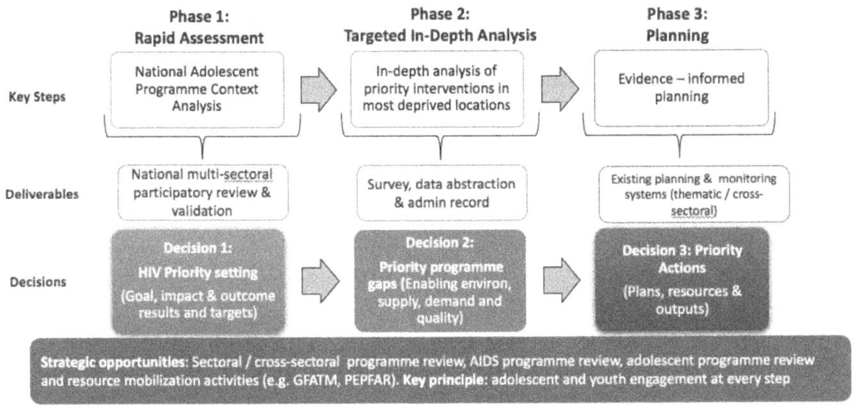

Figure 4.1 All In three-phase country assessment process

The country assessments adopted a three-phase approach (Figure 4.1) building on the broader UNICEF approach to equity-based programming (MoRES) (UNICEF, 2014). Phase I was a rapid assessment of the adolescent programming context. It examined data at the national and sub-national levels to define which adolescent populations were most affected, where they were located, what interventions have been implemented and where are the most significant gaps in terms of quality and extent of coverage to accelerate HIV results. It also included an assessment of the national programme enabling environment focusing on policy and legislation; planning, budgeting and coordination; and adolescent participation and monitoring systems. Phase II was an in-depth analysis of bottlenecks affecting coverage of priority HIV interventions in priority geographic locations identified in Phase I. This analysis enabled an understanding of cause and-effect mechanisms in programming, with the recommended corrective actions. Phase III utilized the evidence generated to inform planning to implement and accelerate corrective actions to address bottlenecks and data gaps and improve intervention coverage, quality and impact (UNICEF, 2016b).

A key feature of these assessments was to encourage countries to recognize potential limitations of existing adolescent-specific data on health. This analysis was supported by a review of data from other sectors such as education, reproductive health and social protection in terms of appropriateness and quality. New sources of data were also identified and concerted efforts were made to seek it out. Personnel in monitoring and evaluation programmes were also mobilized to support data analysis and data advocacy efforts. The assessments allowed for the utilization of data to inform programming, including an in-depth analysis of service delivery level challenges, with necessary recommended actions through the development of work plans.

Standardized tools and guidance, including the Adolescent Assessment and Decision-Makers' (AADM) Tool, supported the country assessment process (UNICEF, 2016a, 2016b), as existing tools did not provide a sufficient level of detail for HIV-specific analysis or programme planning for adolescents. This built on an earlier eMTCT Bottleneck Analysis Tool (UNICEF, 2016b) that was developed to facilitate decentralized planning towards the elimination of mother-to-child transmission. The concepts used in the eMTCT tool (i.e. using data from routine, estimate and household survey sources) were then applied to adolescent programming.

The AADM afforded countries the necessary platform and analytics to validate data, inform the review and analysis of adolescent programming gaps and facilitate the decision-making process in response. The tool collated data across multiple sectors and data sources (administrative and programme data, census data, global/national estimates, household survey data, etc.). In so doing, this process enabled professionals from different sectors and affiliations to look at data across the entire adolescent continuum for the first time. Its interactive dashboard enabled the visualization of data, optimizing data usage and the capacity to monitor the progress of key indicators. This was particularly helpful to visualize and understand the trends and HIV prevalence among the adolescent population groups (10–14 years and 15–19 years) by sex. After piloting the AADM tool, the dashboard was updated to include 20–24-year-olds in response to countries' requests to focus on adolescents transitioning into adulthood. The country dashboards typically showed patterns of very low HIV prevalence among 10–14-year-olds and then a trend of increasing new infections among older adolescents alongside disproportionate levels of HIV prevalence among adolescent girls and young women. These trends in the data allowed for discussions on the type of strategies required for specific age bands of adolescents and young people.

Although the country assessments were defined by a structured systematic approach, individual countries adapted the process and tools to reflect the local nature of HIV epidemics as well as their programmatic and geographic priorities. For example, to reflect its devolved health system structure, Kenya's entire All In assessment had a sub-national approach. In Rwanda, after the Phase I assessment, a national operational plan was immediately prioritized. Some countries did not carry out the whole process and used the AADM for programmatic assessments and analysis on adolescents (e.g. Malawi, Lesotho and Zambia). Stakeholders in these countries noted that the flexible nature of the approach supported their ownership over their assessments.

Engagement and collaboration with key stakeholders

The country assessments brought together key stakeholders within HIV and health; across sectors such as social welfare, ministries of education, youth and development, and justice; and other relevant departments in the ministries of health to coordinate activities for adolescents (UNICEF, 2016c). A number of challenges were noted in these processes. For example, countries found the enrolment process took time to get all the stakeholders on board, stakeholders faced competing priorities, addressing adolescents was new for many and there weren't dedicated experts to lead on it, and countries had limited experience in engaging adolescents. Political will and commitment were critical in the uptake and implementation of All In, with prominent leaders involved in launching and promoting the initiative across the ESA region (UNICEF, 2016c). The government's role in convening stakeholders was instrumental and strengthened their mandate as the lead for adolescent health. They took the lead in coordinating and analysis the data with support from UNICEF, UNAIDS and engagement from UN agencies (including UNESCO, UNFPA, ILO, WHO and UN Women) and key HIV partners in country (UNICEF, 2016c). UNICEF ensured regional colleagues were regularly updated on progress being made in countries in the region, which contributed to the regional visibility and mobilization. Particularly for countries undertaking All In activities in priority districts, the assessment processes facilitated efficient work between national and sub-national departments through having dedicated time to meet and focus on adolescent programming (see Box 4.2 for lessons learnt).

Box 4.2 Lessons learnt: leadership and collaboration

- Political will and leadership from the designated ministry or national authority is critical in driving the assessment process.
- Conducting data assessments at the sub-national level increases ownership and accelerates the assessment process.
- Bringing together a wide range of stakeholders, from different departments and ministries, improves understanding and working relationships.
- Engaging stakeholders from the very beginning of the assessment process is essential to facilitate ownership and commitment.
- Collaborative working between national and sub-national stakeholders ensures sufficient technical support to build capacity and enables the effective review of relevant policies and their implementation.
- Building upon existing technical working groups strengthens leadership and collaboration.
- Engaging M&E as well as programme staff improves future data collection for adolescents.
- Aligning advocacy efforts between multiple stakeholders increases its impact and the probability of a successful response.
- Technical support from joint UN organizations increases political commitment and supports advocacy effort throughout the process.

Through multi-sectoral technical working groups (TWGs), coordinating mechanisms for adolescents were established or strengthened, often for the first time (UNICEF, 2016c; UNICEF, 2018a). The TWGs included a range of government, civil society and implementing partners. They provided a platform for partnership, strengthening knowledge and data sharing, joint planning and the implementation of work plans. Four countries (Botswana, Kenya, Namibia and Mozambique) have also established TWGs at the subnational level. For the majority of countries where TWGs were established as part of All In, these have evolved into formalized structures to support ongoing adolescent programming and to accelerate and drive new initiatives (UNICEF, 2018a).

The multi-sectorial approach provided an opportunity to look beyond HIV-specific data and programmes and to review the broader health, policy and development context for adolescents. This approach contributed to addressing cross-cutting HIV structural drivers. For example, Ethiopia observed the inclusion of adolescent HIV in social protection programming, and in Mozambique, the process led to an evaluation of social norms that create barriers for adolescents living with HIV (ALHIV) to access services. In both Kenya and Ethiopia, other health departments and non-health sectors are starting to focus on adolescent programming (UNICEF, 2018a).

The country-level assessments were meant to complement existing HIV efforts such as the UNAIDS Fast-Track initiative (Joint United Nations Programme on HIV/AIDS, 2015b), PEPFAR's Accelerating Children's HIV/AIDS Treatment (ACT) Initiative (PEPFAR, 2014) and the Eastern and Southern Africa (ESA) Ministerial Commitment on sexuality education and sexual and reproductive health services for adolescents and young people (UNESCO, 2013); as well as new global and regional initiatives on adolescent health and HIV, including the Global Strategy for Women's, Children's and Adolescents' Health (UN, 2015), the PEPFAR DREAMS Initiative (PEPFAR, 2015), the Start Free, Stay Free, AIDS Free Fast Track Framework (PEPFAR et al., 2016) and the Global Accelerated Action for the Health of Adolescents (WHO, 2017). Working and aligning with these initiatives, All In has informed, supported and leveraged resources to expand country progress in addressing the HIV epidemic in adolescents and ensuring that they are at the forefront of the HIV response.

A key focus of All In is the engagement and mobilization of adolescents as leaders and agents of social change (UNICEF, 2016c). The country assessment process strengthened existing mechanisms to engage adolescents in programme design. To facilitate further engagement, the majority of All In ESA countries held consultations, focus groups or adolescent and youth stakeholder meetings and included adolescent representatives in the TWGs (UNICEF, 2016c; UNICEF, 2018a). Mobile technology (U-Report) was also utilized to understand views on sexual and reproductive health (SRH) and HIV interventions. In Botswana and Mozambique (see Box 4.3), the consultations generated countrywide engagement, including from rural areas and groups working with key populations and those with disabilities (UNICEF, 2017b). The consultation held in Rwanda was the first time that adolescents engaged in policy and programming efforts at the national level. At Tanzania's youth stakeholder meetings, adolescents produced a declaration that outlined the key actions and programming requirements that they hoped to see.

Box 4.3 Catalyzing adolescent participation in Mozambique

All In brought together 28 adolescents from 11 provinces across the country to Maputo for an intense debate on improving the HIV response. Mozambique's National AIDS Committee worked to make sure that the young people were in charge of the process: they fostered a safe space for adolescent participation, including the establishment of a youth Steering Committee; selected young facilitators; and relied on local organizations to choose participants.

> They traveled so far to discuss HIV issues, and they were so engaged and involved – they really understood what they were talking about. The adults were the shy ones in the back and the teenagers were in front. There was a power in the air.
>
> —Youth advocate and meeting facilitator, Mozambique

Source: UNICEF (2017b).

Ethiopia and Namibia leveraged existing youth networks, including those for ALHIV, and facilitated the involvement of younger adolescents, who are often overlooked. The All In process in Kenya continues to strengthen the response of the network of young people living with HIV (YPLHIV), with its members leading programming efforts at the sub-national level including HIV testing demand generation (UNICEF, 2018a).

The momentum generated by All In has contributed to and helped sustain adolescent participation in both policy and programming spaces, not only for HIV and SRH but across other health and development areas. Key lessons learnt throughout the process can now inform longer-term engagement with adolescents in the future.

All In country progress in ESA since implementation

The All In strategy has impacted multiple areas of HIV programming for adolescents. Across the ESA region, the strategy has made adolescents more visible, calling attention to their HIV health and well-being. The implementation process was seen by some governments' officials as a breakthrough that helped galvanize attention and focus on adolescents (UNICEF, 2018a). The country assessments also generated and collated data revealing changing dynamics of adolescent epidemiology along the HIV cascade (UNICEF, 2017b, 2018a). This strategic information is now forming the basis of national HIV responses and serving as a critical advocacy tool through the development of adolescent-focused work plans and strategies. As a result, adolescent HIV issues, including the call and need for tailored approaches in accordance with specific age groups (10–14, 15–19 and 20–24 years), are now on the radar of policy-makers and decision-makers, and shifts in programming are being seen (UNICEF, 2016c). The strategic information gathered by the All In country assessments has enabled changes to data collection for adolescents, policy and plans, more targeted adolescent HIV programming and mobilized resources. The following sections describe the progress made in these four pillars of programming.

Strengthening of strategic information

The All In country assessments collated available adolescent data and generated new adolescent data for the first time. This included critical strategic information at the sub-national level that was used immediately to inform adolescent programme planning (UNICEF 2017c, 2018a).

In Kenya and Tanzania, changes were made to key data collection tools to ensure national age disaggregation of data (see Box 4.4). The revision of tools for the national Health Management Information System (HMIS) in Kenya, the Tanzania Health Indicator Survey and the Kenya Population-Based HIV Impact Assessment will ensure the routine availability of adolescent specific data to support targeted programming for this population (UNICEF 2017c, 2018a). In addition, this available adolescent data is being used to strengthen country HIV estimates through Spectrum Estimation and Projection Package modelling. The All In assessments in Botswana also strengthened the strategic information components in the new national programming framework for adolescents and young adults (UNICEF, 2018a).

Box 4.4 Case study: strengthening adolescent strategic information in Kenya – revising tools and systems for disaggregation

In Kenya, the Ministry of Health worked together with other partners to overcome data availability limitations and challenges.

Actions taken:

- Established technical working groups to provide guidance and support
- Decided on the key indicators to assess across the HIV cascade and within other key sectors for adolescents
- Conducted a desk review of reports to identify and map out available denominators and numerators (for the key indicators).

Additional actions to address data gaps:

- Extracted HIV care and treatment data by age from facility electronic medical records and registers to estimate age disaggregated numerators
- Calculated sub-national adolescent HIV estimates using Spectrum EPP modelling by apportioning larger (regional) geographical data to estimate smaller area (county-level) population estimates.

This process and the results pointed to the critical need to strengthen and use strategic information for adolescents. As a result, the national HMIS data collection tools for HIV were revised to allow for age disaggregation.

Source: UNICEF (2017c).

The process was also able to accelerate advocacy efforts in Lesotho, Namibia and Zimbabwe on collecting and reporting age-disaggregated data, with a push to increase funding and capacity to strengthen data collection (UNICEF, 2018a). In Rwanda, where data collection previously allowed for age disaggregation, the data was not analyzed or reported accordingly. Country-level assessments also highlighted the need for continuous reporting of adolescent data (UNICEF, 2018a). See Box 4.5 for lessons learnt on strategic information.

Box 4.5 Lessons learnt: strategic information

- Utilizing a variety of data systems and sources, including primary data collection, provides clarity of programme coverage, needs and data gaps.
- Data gaps can be addressed by actively seeking data from alternative sources to generate new comprehensive data sets.

- The AADM tool can be successfully adapted to the availability of data and the country's context.
- Developing country-specific guidance on how to carry out the sub-national analysis (i.e. what data is available, where it comes from and potential system challenges) supports the analysis to be carried out in other districts.
- There are limitations to the data, in particular the use of denominator estimates. However, future use of the newly revised data collection tools allowing age disaggregation will reduce these limitations.
- Aligning timelines with other data or programming processes provides opportunities to share and advocate for robust data collection on adolescents.

Informing national policy and plans

All In supported the identification of adolescent sub-populations, interventions and geographic areas of focus, facilitating the inclusion of adolescents in relevant policy changes and planning. In Botswana, the process informed the development of a National Programming Framework for Adolescents and Young Adults, which in turn will direct the National HIV Strategic Framework for the next five years (UNICEF, 2018a). Likewise, in Namibia, adolescents now feature prominently in the National Strategic Framework 2017–2019, and its policy on ALHIV is being updated to account for the new data and programme changes generated (UNICEF, 2018a).

The data produced by the country assessments were instrumental in informing national plans in Zimbabwe (Accelerated Action Plan for the national scale-up of antiretroviral treatment [ART] for infants, children and adolescents), Rwanda (National Operational Plan for HIV and Sexual and Reproductive Health among Adolescents and Young Adults) and Ethiopia (Adolescent Sexual and Reproductive Health Plan) (UNICEF, 2017d, 2018a).

In Kenya, Mozambique, Namibia and Botswana, there are targeted adolescent activities planned at the sub-national level, showing that change from the national to local level can be supported (UNICEF, 2018a).

Evidence-informed programming

Given the challenges in generating evidence to inform HIV programming, the country-level assessments enabled more targeted programming for adolescents as a distinct population group with specific needs, the expansion and scale-up of existing adolescent programmes and interventions, improved collaboration for integrated adolescent interventions, better understanding of adolescent programming and importance of age and sub-national data, increased capacity of sub-national implementers and the introduction of new adolescent personnel.

Programmatic changes have been observed across the HIV cascade in Kenya. Priority counties have increased outreach programmes to provide adolescents and young people with HIV and SRH information, expanded HIV testing beyond voluntary counselling and testing (VCT) centres by training of hospital and clinic staff, and increased the provision of psychosocial support in facilities for ALHIV (UNICEF, 2018a). Youth-friendly services have also been revitalized, with key age-specific changes being made to services for ALHIV, such as adolescent-only times or queues. Since the All In country assessment, Namibia has also expanded psychosocial support for ALHIV through support groups and is moving towards national scale-up (UNICEF, 2018a, 2018b). Tanzania has developed an integrated, multi-layered intervention called Cash Plus, which provides a comprehensive package including training, mentorship and services for all adolescents aged 14–19 alongside a cash transfer programme (UNICEF, 2018c). Box 4.6 outlines key programming lessons learnt.

Box 4.6 Lessons learnt: programming

- Scheduling Phase II of the assessment prior to district planning maximizes the impact on programming.
- Allocating sufficient time at the sub-national level to undertake the analysis facilitates joint working and capacity building.
- Adolescent programming capacity at the national level is required to sufficiently support the sub-national analysis as well as ongoing adolescent programming.
- Having a clearly established three-phase country assessment, including supportive guidance tools, offers credibility to the initiative and provides greater confidence for stakeholders invested in the outcomes of the process.
- Sharing assessment results is a critical advocacy tool for improving programmes and strategic information for adolescents.
- Availability of adolescent-specific data offers a powerful advocacy tool to leverage resources.

The capacity of service providers and others working on adolescent health has also improved in terms of their understanding of targeted interventions and the importance of age and sub-national data to inform adolescent programming (UNICEF, 2018a). In Botswana, the Phase II bottleneck analysis in priority districts played a significant role in strengthening the capacity of sub-national level implementers (see Box 4.7) (UNICEF, 2018d). Namibia further supported their bottleneck analysis by providing additional training for both national and district teams on adolescent HIV during Phase II. Lesotho used the assessment outcomes to inform the development of adolescent-specific health and sexuality education training curriculums (UNICEF, 2018a).

A number of countries appointed additional adolescent personnel, including Kenya, Namibia and Mozambique. In Mozambique, funds were provided for technical assistance on adolescent programming to the National AIDS Council; in Namibia, an additional three positions at the national Ministry of Health were created on HIV prevention and treatment (UNICEF, 2018a, 2018b).

Box 4.7 Case study: building adolescent programming capacity at the local level in Botswana

In Botswana, the National AIDS Coordinating Agency (NACA) led the All In assessment, with technical support from UNICEF. Phase II was carried out in participation with sub-national stakeholders: the District AIDS Coordinators, District Health Management Team and representatives from the Ministry of Youth and the Ministry of Education.

Four districts were prioritized based on HIV prevalence, presence of key HIV drivers, geographic and demographic settings and performance of priority interventions. The in-depth analysis of the bottlenecks provided valuable evidence and understanding to inform future sub-national adolescent HIV programming.

Through this process, capacity was built around:

- Awareness of adolescents as a distinct population group requiring targeted programming and intervention
- The importance of age and sub-national data to inform adolescent programming
- Identifying available data and gaps
- The importance of utilizing other sector data
- Understanding of adolescent service delivery gaps and understanding of the implementation bottlenecks
- Sub-national adolescent programme planning.

Source: UNICEF (2018d).

Mobilizing resources

Since the launch of All In in 2015, international and domestic resource investment in adolescent HIV programming has increased in the countries that conducted the assessment. The All In process has assisted programmes to be more targeted and evidence informed while building in routine processes to make it easier for countries to request and allocate funds for these programmes (UNICEF, 2018a). Resources have also been leveraged to implement work plans generated as part of the All In process and for the expansion and scale-up of key adolescent interventions.

Across the region, funds from partners and donors, including UNICEF and UNAIDS, have supported key milestones of the All In country assessments. For Lesotho, partners, including Global Fund and PEPFAR, provided funds to further strengthen strategic information for adolescents (UNICEF, 2018a). In Kenya and Namibia, the integration of adolescent activities into larger international development partner operational plans and initiatives were particularly successful (see Box 4.8) (UNICEF, 2018a, 2018b). In Tanzania and Ethiopia, the All In assessment outcomes were instrumental in mobilizing additional funds for multi-sectoral programme proposals (UNICEF, 2018a). In Mozambique, Namibia and Kenya, funds have been allocated to appoint dedicated adolescent HIV personnel, increasing adolescent technical capacity at the national and sub-national levels (UNICEF, 2018a).

Additionally, All In assessments contributed to leveraging resources from country funding processes for the Global Fund to Fight AIDS, TB, and Malaria (GFATM). More specifically, the country assessment outcomes provided data and the direction to inform the adolescent components of concept notes and proposals for initiatives such as for adolescent girls and young women (AGYW) (UNICEF, 2018a). In Mozambique, assessments expanded understanding of in-school and out-of-school health services for AGYW, thus informing applications to the Global Fund for funding to improve and response to service gaps (UNICEF, 2018a). With the generation of routine adolescent strategic information and changes to key policies and plans, further domestic and international funds for adolescent HIV activities are anticipated, including resources for programme implementation (UNICEF, 2018a).

Box 4.8 Case study: leveraging funds for adolescent HIV programming in Namibia

The All In assessment findings helped Namibia leverage international and domestic resources to advance adolescent HIV programme planning and implementation.

Resources supported:

- Phase II of the assessment to be carried out
- The strengthening of national adolescent HIV technical capacity through three new positions at the national ministry
- Implementation of national and sub-national workplans, including:
    - Integration into larger international development partner operational plans;
    - Expansion and planned national scale up of support groups for adolescents living with HIV;
    - Programming for adolescent girls and young woman and for older adolescents from key populations.

Moving forward: challenges and opportunities

All In has made notable progress for adolescents and young people in ESA, catalyzing the HIV response to not only pay attention to their needs but also take targeted action. Despite this momentum, these populations continue to face barriers to receiving necessary HIV prevention, treatment and care. Most recent data indicate increasing numbers of new HIV infections as well as regional and gender disparities, highlighting the pressing need for continued and sustained efforts in this area (UNICEF, 2017a). For the adolescent HIV and health response, many programmatic challenges across strategic information, policy, planning, implementation and coordination remain.

The implementation of the All In country assessment within the ESA region has been varied. Priority countries, without routine disaggregated data, may need to repeat the initial assessment, which was completed two years ago, while other countries are only now gaining momentum and interest in conducting elements of the assessment. Non-priority countries have yet to conduct the assessments. Ideally these assessments need to be adapted and embedded in systematic monitoring and evaluation efforts that inform ongoing HIV programming for adolescents and young people across the region. The lessons from All In need to be promoted across ESA, where there is an opportunity to improve HIV programming and broader adolescent health. These assessments need to improve on processes and platforms for documenting case studies and results, in addition to facilitating intra- and inter-country peer-to-peer learning. Strengthening technical support will also be critical to building programming capacity and implementing adolescent programmes at national and sub-national levels.

All In has demonstrated the power of disaggregated data, especially at the sub-national level, showing that its routine collection and integration within existing data systems is achievable. However, for many ESA countries at the centre of the HIV epidemic, this granular level of data is still not systematically available. Ongoing advocacy for routine age- and sex-disaggregated data remains of critical importance as an essential requirement for adolescent programming (UNICEF, 2016a, 2016b). The promotion of the AADM tool and the supportive guidance generated (UNICEF, 2016a, 2016b) by All In, together with technical support, are urgently required to strengthen strategic information for this age group. Furthermore, to guarantee meaningful analysis, additional collaborative efforts are needed with national statistics departments to ensure appropriate sample sizes are reached while surveying the adolescent population. Although All In has used programmatic data to inform adolescent HIV programming, further support to data systems specific to adolescents is needed.

Although data across the HIV cascade are becoming more available, gaps remain, with less known about other important adolescent issues that extend beyond HIV, including sexual violence, mental health and substance abuse. These issues are increasingly prevalent and data is important for developing coherent, comprehensive programmes that target this transitional period of adolescence in a more deliberate way (Vreeman, McCoy and Lee, 2017; Lundgren and Amin, 2015). However, limited systematic data collection and analysis is in place, highlighting the need for health and other sector data systems to be adapted and harmonized. This could be achieved through the development of a central data repository for adolescents that is regularly updated, maintained, analyzed and easily accessed by those by the appropriate programme managers. Additionally, new indicators need to be established, including those for adolescents' participation and empowerment, to ensure their evolving contributions and engagement are monitored. For younger adolescents (10–14 years) and adolescent key populations, data are scarce and often anecdotal. Using community-based participatory approaches or implementing community or youth advisory boards that engage adolescents as partners can support relevant, ethically and appropriate research, especially for adolescents from key populations (Auerswald, Akemi Piatt and Mirzazadeh, 2017).

As a result of All In, targeted interventions for adolescents have now been planned and implemented. It is now vital to understand which of these interventions work and why. Ongoing mechanisms for monitoring the effectiveness of programming, including implementation science, should be developed to understand aspects of feasibility and sustainability – ultimately informing on how to take adolescent-targeted interventions to scale (Indig et al., 2017). Ensuring the quality of these interventions at scale demands clear policies and plans as well as tools to facilitate implementation, such as standard operating procedures (WHO, 2015b). Most importantly, targets and benchmarks need to be set to assess progress, facilitating the monitoring of equity in access and use of services by age, sex, geography and other socio-demographics, and programme performance for adolescents across multiple sectors.

Through All In, adolescents have become a prominent group in national policies and plans. Nonetheless, it is important that this population is not only included but that the content takes into account their distinct developmental differences, targeting its response accordingly. Such policy development is dependent on sufficient evidence from programmes and research. Academics have a key role in conducting research that is responsive to national contexts and priorities (WHO and IAS, 2017). Advocacy at the country and regional levels is essential for policies to overcome the ethical and legal challenges and age of consent barriers. These barriers limit access to essential HIV and health services and prevent data collection and analysis – a key priority for understanding and accessing adolescents, especially those between 10–14 years of age.

Coordination and engagement of stakeholders including adolescents were critical to the success of All In. The continuation and strengthening of TWGs will serve to advance collaboration and further facilitate emerging initiatives. The development of ongoing systematic processes that ensure the meaningful participation of adolescents and young people is fundamental. Achieving this demands requires investment and support for the capacity building of national and regional mechanisms and networks of adolescents and young people. Overall, for adolescent well-being – not just health or HIV – a comprehensive multi-sectoral response requires establishing a national institutional framework, as demonstrated by the National AIDS Councils for HIV. This approach could provide an accountability mechanism and platform for adolescent programme planning and house a central database.

With a competitive funding landscape for HIV, there is a need to optimize available resources. A clearly articulated case for investment supported by robust data and targeted programmes will ensure the greatest impact for this population. While All In successfully leveraged resources, there is a requirement for national ownership through domestic fund allocation, thus ensuring that adolescent programmes are embedded in government investments rather than ad hoc external funding initiatives.

Conclusion

All In has demonstrated that collating available adolescent-specific data – and in a number of countries, generating new data for the first time – is possible. The program has been at the forefront in supporting sustainable long-term change in national adolescent programming within the ESA region. This change places adolescents and young people at the centre of HIV programming and decision-making. The All In country-level assessments have indicated the need for comprehensive multi-sectoral focus on adolescents. They have catalyzed engagement and collaboration across multiple sectors in an inclusive and coordinated way, providing a visible and structured mechanism for the engagement and participation of adolescents in HIV and SRH issues.

The data collated and generated though the country assessments initiated important discussions and led to improvements in national data collection tools to allow for routine age and sex disaggregation, including at the sub-national level. This collation of data and improvements in some national data systems catalyzed the targeting of HIV interventions, the inclusion of adolescents in programming discussions and development, the development of adolescent-specific operational plans and the inclusion of adolescent interventions in national strategic plans. It also helped make a strong case for investment in adolescent HIV and leveraged additional resources from both government and other partners.

Above all, All In facilitated a differentiated approach to HIV for adolescents and generated a momentum that must be sustained. We learned that having adolescent-specific data is critical to designing and implementing programmes that are responsive to the unique needs of adolescents living with, at risk of and affected by HIV. It is vital that we share the lessons and steps taken so that programmes review, use and generate data on adolescents to strengthen the HIV response, and that these processes are routine and systematically part of our HIV review to strengthen HIV strategies and responses. Without a persistent, coordinated response that builds upon the insights and successes of All In, improving adolescents' health and wellbeing and ending the AIDS epidemic for this population will not be realised by 2030.

Authors' note

Conflicts of interest and sources of funding: Funding for this project was provided by core UNICEF funds for HIV (regular resources and funds through the unified budget, results and accountability framework).

Acknowledgements

This chapter brings together information and data from the All In process, which was implemented by the UNICEF regional office for ESA under the leadership of Anurita Bains and with technical support from Renato Pinto and colleagues in the country offices. Tyler Porth and Priscilla Idele were instrumental in development of the assessment tools, data quality assurance and technical assistance to countries. The chapter was compiled by Alice Armstrong and forms part of a series of case studies, blogs and videos showcasing the progress of individual countries and the impact of the All In country assessments in ESA.

The chapter includes contributions from All In country assessment reports as well as in-person and virtual interviews with 43 key government and UNICEF personnel and implementing organizations at the national and sub-national levels. Special thanks to all for their time, insights and technical contributions.

References

Auerswald, C., Piatt, A. and Mirzazadeh, A., 2017. *Research with Disadvantaged, Vulnerable and/or Marginalized Adolescents.* Innocenti Research Briefs no. 06, UNICEF Office of Research – Innocenti, Florence.

Ferrand, R., Corbett, E., Wood, R., Hargrove, J., Ndhlovu, C., Cowan, F., Gouws, E. and Williams, B., 2009. AIDS among older children and adolescents in Southern Africa: Projecting the time course and magnitude of the epidemic. *AIDS*, 23(15), pp. 2039–2046.

Govender, K., Masebo, W., Nyamaruze, P., Cowden, R., Schunter, B. and Bains, A., 2018. HIV prevention in adolescents and young people in the Eastern and Southern African region: A review of key challenges impeding actions for an effective response. *Open AIDS Journal*, 12, pp. 53–67.

Grimsrud, A., Balkan, S., Casas, E., Lujan, J., Van Cutsem, G., Poulet, E., Myer, L. and Pujades-Rodriguez, M., 2014. Outcomes of antiretroviral therapy over a 10-year period of expansion. *JAIDS Journal of Acquired Immune Deficiency Syndromes*, 67(2), pp. e55–e66.

Hodgson, I., Ross, J., Haamujompa, C. and Gitau-Mburu, D., 2012. Living as an adolescent with HIV in Zambia – lived experiences, sexual health and reproductive needs. *AIDS Care*, 24(10), pp. 1204–1210.

Idele, P., Gillespie, A., Porth, T., Suzuki, C., Mahy, M., Kasedde, S. and Luo, C., 2014. Epidemiology of HIV and AIDS among adolescents. *JAIDS Journal of Acquired Immune Deficiency Syndromes*, 66, pp. S144–S153.

Indig, D., Lee, K., Grunseit, A., Milat, A. and Bauman, A., 2017. Pathways for scaling up public health interventions. *BMC Public Health*, 18(1).

Joint United Nations Programme on HIV/AIDS, 2015a. *Interagency Working Group on Key Populations. Young Key Populations Technical Brief Series.* Geneva: UNAIDS. Available at: www.nswp.org/resource/young-key-populations-and-hiv-technical-briefs [Accessed 5 February 2018].

Joint United Nations Programme on HIV/AIDS, 2015b. *Fast-Track – Ending the AIDS Epidemic by 2030.* Geneva: UNAIDS. Available at: www.unaids.org/en/resources/documents/2014/JC2686_WAD2014report [Accessed 5 February 2018].

Joint United Nations Programme on HIV/AIDS and United Nations Children's Fund, 2015. *All in to End the Adolescent Aids Epidemic Launch Document.* Geneva: UNAIDS. Available at: https://childrenandaids.org/all-in-to-endadolescentAIDS [Accessed 5 February 2018].

Lamb, M., Fayorsey, R., Nuwagaba-Biribonwoha, H., Viola, V., Mutabazi, V., Alwar, T., Casalini, C. and Elul, B., 2014. High attrition before and after ART initiation among youth (15–24 years of age) enrolled in HIV care. *AIDS*, 28(4), pp. 559–568.

Li, R., Jaspan, H., O'Brien, V., Rabie, H., Cotton, M. and Nattrass, N., 2010. Positive futures: A qualitative study on the needs of adolescents on antiretroviral therapy in South Africa. *AIDS Care*, 22(6), pp. 751–758.

Lowenthal, E., Bakeera-Kitaka, S., Marukutira, T., Chapman, J., Goldrath, K. and Ferrand, R., 2014. Perinatally acquired HIV infection in adolescents from sub-Saharan Africa: A review of emerging challenges. *Lancet Infectious Diseases*, 14(7), pp. 627–639.

Lundgren, R. and Amin, A., 2015. Addressing intimate partner violence and sexual violence among adolescents: Emerging evidence of effectiveness. *Journal of Adolescent Health*, 56(1), pp. S42–S50.

MacPherson, P., Munthali, C., Ferguson, J. et al., 2015. Service delivery interventions to improve adolescents' linkage, retention and adherence to antiretroviral therapy and HIV care. *Tropical Medicine & International Health*, 20(8), pp. 1015–1032.

Mellins, C. and Malee, K., 2013. Understanding the mental health of youth living with perinatal HIV infection: Lessons learned and current challenges. *Journal of the International AIDS Society*, 16(1), p. 18593.

Nachega, J., Hislop, M., Nguyen, H., Dowdy, D., Chaisson, R., Regensberg, L., Cotton, M. and Maartens, G., 2009. Antiretroviral therapy adherence, virologic and immunologic outcomes in adolescents compared with adults in Southern Africa. *JAIDS Journal of Acquired Immune Deficiency Syndromes*, 51(1), pp. 65–71.

Napierala Mavedzenge, S., Doyle, A. and Ross, D., 2011. HIV prevention in young people in sub-Saharan Africa: A systematic review. *Journal of Adolescent Health*, 49(6), pp. 568–586.

President's Emergency Plan for AIDS Relief, 2014. *PEPFAR's Accelerating Children's HIV/AIDS Treatment (ACT) Initiative*. Available at: www.pepfar.gov/partnerships/ppp/dreams/ [Accessed 14 February 2018].

President's Emergency Plan for AIDS Relief, 2015. *DREAMS: Working Together for an AIDS-Free Future for Girls and Women*. Available at: www.pepfar.gov/partnerships/ppp/dreams/ [Accessed 14 February 2018].

President's Emergency Plan for AIDS Relief, Joint United Nations Programme on HIV/AIDS, United Nations Children's Fund, World Health Organization, 2016. *Start Free, Stay Free, AIDS Free. A Super-fast-track Framework for Ending AIDS among Children, Adolescents and Young Women by 2020*. Geneva: UNAIDS. Available at: https://free.unaids.org [Accessed 14 February 2018].

Slogrove, A., Mahy, M., Armstrong, A. and Davies, M., 2017. Living and dying to be counted: What we know about the epidemiology of the global adolescent HIV epidemic. *Journal of the International AIDS Society*, 20(0).

United Nations, 2015. *Every Woman, Every Child. Global Strategy for Women's, Children's, and Adolescents' Health (2016–2030): Survive, Thrive, Transform*. New York: UN. Available at: www.who.int/pmnch/media/events/2015/gs_2016_30.pdf [Accessed 5 February 2018].

UNICEF, 2011. *Opportunity in Crisis: Preventing HIV from Early Adolescence to Young Adulthood*. New York: UNICEF. Available at: www.unicef.org/publications/index_58708.html [Accessed 5 February 2018].

UNICEF, 2013. *Towards an AIDS-Free Generation Children and AIDS: Sixth Stocktaking Report, 2013*. New York: UNICEF. Available at: www.unicef.org/publications/index_70986.html [Accessed 5 February 2018].

UNICEF, 2014. *Formative Evaluation of UNICEF's Monitoring Results for Equity System (MoreS): From Evidence to Equity*. New York: UNICEF. Available at: www.unicef.org/evaldatabase/files/2120-UNICEF-MoRES_2015-LR(1).pdf [Accessed 5 February 2018].

UNICEF, 2015. *Synthesis Report of the Rapid Assessment of Adolescent and HIV Programme Context in Five Countries: Botswana, Cameroon, Jamaica, Swaziland and Zimbabwe*.

New York: UNICEF. Available at: www.childrenandaids.org/synthesis-report-rapid-assessment-adolescents [Accessed 5 February 2018].

UNICEF, 2016a. *Collecting and Reporting of Sex- and Age-Disaggregated Data on Adolescents at the Sub-National Level.* New York: UNICEF. Available at: https://childrenandaids.org/collecting-reporting-sex-age-disaggregated-data [Accessed 5 February 2018].

UNICEF, 2016b. *Guidance on Strengthening the Adolescent Component of National HIV Programmes through Country Assessments.* New York: UNICEF. Available at: https://childrenandaids.org/guidance-on-strengthening-adolescent-component [Accessed 5 February 2018].

UNICEF, 2017a. *Children and AIDS: Statistical Update.* New York: UNICEF. Available at: https://data.unicef.org/resources/children-aids-statistical-update [Accessed 14 February 2018].

UNICEF, 2017b. *Adolescent Participation in Mozambique: Blog.* Kenya: UNICEF. Available at: https://childrenandaids.org/node/467 [Accessed 14 February 2018].

UNICEF, 2017c. *Strengthening Adolescent Strategic Information: Revising Tools/Systems for Disaggregation Case Study.* Kenya: UNICEF. Available at: https://childrenandaids.org/node/469 [Accessed 14 February 2018].

UNICEF, 2017d. *Developing an Adolescent Operational Plan – Rwanda: Blog.* Kenya: UNICEF. Available at: https://childrenandaids.org/node/468 [Accessed 14 February 2018].

UNICEF, 2018a. *All In Country Assessments: Catalysing the HIV Response for Adolescents in East and Southern Africa.* Kenya: UNICEF. In press.

UNICEF, 2018b. *Leveraging Resources for Adolescent HIV Programming: Namibia Case Study.* Kenya: UNICEF. In press.

UNICEF, 2018c. *Cash Plus: Ensuring Healthy Futures for Tanzania's Adolescents: Blog.* Kenya: UNICEF. In press.

UNICEF, 2018d. *Building Adolescent Programming Capacity at Sub-national Level: Botswana Case Study.* Kenya: UNICEF. In press.

United Nations Children's Fund and Joint United Nations Programme on HIV/AIDS, 2016c. *A Progress Report: All in to End the Adolescent AIDS Epidemic.* New York: UNICEF. Available at: www.childrenandaids.org/UNAIDS-UNICEF_all-in-progress-report_2017 [Accessed 5 February 2018].

UNESCO, 2013. *Eastern and Southern Africa Commitment.* Paris: UNESCO. Available at: http://youngpeopletoday.net/wp-content/uploads/2014/12/ESACommitment-Progress_AnnualReport-DIG- ITAL.pdf [Accessed 5 February 2018].

Vreeman, R., McCoy, B. and Lee, S. (2017). Mental health challenges among adolescents living with HIV. *Journal of the International AIDS Society*, 20(0).

WHO, 2006. *Preventing HIV/AIDS in Young People: A Systematic Review of the Evidence from Developing Countries. UNAIDS Interagency Task Team on HIV and Young People.* Geneva: WHO. Available at: www.who.int/maternal_child_adolescent/documents/trs_938/en/ [Accessed 14 February 2018].

WHO, 2013. *HIV and Adolescents: Guidance for HIV Testing and Counselling and Care for Adolescents Living with HIV.* Geneva: WHO. Available at: www.who.int/hiv/pub/guidelines/adolescents/en/ [Accessed 5 February 2018].

WHO, 2014a. *Health for the World's Adolescents. A Second Chance in the Second Decade.* Geneva: WHO. Available at: www.who.int/maternal_child_adolescent/topics/adolescence/second-decade/en/ [Accessed 5 February 2018].

WHO, 2014b. *Consolidated Guidelines on HIV Prevention, Diagnosis, Treatment and Care for Key Populations.* Geneva: WHO. Available at: www.who.int/hiv/pub/guidelines/keypopulations/en/ [Accessed 5 February 2018].

WHO, 2015a. *Consolidated Strategic Information Guidelines for HIV in the Health Sector.* Geneva: WHO. Available at: www.who.int/hiv/pub/guidelines/strategic-information-guidelines/en/ [Accessed 5 February 2018].

WHO, 2015b. *Global Standards for Quality Health Care Services for Adolescents.* Geneva: WHO. Available at: www.who.int/maternal_child_adolescent/documents/global-standards-adolescent-care/en/ [Accessed 5 February 2018].

WHO, 2017. *Global Accelerated Action for the Health of Adolescents (AA-HA!): Guidance to Support Country Implementation. Summary.* Geneva: WHO. Available at: www.who.int/maternal_child_adolescent/topics/adolescence/framework-accelerated-action/en/ [Accessed 14 February 2018].

World Health Organization and International AIDS Society, 2017. *A Global Research Agenda for Adolescents Living with HIV.* Geneva: WHO. Available at: www.who.int/hiv/pub/toolkits/cipher-research-adolescents-living-with-hiv/en/ [Accessed 5 February 2018].

World Health Organization and Royal Tropical Institute, 2012. *The Voices, Values and Preference of Adolescents on HIV Testing and Counselling: Consultation for the Development of the World Health Organization HIV Testing and Counselling Guidelines for Adolescents.* Amsterdam: KIT. Available at: http://apps.who.int/iris/bitstream/10665/95143/1/WHO_HIV_2013.135_eng.pdf [Accessed 5 February 2018].

5 Three billboards to support ethical-legal adolescent HIV prevention research in Eastern and Southern Africa

Ann E. Strode and Catherine M. Slack

Introduction

It is a universally accepted legal norm that children (individuals under the age of 18) have fundamental human rights, like adults, and these rights may only be limited in justifiable circumstances (United Nations General Assembly: Convention on the Rights of the Child [CRC], 1989; Teddy Bear Clinic for Abused Children and Another v Minister of Justice and Constitutional Development, 2013). The South African Constitutional Court has succinctly set out the rationale for this approach by stating:

> Every child has his or her own dignity. If a child is to be constitutionally imagined as an individual with a distinctive personality, and not merely as a miniature adult waiting to reach full size, he or she cannot be treated as a mere extension of his or her parents.
>
> (*S v M*, 2007, p. 11)

The Convention on the Rights of the Child (CRC) is premised on the principle that all children are right bearers with inherent dignity (United Nations General Assembly, 1989). It is underscored by four principles, namely the right of every child to not be discriminated against; to survival and development; to have their best interests accounted for; and to be involved in decision-making which impacts them (United Nations General Assembly, 1989). These principles ought to inform the way in which we approach all public health programming for children, including the development of new HIV prevention interventions.

There is a critical need to evaluate whether HIV prevention modalities are safe and effective for use in a sub-set of children, namely, adolescents (Abdool-Karim and Dellar, 2014). Adolescents are often defined as persons aged 10–19 and this broad definition is widely accepted, even though it does not fit neatly with legal definitions that end childhood at 18 (United Nations General Assembly, 1989). In this chapter, we will highlight the complexities of undertaking HIV prevention research with persons who have evolving capacity to make health-related choices and are accorded special protections in law.

Prior work has examined how the principles in the CRC can be utilized to consider thoughtful involvement of adolescents in HIV prevention studies (Busza et al., 2016). This chapter builds on that work by critically discussing the legal and ethical complexities of involving adolescents in HIV prevention studies in Eastern and Southern Africa (ESA).

Inspired by the title of the 2017 Hollywood film (*Three Billboards outside Ebbing, Missouri*), this chapter first highlights that including adolescents in HIV prevention studies is legally and ethically justified; second, it emphasizes that the legal ethical complexities of involving them are resolvable; and third, it outlines how various stakeholders can "come to the table" to promote adolescent enrolment in HIV prevention trials.

Billboard 1 – adolescent HIV prevention research is legally and ethically justified

A fundamental human right is, as the International Covenant on Economic, Social and Cultural Rights (ICESCR) records: everyone is entitled to "the highest attainable standard of physical and mental health" (United Nations Office of the High Commissioner for Human Rights [OHCHR], 1966, p. 4). The CRC uses the same terminology when describing children's rights (United Nations General Assembly, 1989). The African Charter on Human and People's Rights (ACGPR) formulates this in a similar manner, stating that all people have the right to the "best attainable state of physical and mental health" (African Commission on Human and Peoples' Rights [ACHPR], 1981, p. 3). It is argued that to achieve this goal (of "best" or "highest" "attainable standard" of healthcare), ongoing research is required to develop and improve interventions, treatments and services.

Furthermore, when research is undertaken, everyone has the right to benefit from it. Article 15 of the ICESCR states that everyone is entitled to "enjoy the benefits of scientific progress and its applications" (OHCHR, 1966, p. 5). Recently, this has been referred to as a "right to science" (Scanlon et al., 2017). It is suggested that the right has three core elements, all of which place obligations on the state (Scanlon et al., 2017). These elements are, first, an obligation on the state to ensure everyone benefits from science; second, a right to contribute to scientific advances and a freedom to undertake research; and third, a right to be involved in scientific decision-making (Scanlon et al., 2017).

The CRC does not itself expressly refer to a child's rights regarding research or science. However, point 29 of the General Comment No. 3 (2003) on HIV/AIDS and the Rights of the Child issued by the Committee on the Rights of the Child emphasizes:

> Consistent with article 24 of the Convention, State parties must ensure that HIV/AIDS research programmes include specific studies that

> contribute to effective prevention, care, treatment and impact reduction for children.
>
> (p. 23)

General Comment No. 5 of 2003 asserts further that states should ensure that this is done in a particular way:

> The Committee emphasizes that, in many cases, only children themselves are in a position to indicate whether their rights are being fully recognized and realized. Interviewing children and using children as researchers (with appropriate safeguards) is likely to be an important way of finding out, for example, to what extent their civil rights, including the crucial right set out in article 12, to have their views heard and given due consideration, are respected within the family, in schools and so on.
>
> (UN Committee on the Rights of the Child [CRC], 2003, p. 41)

The approach in this General Comment reflects a shift towards protecting children *from unsafe, ineffective interventions* through data obtained from children themselves, via rigorous studies, and away from protecting children *from research participation per se* (Nelson et al., 2010). The General Comments quoted above show that the Committee on the Rights of the Child (the body which ensures implementation of the CRC) interprets the health rights within the CRC to include child participation in research.

Likewise, there are ethical arguments for including adolescents in HIV prevention trials that can be made through the application of key ethical principles – beneficence and justice, based on various international ethical guidelines.

The principle of *beneficence* motivates the inclusion of children in research because it requires researchers to strive for the greater good. In the case of HIV prevention research, this point has been argued because HIV is a significant health threat and health challenge for many adolescents, including in Africa:

> Beneficence provides an ethical basis for conducting research that may improve health and a basis for maximizing the benefit of research and minimizing its risk. Research with adolescents may have important benefits to individual adolescents, and it may benefit adolescents as a group as well.
>
> (Santelli et al., 2003, p. 398)

Accordingly, the ethical principle of beneficence as grounds to promote the welfare of enrolled children, and to consider benefits to "children as a social group . . . through the implementation of evidence-based policy-practice" is a recommended consideration for researchers (UNICEF, 2013, p. 17).

The ethical principle of non-maleficence (to *avoid harm*) can also be invoked to enable inclusion of children/adolescents in research. For example, not testing products on adolescents can result in their exposure to interventions that are potentially ineffective and possibly harmful:

> In general, this lack of information results in higher risks for . . . adolescents from being exposed to interventions where little is known about their specific effects or safety in this population. Therefore, it is imperative to involve . . . adolescents in research.
>
> (Council for International Organizations of Medical Sciences [CIOMS], 2016, p. 66)

Also, the ethical principle of *justice* underpins efforts to include adolescents in research, as it requires adolescents to be treated equally:

> The principle of justice demands a fair sharing of both risks and benefits. If certain groups of persons are systematically excluded from participation in research, these groups may not share in the beneficial results of that research. Promoting full participation by groups that historically have been excluded from research and its benefits is founded on the principle of justice. The interests of justice demand that adolescents . . . not be excluded from participation in research that may have direct or indirect benefit.
>
> (Santelli et al., 2003, p. 398)

Another ethical principle that is relevant is that of *respect for persons* (Santelli et al., 2003), which encourages researchers to show respect for the evolving ability of adolescents to make decisions about participation in research and to recognize adolescent limitations in judgement when consent approaches are designed.

When international ethical-legal principles are applied in the context of HIV prevention, it is argued that enrolling adolescents in such research is justified both legally and ethically. First, using the Scanlan, Macnaughton and Sprague approach it is submitted that countries have a responsibility to ensure that the highest attainable standard of healthcare is provided to children. As stated previously, adolescents are at an increased risk of contracting HIV and interventions are necessary to address their particular vulnerability to infection (Bekker et al., 2015; Hosek and Zimet, 2010; Shah et al., 2018; Osmanov, 2007). More specifically, adolescent behaviours place them at risk of HIV (e.g. early sexual debut, inconsistent condom use). Features of adolescence may also heighten their HIV risk (e.g. sensation-seeking). Structural factors may impact their risk (e.g. inadequate frameworks for their access to services). Adolescents constitute a key population for HIV intervention including for biomedical approaches (Hosek and Zimet, 2010; Wilson et al., 2010).

Extrapolation of data from adult studies (e.g. on safety, acceptability, efficacy) may be very difficult. Even where such extrapolations may be made, some studies will be necessary to answer specific questions of safety, feasibility, acceptability or adherence in the adolescent group given the differences in the way adolescence may react to, metabolize or respond to interventions only tested in adults. Also, regulatory approval will likely require data from this group (for "youth labelling indications," i.e., detail in the package insert which describes dosage and possible side effects for young people). Ideally this should be concurrent with adult product licensure to prevent off-label use (Kapogiannis et al., 2010), where adolescents make use of prevention products in an manner unsupported by evidence or regulatory approval.

In summary, it is argued that failing to address the needs of adolescents for HIV prevention violates their right to the highest attainable standard of healthcare as provided for in both the CRC and the ICESCR. This argument is supported by the wording in Article 24(2)(f) of the CRC that requires state parties to "develop preventive health care" as part of a child's right to health (CRC, 2003, p. 172). Arguably, preventive healthcare cannot be developed without research involving adolescents. This interpretation of Article 24 in the CRC is confirmed by General Comments 3 and 5, referred to earlier, both of which require research to ensure the promotion of children's right to health.

The legal rights–based argument – that research is an essential element of the right to ensure the highest attainable standard of health – is supported by the approach in ethics guidelines in many countries. South African ethics guidelines remind researchers that while adolescents should not bear research burdens unnecessarily, adolescents "are entitled to improved health care based on findings drawn from rigorous research conducted in the child population" (South Africa Department of Health [SA DOH], 2015, p. 28). Researchers are also encouraged to avoid the systematic exclusion of "vulnerable participants because to do so is unfairly discriminatory and vulnerable persons are potential beneficiaries of relevant research" (SA DOH, 2015, p. 8). This ethical approach is similar to the legal one, as it is premised on obligations to achieve a high standard of health.

Second, failing to undertake adolescent HIV prevention studies, and excluding adolescents as participants, violates adolescents' rights to equality. It would be wrong for adults to "enjoy the benefits of scientific progress" while adolescents do not, insofar as they access interventions with little safety or effectiveness data for their age category (OHCHR, 1966, p. 5; Strode et al., 2014).

Third, using the Scanlan et al. approach, it is submitted that a core part of the right to science is to participate in its development (Scanlon et al., 2017). Excluding adolescent participants from studies of HIV prevention means that we violate one of the one core principles underpinning the CRC, that of child participation. This impacts directly on the interventions we are trying to develop for this age category. Ivan-Smith and Johnson (1998) have stated that vital information is needed in order to develop solutions that will address adolescent concerns.

It also undermines adolescents' right to dignity (*S v M*, 2007). The CRC recognizes that every child has inherent worth (United Nations General Assembly, 1989). Delaying adolescents access to potentially life-saving interventions to prevent HIV violates their dignity as it shows a lack of commitment to addressing their particular needs, implying they are of less value in a national HIV prevention programme.

Likewise, ethics guidance suggests a need to recognize the "positive benefits that well-conducted clinical research can bring, and the dangers of providing healthcare that is not underpinned by a solid evidence base" (Nuffield Council on Bioethics, 2015, p. 80).

Billboard 2 – stakeholders must prepare for complexities related to adolescent capacity and adolescent behaviour

It is evident that adolescent enrolment in HIV prevention studies is critical, yet features of adolescence may potentially heighten risk of study-related harm and potentially undermine comprehension required for agreement to take part. For example, sensitivity to peer evaluation may heighten their experiences of stigma from trial participation, or deficiencies in abstract reasoning or conceptual thinking and experiential immaturity may compromise their ability to understand research and research-related risks (MacQueen and Abdool-Karim, 2007). Furthermore, HIV prevention studies may involve invasive procedures with the potential for risk and burden. Adolescents may undergo sexual risk assessments, contraceptive compliance assessments, STI and/or HIV testing and product administration (Bekker, 2014, 2015).

In ESA, the enrolment of adolescents in HIV prevention studies is not a simple endeavour. Complexities relate to regulatory frameworks that do not adequately address issues relating to the *study population* (adolescents). Some frameworks also provide insufficient guidance on complexities related to the *study questions and procedures* (e.g. sensitive, stigmatized behaviours related to sexual activity or identity, such as same-sex behaviour). The following sections describe some of these complexities and ways in which researchers, research ethics committees and other stakeholders can respond to them.

Adolescent capacity

The complexity with involving persons under the age of 18 in studies is that they lack *full legal capacity* (United Nations General Assembly, 1989; World Health Organization [WHO], 2018). This generally necessitates the assistance of an adult entrusted with decision-making authority, which is usually the parent or guardian (Strode et al., 2010; WHO, 2018). It is generally recognized that parents/guardians generally are the individuals who would have knowledge of what their child needs are, would protect them from risks and hazards and would protect their interests (Santelli et al., 2017), given adolescents' inexperience regarding decision-making in real-world situations (Santelli et al., 2003). This has led to many countries requiring parental/guardianship permission for adolescent participation in studies (CIOMS, 2016).

Responses to lack of adolescent capacity are reflected in the ethical-legal frameworks of several ESA countries, where adolescents are only able to participate in health research with parental or guardianship consent (Grant and Patel, 2016). Table 5.1 provides information from four countries to illustrate this point.

Table 5.1 shows that in some ESA countries hosting prevention studies, the legal framework narrowly confines acceptable consent strategies to parental/guardianship consent. This consent strategy means dual decision-making (parental permission and adolescent assent), and it is not straightforward because:

1 Some adolescents may not be cared for on a day-to-day basis by their parents or legal guardians (Strode and Slack, 2011).
2 The values and preferences of both parties may not be aligned.
3 There may be power disparities between children and adults, and some societies may place a high social value on obedience, which might tempt adolescents to align their decisions to parental preferences over their own.
4 Most critically, many adolescents generally do not want their parents to know about sexual activity or sexual orientation that might attract parental disapproval or sanction (Abdool-Karim and Dellar, 2014; Gilbert et al., 2015; Hosek and Zimet, 2010; Knopf et al., 2017; Shah et al., 2018; Wallace et al., 2018).

RECs reviewing trials in such settings may be sympathetic to the above problems; nevertheless, they face an ethical-legal dilemma in that they are required to act ethically *and* to comply with legal obligations. Where there

Table 5.1 The legal age of consent to health research in selected ESA countries

Country	*Age of independent consent to health research*
Ethiopia	18
Kenya	18
Mozambique	21
South Africa	18

is a conflict between law and ethics the REC ought to seek advice on the way forward. A principled position should be developed and institutional support sought to ensure consistency in REC decision-making.

The situation is also complex because although children do not have full legal capacity until they are 18, their capacity is constantly developing. The CRC recognizes that (a) as adolescents get older, *their capacity evolves*; and (b) even where adolescents lack full legal capacity, *they ought to be involved in decisions that affect them* (United Nations General Assembly, 1989; WHO, 2018).

Some countries have acknowledged this and passed legislation that recognizes the capacity of children under the age of 18 to consent independently to various sexual and reproductive health interventions (Shah et al., 2018). However, other countries, particularly in ESA, have been slow to pass laws that provide adolescents the right to consent independently to sexual and reproductive interventions (see Table 5.2). Where the law is silent on this issue, it is presumed that adolescents in such settings will require parental or guardianship consent for the listed interventions.

Reading Tables 5.1 and 5.2 together, this means that in some ESA countries hosting prevention studies, *parents are required to give permission for both enrolment and various study-related components.* In such instances, adolescent participants will have little expectation of privacy for components where parents have given permission. However, study participation itself may be even less appealing for adolescents, who may not wish their parents to consent for and receive information about sensitive components such as STI or HIV testing or contraception use (Hosek and Zimet, 2010; Strode and Essack, 2017); this may deter them from enrolment.

Table 5.2 Ages of consent in selected ESA countries to medical treatment, contraceptives and HIV testing

Country	*Medical treatment*	*Contraceptives*	*HIV testing*
Botswana	16	16	16
DRC	Unclear	Unclear	18
Ethiopia	18	18	15 (policy)
Kenya	Unclear	Unclear	18
Lesotho	12	12	12
Malawi	–	–	13
Mozambique	–	–	16
Namibia	14	–	14
Rwanda	–	15	15
South Africa	12	12	12
Eswatini	12	12	12
Tanzania	–	–	18
Uganda	–	–	12
Zambia	–	–	16
Zimbabwe	–	–	16

Source: Grant and Patel (2016).

Again reading Tables 5.1 and 5.2 together, this also means that in some ESA countries, parents are required to give permission for enrolment into HIV prevention studies but are *not* required to give permission for various components adolescents will likely receive in such studies. For example, in three countries adolescents require parental consent for study enrolment below age 18 but *can self-consent* to HIV testing below age 18. These are Ethiopia (HIV testing 15, research 18), Mozambique (HIV testing 16, research 21) and South Africa (HIV testing 12, research 18). In such instances, careful thought must be given as to how researchers will respect adolescents' rights to consent to certain sexual and reproductive components within the context of research where parental consent has been sought for enrolment.

Adolescent behaviour

Another category of ethical-legal complexities relates to the adolescent behaviours that may be uncovered or explicitly researched during studies of HIV prevention. These complexities often flow from an intersection between the research questions and procedures on the one hand and the criminal law on the other hand. Some HIV prevention studies might enrol at-risk or high-risk adolescents to answer key questions about the safety, tolerability or efficacy of products for HIV prevention. In such studies, sexual activity may be an eligibility criterion for enrolment. Even if this is not the case, the research team may come to know (in some way or another) about *adolescent sexual activity* (e.g. through behavioural questionnaires, in-depth interviews, tests or examinations, or even inadvertent disclosure) (Strode and Slack, 2009). In many countries, persons cannot lawfully consent to sex below the age of 18, for example in Ethiopia, Kenya, Mozambique, Rwanda, Tanzania and Uganda (see Table 5.3). In such instances, researchers should establish if there are mandatory reporting obligations on researchers to report adolescent participants who are breaking the law by engaging in underage but consensual sexual activity. Here researchers may be concerned that they will not be able to provide adolescent participants with directed prevention counselling that they are expected to provide (cf. United Nations Programme on HIV/AIDS [UNAIDS] and World Health Organization [WHO], 2012) because adolescents will understandably not make full disclosures of their risks when such risks relate to criminal activity.

This situation holds true for South Africa, where we have outlined several complexities which result from mandatory reporting obligations in the Sexual Offences Act, which require persons who know about a sexual offence against a child to report this to the police. (Bhamjee et al., 2016; Strode and Slack, 2009, 2013; Strode et al., 2013; Strode et al., 2014; Slack et al., 2007a; 2007b; Parliament of South Africa, 2007). If strictly applied, several harms may accrue to adolescent participants.

Adolescent participants might divulge other behaviours that are criminal offences, such as same-sex behaviour. Researching illegal behaviour

Table 5.3 Ages of consent to sex in selected ESA countries

Country	*Sex*
Botswana	16
DRC	14 (females); 18 (males)
Ethiopia	18
Kenya	18
Lesotho	16
Malawi	13 (females); 12 (males)
Mozambique	18 (females); age for males unclear
Namibia	16
Rwanda	18
South Africa	16
Eswatini	16
Tanzania	18
Uganda	18
Zambia	16
Zimbabwe	16

Source: Grant and Patel, 2016.

Table 5.4 Same-sex behaviour in selected ESA countries

Country	*Illegal?*
Botswana	No
Ethiopia	Yes
Kenya	Yes
Lesotho	Yes
Malawi	Yes
Namibia	Yes
Eswatini	Yes
Uganda	Yes
Zambia	Yes
Zimbabwe	Yes

Source: Grant and Patel, 2016; *Motshidiemang, L. v Attorney General and Lesbian, Gays and Bisexuals of Botswana 2019.*

is not unethical per se; however, where such behaviours triggers mandatory reporting to authorities, this poses a complex ethical-legal dilemma. Table 5.4 shows that same-sex sexual behaviour is an offence in several countries in ESA. In such settings, potential adolescent participants might be deterred from enrolling in research that identifies such "criminal" behaviour. Researchers may be anxious that if they do not comply with mandatory reporting obligations they might attract criminal sanctions for themselves, but if they do report, then considerable sanctions might accrue to their participants. Here the interests of adolescent participants are pitted against legal obligations (Bhamjee et al., 2016). Researchers and RECs in such settings may not have access to national ethics guidelines that provide thoughtful responses to mandatory reporting dilemmas. RECs themselves may be concerned about their own liability if they approve research with an ethically grounded approach that is inconsistent with the law (Strode et al., 2018).

Billboard 3 – stakeholders can advance adolescent HIV prevention research

The success of clinical trials of HIV prevention products requires cooperation between multiple stakeholders with various expertise and interests (United Nations Programme on HIV/AIDS [UNAIDS] and AIDS Vaccine Advocacy Coalition [AVAC], 2011), and nowhere is this more obvious than in adolescent trials. Next we set out the roles that should be played by a wide range of stakeholders in order to promote the rights of adolescents to benefit from the ever-evolving science of HIV prevention.

Ethics guideline developers

Guideline developers should ensure that national ethics guidelines encourage the inclusion of adolescents in critical research. More specifically, ethics guidelines should explicitly address the conditions under which *waivers of parental consent* will be allowed. For example, the Kenyan national guidelines (National AIDS and STI Control Program [NASCOP], 2015) allow this when parental consent is not a "reasonable requirement" or where it will be "inappropriate," such as in studies involving gay or transgender persons (p. 24). An international ethics document from WHO (2018) refers to conditions such as study sensitivity (e.g. sexual activity) and appropriate risk thresholds. Also, national ethics guidelines should address the *issue of adolescent privacy*; for example, the Kenyan national guidelines (NASCOP, 2015, p. xiii) argue that privacy for "some components" (e.g. family planning) must be maintained even when a parent gives permission for enrolment. Furthermore, national guidelines must address ethical approaches to *mandatory reporting* of underage sex and other illegal behaviour. For example, Kenyan guidelines assert that adolescents should understand the "possibility of such [mandatory] reporting" (NASCOP, 2015, p. xiii). In our view, guidelines should explicitly recommend an ethical approach that mitigates against research-related negative social impacts presented by mandatory reporting and its attendant criminal sanctions. For example, the South African Department of Health (2015) national ethics guidelines call for researchers to avoid "thoughtless reporting" (p. 35) to authorities. Guideline developers should ensure that there is a balance between child participation (United Nations General Assembly, 1989), child protection (United Nations General Assembly, 1989) and research facilitation (Strode, 2015).

RECs or IRBs

RECs may need to review and approve alternate *consent approaches*, where parental consent will be a significant impediment to the enrolment of high-risk adolescents (Wallace et al., 2018). Where parental waivers are allowed in national ethics guidance but not in law, then RECs must prepare for a complex ethical-legal dilemma, and we recommend they should approve consent strategies in line with national ethics norms (Strode et al., 2018). We argue that this is appropriate as their primary function is to act ethically and to protect research participants from harm. Nevertheless, they must accept responsibility for this approach and be able to justify their deviation from the law in line with national ethics guidance (Strode et al., 2018). In addition, RECs should fully engage with and review ethical approaches to *mandatory reporting*. In prior papers we have laid out various components of an ethical approach to South African reporting requirements (Bhamjee et al., 2016; Slack et al., 2007b; Strode et al., 2013; Strode and Slack, 2009, 2013). REC members should vigorously debate the nature and extent of reporting obligations within the context of each HIV prevention study to establish whether reporting will protect adolescents or simply trigger criminal sanctions and further alienation from support. RECs should consider whether there are sufficient protections outlined in the protocol for adolescents engaged in risk behaviour (e.g. through onsite counselling and referral) given the REC's central role in promoting the rights and welfare of participants (Amdur and Bankert, 2011). RECs should carefully balance their core mandate with societal needs to respond to "criminal" behaviour.

In general, RECs should have members that are fluent in laws affecting children and the limitations of such laws, as well as the likely negative impacts on enrolment in socially valuable, otherwise ethical research. RECs should have members prepared to debate and explicitly adopt approaches to adolescent enrolment that are thoughtful, well grounded in relevant ethics principles, and transparently accessible by researchers. REC members should be guided by their primary role to protect research participants rather than adopt the role of "law enforcement." RECs may well find themselves in an ethical-legal conflict regarding consent and reporting approaches (Strode and Slack, 2015; Strode et al., 2018), and in such instances they should seek reassurance about their collective liability if they approve approaches that are inconsistent with the law but are ethical (Strode et al., 2018). The institutions that host RECs should have insurance that protects REC members in the event of a delictual claim for damages resulting from an REC decision (Strode et al., 2018).

Researchers

As discussed earlier, adolescents may reluctant for their parents to know about sexual activity or orientation (Hosek et al., 2016; Pettifor et al., 2018), therefore parental consent may present a considerable barrier to the enrolment of high-risk youth or sexual or gender minority youth (Gilbert et al., 2015; Knopf et al., 2017; WHO, 2018). This concern will exist even where the interviews are conducted in a private space, as it relates to parental knowledge of the nature of the study and its enrolment criteria.

In such instances researchers should explore whether the ethical framework (i.e. national ethics guidelines) will support a waiver of parental consent, even where local laws mandate parental consent, thus allowing self-consent by older adolescents (Strode et al., 2018). For example, South African and Kenyan national guidelines allow such waivers under some instances (SA DOH, 2015; NASCOP, 2015). In South Africa, the REC requires evidence of engagement with community stakeholders, which is also recommended by WHO (2018). In addition, researchers should engage with the responsible REC regarding the optimal *consent approach*. Where the availability of parents/guardians is an impediment, then seeking to secure permission from an alternative proxy consenter such as a caregiver may be appropriate (Strode and Slack, 2009). However, it is not clear whether adolescents would perceive the involvement of caregivers as a similar deterrent.

With parental waivers and self-consent strategies, researchers must consider "decisional supports" (Knopf et al., 2017) to provide adolescents with additional protections in their decision-making (Gilbert et al., 2015). Adolescents who *self-consented* to a PrEP trial reported feeling well informed and volunteering freely, yet some wished for additional support at enrolment, which supports the inclusion of such supports (Knopf et al., 2017). This means that researchers should enable adolescents to discuss their decisions with trusted adults (Shah et al., 2018), even chosen by adolescents (Santelli et al., 2017). Researchers should assess capacity for self-consent and carefully assess comprehension of study concepts (Santelli et al., 2003). They should tailor consent processes to target deficiencies in decision-making, such as susceptibility to peer pressure and favouring of short-term rewards over long-term risks (Shah et al., 2018).

Where parental involvement in enrolment will be the consent approach, a *privacy strategy* must be delineated, that is, which information parents will be informed about. It is clear that children, like adults, have a right to privacy (United Nations General Assembly, 1989), but adult expectations about access to private information must be fully clarified. It follows that some parents may refuse permission for their child's enrolment if the privacy strategy means parents may not be directly informed for components to which adolescents self-consent, as set out elsewhere (Strode and Essack, 2017; Bhamjee et al., 2016; Strode and Slack, 2011, 2013; Strode et al., 2010; Slack et al., 2007a). Careful development of a privacy strategy may well facilitate adolescent enrolment. Also, researchers need to plan an ethical approach to *mandatory reporting*, namely, an approach that is engages fully with the law that criminalizes the behaviour and any attendant requirements to report this to authorities; in other words, the approach should not merely ignore such requirements or demonstrate ignorance of them (Bhamjee et al., 2016). The approach should carefully justify not reporting such consensual behaviour to authorities by invoking ethical principles to promote the welfare of enrolled participants and to avoid research-related harms to them, and the approach should ensure that adolescents engaged in at-risk behaviour receive appropriate help and services for at-risk behaviour (Bhamjee et al., 2016). Researchers should set this out in an application to RECs for a waiver of reporting obligations, as set out elsewhere (Bhamjee et al., 2016).

Adolescents

Adolescents should understand the personal implications of approaches to consent, privacy and mandatory reporting to be used in the study. To meet obligations for "community" or stakeholder engagement (UNAIDS-AVAC, 2011), adolescent representatives should be engaged by the research team to get their insights about the problem of privacy and mandatory reporting, and possible remedies in the form of sensitive ethically nuanced approaches. That is, adolescents should offer their expertise to the research team regarding possible impediments to enrolment and retention. Here adolescent representatives should be engaged by researchers who are trained to interact with this group and who will carefully document their outreach (UNAIDS-AVAC, 2011). Adolescent representatives should be engaged early, so their input is obtained prior to protocols and protocol approaches being finalized or polished. Researchers should obtain inputs regarding how to make the consent, privacy and reporting strategies more acceptable. The participation of adolescents *in the research process* is underscored in some ethics guidelines (NASCOP, 2015), and our recommendation logically extends their participation to *the design of ethical approaches.* This is also consistent with their rights as described in the CRC (1989) and with recommendations from commentators (Pettifor et al., 2018).

Policy-makers

Knee-jerk compliance with reporting laws may draw adolescents (or their partners) into the criminal justice system in a way that attracts potential physical or social harm to participants (Bhamjee et al., 2016; Strode et al., 2013; Strode and Slack, 2009, 2013). Policy-makers should carefully consider amendments to reporting requirements that might deter adolescents from research and may undermine their rights to benefit from scientific progress through their enrolment in socially valuable research (Bhamjee et al., 2016). Policies are needed which underscore the importance of adolescent involvement in HIV prevention research.

Advocates or activists

HIV prevention advocates in such settings are uniquely placed to ask difficult questions about how national HIV prevention research agendas are thoughtfully accommodating adolescents. Where laws are identified that hamper such progress, there is no better-placed group to argue for their amendment. Such groups have the skills and voice to advocate for more HIV prevention research involving adolescents so as to ensure that their rights to science are fulfilled, and for reform to laws that impede such rights.

Conclusions

Adolescents have rights to benefit from scientific advances, as set out in international documents like the CRC. Enrolling them entails consideration of the complications that can arise for study design and implementation. Our message is that such enrolment is feasible with adequate thought and preparation. Adolescent enrolment is also important enough to justify the considerable efforts that must be made to accommodate them. Various stakeholders should recognize their unique contributions to facilitating such enrolment. We reserve the final word for the importance of RECs in such settings, who are required to evaluate whether adolescent protocols are "ethically acceptable" (CIOMS, 2016, p. 8) while often situated in an imperfect legal framework – which necessitates that RECs make sometimes uncomfortable decisions to approve balanced, nuanced, well-justified ethical approaches.

References

2013. Teddy Bear Clinic for Abused Children and Another v Minister of Justice and Constitutional Development. ZACC 35.

2019. *Motshidiemang, L. v Attorney General and Lesbian, Gays and Bisexuals of Botswana 2019*. High Court of Botswana held at Gabarone.

Abdool-Karim, Q. & Dellar, R. 2014. Inclusion of adolescent girls in HIV prevention research – an imperative for an AIDS-free generation. *Journal of the International AIDS Society*, 17.

African Commission on Human and Peoples' Rights [ACHPR] 1981. *African Charter on Human and Peoples' Rights*. Organization of African Unity (OAU).

Amdur, R. & Bankert, E. 2011. *Institutional Review Board Member Handbook*. Sudbury, MA: Jones and Bartlett Publishing.

Bekker, L.-G., Gill, K. & Wallace, M. 2015. Pre-exposure prophylaxis for South African adolescents: What evidence? *South African Medical Journal*, 105, 907–911.

Bekker, L.-G., Slack, C., Lee, S., Shah, S. & Kapogiannis, B. 2014. Ethical issues in adolescent HIV research in resource-limited countries. *JAIDS Journal of Acquired Immune Deficiency Syndromes*, 65, S24–S28.

Bhamjee, S., Essack, Z. & Strode, A. E. 2016. Amendments to the sexual offences act dealing with consensual underage sex: Implications for doctors and researchers. *South African Medical Journal*, 106, 256–259.

Busza, J., Strode, A., Dauya, E. & Ferrand, R.A. 2016. Falling through the gaps: How should HIV programmes respond to families that persistently deny treatment to children? *Journal of the International AIDS Society*, 19, 20789.

Council for International Organizations of Medical Sciences [CIOMS] 2016. *International Ethical Guidelines for Health-related Research Involving Humans*. Geneva: CIOMS.

Gilbert, A.L., Knopf, A.S., Fortenberry, J.D., Hosek, S.G., Kapogiannis, B.G. & Zimet, G.D. 2015. Adolescent self-consent for biomedical human immunodeficiency virus prevention research. *Journal of Adolescent Health*, 57, 113–119.

Grant, C. & Patel, P. 2016. *UNDP Age of Consent Research Inception Report*. Unpublished.

Hosek, S.G., Celum, C., Wilson, C.M., Kapogiannis, B., Delany-Moretlwe, S. & Bekker, L.G. 2016. Preventing HIV among adolescents with oral PrEP: Observations and challenges in the United States and South Africa. *Journal of the International AIDS Society*, 19, 21107.

Hosek, S.G. & Zimet, G.D. 2010. Behavioral considerations for engaging youth in HIV clinical research. *JAIDS Journal of Acquired Immune Deficiency Syndromes*, 54, S25–S30.

Ivan-Smith, E. & Johnson, V. 1998. The way forward. *In:* Johnson, V., Ivan-Smith, E., Gordon, G., Scott-Villiers, P. & Pridmore, P. (eds.) *Stepping Forward: Children and Young People's Participation in the Development Process*. Intermediate London: Technology Publications.

Kapogiannis, B.G., Handelsman, E., Ruiz, M.S. & Lee, S. 2010. Introduction: Paving the way for biomedical HIV prevention interventions in youth. *JAIDS Journal of Acquired Immune Deficiency Syndromes*, 54, S1–S4.

Knopf, A.S., Ott, M.A., Liu, N., Kapogiannis, B.G., Zimet, G.D., Fortenberry, J.D. & Hosek, S.G. 2017. Minors' and young adults' experiences of the research consent process in a phase II safety study of pre-exposure prophylaxis for HIV. *Journal of Adolescent Health*, 61, 747–754.

Macqueen, K.M. & Abdool-Karim, Q. 2007. Practice brief: Adolescents and HIV clinical trials: Ethics, culture, and context. *Journal of the Association of Nurses in AIDS Care*, 18, 78–82.

National AIDS and STI Control Programme (NASCOP) & Kenya Medical Research Institute (KEMRI). 2015. *Guidelines for Conducting Adolescent HIV Sexual and Reproductive Health Research in Kenya*. Kenya: Government of Kenya.

Nelson, R.M., Lewis, L.L., Struble, K. & Wood, S.F. 2010. Ethical and regulatory considerations for the inclusion of adolescents in HIV biomedical prevention research. *JAIDS Journal of Acquired Immune Deficiency Syndromes*, 54, S18–S24.

Nuffield Council on Bioethics. 2015. *Children and Clinical Research: Ethical Issues*. London: Nuffield Council on Bioethics.

Osmanov, S. 2007. Executive summary and recommendations from WHO/UNAIDS and AAVP consultation on: 'The inclusion of adolescents in HIV vaccine trials', 16–18 March 2006 in Gaborone, Botswana. *AIDS (London, England)*, 21, W1–W10.

Parliament of South Africa. 2007. Criminal Law (Sexual Offences and Related Matters) Amendment Act.

Pettifor, A., Stoner, M., Pike, C. & Bekker, L.-G. 2018. Adolescent lives matter: Preventing HIV in adolescents. *Current Opinion in HIV and AIDS*, 13, 265.

Santelli, J.S., Haerizadeh, S. & McGovern, T. 2017. *Inclusion with Protection: Obtaining Informed Consent When Conducting Research with Adolescents*. Innocenti Research Briefs no. 2017-05. Florence: UNICEF Office of Research.

Santelli, J.S., Rogers, A.S., Rosenfeld, W.D., Durant, R.H., Dubler, N., Morreale, M., English, A., Lyss, S., Wimberly, Y. & Schissel, A. 2003. Guidelines for adolescent health research: A position paper of the society for adolescent medicine. *Journal of Adolescent Health*, 33, 396–409.

Scanlon, M.L., Macnaughton, G. & Sprague, C. 2017. Neglected population, neglected right: Children living with HIV and the right to science. *Health and Human Rights*, 19, 169.

Shah, S.K., Allison, S.M., Kapogiannis, B.G., Black, R., Dawson, L. & Erbelding, E. 2018. Advancing Independent Adolescent Consent for Participation in HIV Prevention Research. *Journal of Medical Ethics*, 44, 431–433.

Slack, C., Strode, A., Fleischer, T., Gray, G. & Ranchod, C. 2007a. Enrolling adolescents in HIV vaccine trials: Reflections on legal complexities from South Africa. *BMC Medical Ethics*, 8, 5.

Slack, C., Strode, A. & Mamashela, M. 2007b. Ethical-legal challenges in adolescent HIV vaccine trials: Research and the law. *Southern African Journal of HIV Medicine*, 2007, 12–13.

South Africa Department of Health [SA DOH] 2015. *Ethics in Health Research: Principles, Processes and Structures*. Pretoria: Department of Health.

Strode, A. 2015. A critical review of the regulation of research involving children in South Africa: From self-regulation to hyper-regulation. *Journal of South African Law/Tydskrif vir die Suid-Afrikaanse Reg*, 2015, 334–346.

Strode, A. & Essack, Z. 2017. Facilitating access to adolescent sexual and reproductive health services through legislative reform: Lessons from the South African experience. *South African Medical Journal*, 107, 741–744.

Strode, A., Richter, M., Wallace, M., Toohey, J. & Technau, K. 2014. Failing the vulnerable: Three new consent norms that will undermine health research with children. *Southern African Journal of HIV Medicine*, 15, 46–49.

Strode, A., Singh, P., Slack, C. & Wassenaar, D. 2018. Research ethics committees in a tight spot: Approving consent strategies for child research that are prima facie illegal but are ethical in terms of national guidelines. *South African Medical Journal*, 108, 828–832.

Strode, A. & Slack, C. 2009. Sex, lies and disclosures: Researchers and the reporting of under-age sex: Opinion. *Southern African Journal of HIV Medicine*, 10, 8–10.

Strode, A. & Slack, C. 2011. Using the concept of 'parental responsibilities and rights' to identify adults able to provide proxy consent to child research in South Africa. *South African Journal of Bioethics and Law*, 4, 69–73.

Strode, A. & Slack, C. 2013. Child privacy rights: A 'Cinderella' issue in HIV-prevention research. *Southern African Journal of HIV Medicine*, 14, 108–110.

Strode, A. & Slack, C. 2015. Child research in South Africa: How do the new regulations help? *South African Medical Journal*, 105, 899–900.

Strode, A., Slack, C. & Essack, Z. 2010. Child consent in South African law: Implications for researchers, service providers and policy-makers. *South African Medical Journal*, 100.

Strode, A., Toohey, J., Slack, C. & Bhamjee, S. 2013. Reporting underage consensual sex after the Teddy Bear case: A different perspective. *South African Journal of Bioethics and Law*, 6, 45–47.

S V M 2007. ZACC 18.

UN Committee on the Rights of the Child [CRC] 2003. General comment no. 5 (2003): General measure of implementation of the Convention on the Rights of the Child.

UNICEF. 2013. *Ethical Research Involving Children.* Florence: UNICEF Office of Research – Innocenti.

United Nations General Assembly. 1989. Convention on the rights of the child: Adopted and opened for signature, ratification and accession by General Assembly Resolution 44/25 of 20 November 1989.

United Nations Office of the High Commissioner for Human Rights [OHCHR]. 1966. International covenant on economic, social and cultural rights: Adopted and opened for signature, ratification and accession by General Assembly resolution 2200A (XXI) of 16 December 1966, entry into force 3 January 1976, in accordance with article 27.

United Nations Programme on HIV/AIDS [UNAIDS] & AIDS Vaccine Advocacy Coalition [AVAC]. 2011. *Good Participatory Practice: Guidelines for Biomedical HIV Prevention Trials.* Geneva: UNAIDS.

United Nations Programme on HIV/AIDS [UNAIDS] & World Health Organization [WHO]. 2012. *Ethical Considerations in Biomedical HIV Prevention Trials* [Additional Guidance Point Added in 2012]. Geneva: UNAIDS.

Wallace, M., Middelkoop, K., Smith, P., Pike, C., Bennie, T., Chandia, J., Churchyard, G., Gray, G., Latka, M. & Mathebula, M. 2018. Feasibility and acceptability of conducting HIV vaccine trials in adolescents in South Africa: Going beyond willingness to participate towards implementation. *South African Medical Journal,* 108, 291–298.

Wilson, C. M., Wright, P. F., Safrit, J. T. & Rudy, B. 2010. Epidemiology of HIV infection and risk in adolescents and youth. *Journal of Acquired Immune Deficiency Syndromes (1999),* 54, S5.

World Health Organization [WHO]. 2018. *Guidance on Ethical Considerations in Planning and Reviewing Research Studies on Sexual and Reproductive Health in Adolescents.* Geneva: World Health Organization.

6 Protecting the vulnerable

Human and health security beyond citizenship, exploring the rationale and the possibilities for adolescents

Annamarie Bindenagel Šehović

Introduction

Contemporary pressures of climate change and migration are abetting the spread of infectious diseases including HIV, Ebola and tuberculosis (TB). As such, HIV is one of a series of re-emerging infectious diseases (EIDs) that pose significant external threats to health security in Eastern and Southern Africa (ESA). Additional internal health threats include detrimental social determinants of health and exclusionary practices, such as denial of treatment and care to non-citizens (CDC, 2018; WHO, 2018). Taking this into account, this chapter develops a threefold proposal for improved HIV prevention and treatment. First, it identifies how a human-centric approach beyond citizenship would better capture the intermingled risks and vulnerabilities that impact individual and population health security. Second, the chapter develops initial ideas towards targeted prevention and treatment interventions aimed at addressing adolescent vulnerabilities. Third, it offers policy sketches aimed at supporting health claims across borders in ESA, reaching beyond citizenship to provide and protect human health security in the region.

While the biological fact remains that any person can become infected with any of these diseases, those most affected are vulnerable populations. In ESA these include marginalized groups such as people who sell sex, LGBTI and MSM, but more widely also adolescents, who represent a particularly vulnerable group. Members of such marginalized and vulnerable communities are excluded from access to provisions and protections of health as part of the paradigm of human security (Paris, 2001), whether out of apathy, fear or jurisdiction or through (deliberate) neglect. On the brink of adulthood, adolescents represent a doubly vulnerable group, both biologically as well as legally, as they often lack the full rights accorded to them by adult citizenship. Likewise caught in such a double vulnerability are migrants and refugees. As Kofi Annan once said, adolescents are inarguably at the

> forefront of global change and innovation. Empowered, they can be key agents for development and peace. If, however, they are left on

society's margins, all of us will be impoverished. Let us ensure that all young people have every opportunity to participate fully in the lives of their societies.

(2014)[1]

Yet such adolescent success is not a foregone conclusion.

Adolescents face inclusion challenges in reaching their potential, faced as they are with twin challenges of particular biological vulnerability to EIDs and limited access to legal (and thereby medical) access to prevention measures and provisions to protect themselves. As such, adolescents represent a particularly vulnerable group, caught on the cusp between child protections and adult citizenship claims, including to health and educational provisions and protections. Without, or with incomplete claims, members of marginalized and vulnerable communities, among them adolescents, are excluded from access to provisions and protections of health as part of human security.

Against that backdrop, this chapter analyzes the unique challenges of vulnerable adolescent populations as these relate to HIV prevention and treatment access. It pays special heed to the "double vulnerability" of non-citizenship and compromised citizenship among this cohort.

This chapter asks three questions: What role(s) might citizenship status play in adolescent vulnerability? Might (lack of) formal citizenship make adolescents doubly vulnerable, legally and socially, to HIV, because (non-) citizenship enables or alternatively thwarts access to preventive and curative health services? How might it be possible to protect the health of vulnerable adolescent populations across borders and "beyond citizenship"?

The chapter rests on the theoretical pillar of human security. Human security puts the security of individuals at the centre of its analysis. This stands in contrast to the 1990s securitization argument, which framed HIV as a threat to state security (Buzan et al., 1998). Human security prioritizes individual security, rendered in access to adequate food, health and environmental protection among other elements, above those of territorial integrity traditionally used to define state security. The human security lens brings not just citizens in designated territories into focus but also the vulnerable, including non-citizens, beyond borders. By invoking the human security paradigm and adapting it to the particular situation facing adolescents contending with HIV in ESA, this chapter aims to analyze and offer initial responses to provide for and protect vulnerable populations beyond borders.

The chapter proceeds as follows: The background section introduces the framework of human and health security in more detail. This includes a discussion of the limits to the reach of the human security paradigm posed by age as well as by citizenship, where full citizenship is gained upon legal maturity (18 years of age in some countries, and 21 in others). This has significant ramifications in terms of the legal residency status of immigrants from Zimbabwe to South Africa and, for adolescents in South Africa, rights of access to education and healthcare services. The following sections present an analysis of the intersection of health security, marginalization, HIV vulnerability and adolescents in ESA, foremost in South Africa and Zimbabwe. These take into account the threat of the rising burden of infectious disease in the region and the inherent, biological vulnerability of adolescents and young adults (AYA), as well as the legal and social risks posed by (non-)citizenship. Finally, the chapter offers initial operational ideas to address the "double vulnerability" of adolescents and (non-)citizenship.

Background

Substantial research has gone into the nexus of state and human and health security outlined earlier (Šehović, 2018). Its argument rests on a centuries-long tradition of Westphalian sovereignty theory in which the state increasingly acquired responsibilities for human rights and human security. Human security was first explicitly named in the 1994 United Nations Development Programme Report: *New Dimensions of Human Security* (UNDP, 1994).

While this chapter prioritizes human security and health security, their relationship to state security is worth mentioning for two reasons. First, population health affects the integrity of the state (Howell, 2014). Second, as introduced earlier, health risks can emerge both externally and internally, and by definition then state security from both within and outside. In addition, among these risks, and significant for the analysis presented here, EIDs, while adversely affecting vulnerable populations, make no distinction between citizens and non-citizens, that is, those within or outside of the state. Instead, the insecurities and the social determinants of health are paramount both to vulnerability and to its countermeasures. This makes rethinking health security beyond borders and as applied to (non-)citizens so necessary. Since adolescents constitute an (over-)represented population both at territorial (as migrants and refugees) and at legal (between childhood and adulthood) borders, and as part of a "youth bulge" – a critical component of the future human and state health in ESA – this chapter focuses on their unique vulnerabilities to HIV infection and interventions.

Population at risk categories: human health security/ adolescents and HIV

The following matrix illustrates the categories of analysis focusing on the first question this chapter addresses: What role(s) might citizenship status play in adolescent vulnerability?

Citizen adolescents	Non-citizen adolescents
Citizen adolescents/HIV	Non-citizen adolescents/HIV

In order to shed light on these categories, the following two sub-sections outline human and health security in more detail.

Human security

As outlined earlier, human security is a human-centric focus of security. It emphasizes the duality of individual and universal human rights. The premise that all individuals everywhere have the same human rights underpins the UN Charter and the WHO Constitution. However, states – and member states of these international organizations – are those tasked with providing and protecting human rights and thus human security.

The 1994 UNDP report and Jorge Nef (1999) identify seven dimensions of human security, each of them with echoes in the UN definitions of human as well as political and social, cultural and economic rights (Nef, 1999). These seven dimensions are economic security, food security, health security, environmental security, personal security, community security and political security. Many of these components have only vague conceptualizations, let alone legal definitions. The sole exception pertains to provisions of asylum for refugees, but only in relation to political conflicts such as civil wars. Economic or health insecurities, including those of people forced to migrate due to climatic catastrophes, are not protected under current international laws governing refugees. Some countries in ESA including South Africa, do have human security–inspired protections that include, for example, the rights to health and education (Constitution of South Africa, 1996). However, while the scope of human rights has seemingly expanded, their realization remains inextricably tied to the state (Šehović, 2018).

This is evident in the response to HIV and AIDS. AIDS activists expanded the claims of human health rights to include those of men who have sex with men (MSM), babies exposed to the virus in utero and during birth, and mothers through prevention of mother-to-child transmission (PMTCT). Yet, as a rule, non-citizens are not summarily afforded such protections.

Historically with regard to state responsibilities, "vulnerable populations" have been conceived of as widows and orphans. This conception informed the anticipation of millions of "orphans and vulnerable children" (OVC) at the outset of the HIV epidemic. Though these numbers have not emerged as a threat to state stabilization, the idea of vulnerable populations has broadened its cache. Initially including primarily girls and young women, and OVCs, vulnerable populations now includes adolescents more broadly. This chapter argues further that non-citizens constitute another vulnerable group as they lack the ability to claim their human rights and human security from a(ny) state. Turning this human security lens on health security makes it possible to highlight the vulnerabilities of adolescents to assess the exclusions of sub-populations, including adolescents and non-citizens, from state responsibilities for health security.

Health security

Health security refers to the availability of and access to means of health at the population level. It invokes protection in the form of prevention from external but also internal risks. It can also include provision of treatment and care in the case of disease infection. Health security is not a guarantee of health or carte blanche for all care, treatment and intervention. It is a strong foundation for promoting the right to health for all who reside in a country. Health security is also increasingly embedded in national constitutional provisions, such as in the Constitution of the Republic of South Africa (Constitution, 1996), as well as in international regulations aimed towards securing health for all. Against the backdrop of both rising levels of EIDs and of the burden of disease, growing recognition of the roles played by the social determinants of health, and ever-increasing capabilities (medical as well as political and economic) to respond to global disease threats, health security has started to evolve from a strategic concept to a policy priority.

Among the most prominent health security policies are the International Health Regulations (IHR; 2005), under which states pledge to upgrade their health facilities and capabilities. However, though ostensibly binding, the IHRs have few enforcement mechanisms beyond shaming noncompliant states. Individuals can sue their governments in states where provisions for health (security) have been rendered in law. This has been done most famously in Brazil, South Africa and Thailand. The lack of these mechanisms highlight the citizen-state relationship and expose the lack of rights and health security claims available to non-citizens.

At times, non-state actors (NSAs) can step into a void left between citizens and states failing to live up to their responsibilities. NSAs can also take measures to include non-citizens. This has been the case during some of the response to the HIV epidemics in ESA. NSAs have provided care and treatment until public pressure and donor financing stepped in to bridge the gap between states and their infected and affected citizens' needs and their treasuries. Non-citizens with access to identity documents or selectively targeted as belonging to identified and prioritized groups also benefitted. Yet a larger effort to include non-citizens did not emerge and remains a blind spot. Two developments emphasize this: first, according to interviews with the director of the German Chamber of Commerce in South Africa, a consensus seems to exist that private actors will "never again" mobilize a response such as they did to HIV in the 1990s.[2] This reinforces the state as the only actor responsible for health security, which threatens to exclude non-citizens from its provisions and protections. Second, as resident non-citizens are embedded in the society of where they live, the health security of the citizen population is instrinsically and inextricably tied to theirs. Arguing for the inclusion of non-citizens among vulnerable populations with regard to HIV and health security is not meant to be a case for the medicalization of security (Elbe, 2010), wherein security issues, including migrants and refugees framed as such, are met with medical responses. Instead, it is an argument for reconceiving vulnerability to include not only medical but also legal elements of human security. The next section applies this analysis to adolescents in ESA.

Analysis: the critical case of adolescents

As noted earlier, adolescents in ESA today are coming of age in a rapidly changing world. They are part of the change. The challenges they face include a demographic bulge, climate change, economic and educational constraints and the promise and pressures of migration, both outward and inward – to stay or to go. In the midst of all of these transitions, adolescents are uniquely exposed and vulnerable to the risks of EIDs. In order for adolescents to cope and adapt, they need information pertinent to counter their vulnerabilities and also to claim their rights, including their right to health security. This makes their health dependent upon themselves but also upon the institutional structures, including their citizenship status and their claimant state.

This section explores the intersection of biological vulnerabilities of adolescence and the risk posed by the ongoing HIV epidemic in the region vis-à-vis the additional factor of non-citizenship or compromised citizenship. In doing so, it seeks to answer the second question posed earlier in the chapter: Might (lack of) formal citizenship make adolescents doubly vulnerable, legally and socially, to HIV because (non-)citizenship enables or alternatively thwarts access to preventive and curative health services? First, the section outlines the status of adolescents and young adults in ESA and their biological vulnerability to HIV infection, and then seeks to answer the key questions posed above. It is imperative at the outset to recognize that adolescents, by virtue of their biological and social vulnerability, are uniquely susceptible to EID and especially HIV infection. Second, the section focuses on their "double vulnerability" with the additional risk of non-citizenship or compromised citizenship. In 2016, UNAIDS estimated the adolescent population of ESA at 1.3 million.[3] UNICEF's estimate for the same year was 1.48 million young people (aged 20–24) living with HIV in the region. The definitions are at times overlapping and at times exclusive. Among these there are an estimated 610,000 new HIV infections among young people between the ages of 15 and 24, and 260,000 new infections among adolescents between the ages of 15 and 19 (UNICEF, 2017a, 2017b). Some of these will migrate within the region; others will belong to communities with many migrants. This movement has both social impacts and health consequences, including in the form of the spread of disease. Indeed, the initial spread of HIV from Eastern to Southern Africa can be traced back to migration from the trading ports in Kinshasa in Congo, down the Zambezi River, to the mines in South Africa (Iliffe, 2006). Likewise in a contemporary comparison, in South America, incidences of malaria, measles, diphtheria and tuberculosis are on the rise, especially at the borders of Venezuela. As an estimated 1.6 million people (World Migration Report, 2015), many of them young people, migrate into neighbouring countries such as Colombia, Ecuador, Peru, and Brazil, without provisions for access to medical care to contain and treat these diseases, they are likely to spread.

Even in their own countries, adolescents and young adults (AYA) often have circumscribed citizenship rights: neither children nor adults, they exist on the cusp of child rights' protections and adult citizenship. They are socially, educationally and economically dependent upon both familial and state ties for their preparation and protection into adulthood. This vulnerability is even more pronounced among foreigners or non-citizens, and is magnified by the lack of and difficulties in securing citizenship, which curbs their access to the protections and provisions of citizenship.

The intersection of adolescent biological and social vulnerability

Adolescent vulnerability is accentuated by biology and social position. Biologically, adolescents are at their prime both in terms of physical fitness and their immune response (Govender et al., 2017). They are also at a moment of experimentation, sexually and otherwise, putting them at heightened risk of HIV infection among other sexually transmitted illnesses.

It is worth noting that this biological and social moment of transition and experimentation can promote a certain nonchalance with regard to an unseen and unknown risk of infection. Exacerbating vulnerabilities are the lack of sexual education, non-use of condoms, inter-generational sexual relationships (known to introduce HIV into adolescent populations), and experience of peer and cross-generational violence. This moment coincides with and can be reinforced both by the access and availability of treatments and by the lack thereof.

Evidence of an attitude of nonchalance can be found in high rates of adolescent abuse of anti-retroviral drugs (ARVs), including the recreational combination of various drugs, including ARVs, especially among migrant adolescents (Timol, 2017).[4] Pupils, including marginalized, non-citizen adolescents, many of them migrants from as far north as Djibouti, Sudan and South Sudan into the outskirts of Cape Town, South Africa, attempt to learn in schoolrooms of 30 pupils speaking 13 languages (Timol, Cape Town, 2017). As non-citizens, their access to the matriculation exam is uncertain – and with it, their future. Consequently, HIV prevalence, nonchalance and future insecurity contrive to create a situation of exacerbated vulnerabilities. That has consequences for the HIV epidemics, but also for the human and health security of the ESA region.

Indeed, despite a broad range and decades of intervention efforts, including increased access to biomedicine and continual efforts to normalize HIV infection as a chronic condition, the HIV epidemics in ESA continue to rage. On the one hand, this might be attributed to the course of HIV infection and prevalence between Eastern and Southern Africa. The earlier peak of the epidemic in eastern Africa reduced the populations of HIV-positive persons in those countries before national treatment programmes were implemented, drastically reducing prevalence rates (WHO, 2017; compare UNAIDS, 2008). In contrast, in southern and especially South Africa, HIV epidemics peaked later and closer to initial campaigns for access to treatment arrived (ca. 2004), resulting in higher prevalence rates (Kharsany et al., 2018). Setting the stage for complications to come, however, rates of tuberculosis infection and (co-)infection with HIV have been climbing especially in South and Southern Africa.[5]

Adolescents' abilities to address these deficiencies – in information, in education, in physical protection – are dependent upon the adults' as well as adolescents' social and political power, which is limited by their lack of adult citizenship. Adolescents and young adults (AYA) can formally engage – contributing to and benefiting from – the societies in which they come of age only if legally recognized and afforded practical and legal access to health, education, economic and political systems. If and where such access is not available, AYA knowledge, access and uptake of healthcare, and of associated social support mechanisms to improve their social determinants of health, including educational and employment opportunities, is substantially limited. The consequences, notably infection with HIV, impact both AYA individually and the communities in which they reside, affecting citizens and non-citizens alike.

The situation of those without citizenship, foreign as opposed to adolescent citizens, is that they are left outside of the citizen-state responsibility nexus. Yet many such AYAs have only ever known one community. For example, over notably the last decade, young Zimbabweans have been migrating to South Africa and raising their non-citizen families there. In other cases, children and adolescents have been crossing the porous border into South Africa with and without legal and legally resident guardians. For the duration of time that these children and adolescents are under the age of 18 and reside with a legal guardian who is a legal resident in South Africa, they can remain and they can access educational and health services, with one caveat that has concrete implications on their future: these adolescents and young people cannot take the matriculation examination – the gateway to higher education – before first resolving their own legal residency status.[6]

This process can involve relinquishing, for example, Zimbabwean citizenship (assuming it can be established in the first instance) and applying for refugee status in South Africa. The decision of such a process can take years.[7] In the interim, adolescents faced with such a "choice" are left in legal limbo with a cascade of consequences that reinforce their marginalization and vulnerabilities. Without legal status, such adolescents cannot complete their secondary education and, therefore, cannot pursue tertiary education, nor can they legally work. When they turn 18, the legal protections they were entitled to as minors are rescinded, leaving them in legal, social and economic limbo.

If an AYA can establish legal residency via either one of these routes, though (s)he remains a non-citizen, (s)he can access most health and other benefits afforded the citizen population. Adolescents without legal guardians become wards of the state with access to health and education until they turn 18. Such adolescents are often assigned to social services' communal residences, which can raise their vulnerability to sexual exploitation and inconsistent educational access and oversight (Blignaut, 2017). Overall, without legal protections, the incentive to study is reduced and the incentive to practice safe sex is lowered (Interviews with female secondary students, Pretoria, April 2017).

Combined, all these elements increase the risk of adolescent HIV infection. They challenge current prevention and intervention policies and protocols to take into account not only adolescent biological and social vulnerabilities but also the "double vulnerability" contained in citizenship status. This creates a "perfect storm" contributing to making HIV prevention and treatment for adolescents – and especially non-citizen adolescents – an uphill battle.

Double vulnerability: adolescents/citizenship/HIV prevention

The protection and preparation of adolescents and young adults for their and their societies' future against the backdrop of ongoing HIV epidemics and EIDs in ESA depends to a large extent on state responsibility and citizenship claims which facilitate access to health provisions and protections. States, delineated by political boundaries yet with porous borders, are increasingly faced with the task of assessing rights, including health rights, to (non-)citizens. This makes it imperative to address the health vulnerabilities of adolescents beyond borders.

The case for doing so can be broken down into four counts:

1 People under age 15 constitute 40% of the continent's population (AU, 2017), and as such the single largest sub-population of national populations in most countries in the region. Including different definitions of young adults, even when restricting consideration to adolescents and young adults (10–24 years), this key population likely makes up the largest sub-population on the continent (Katz et al., 2013).
2 Adolescents and young adults are now recognized as a key population in the sense of being one of the several populations most at risk of HIV infection (others are people who sell sex, MSM and migrants, many of which also include large proportions of AYA).
3 External state and NSA actors are unlikely to commit again to a multi-generational investment in response to a health crisis. This is due to lower levels of international funding support since the 2008 financial crisis and also to a shift in focus after the "grand decade of global health" (2000–2010). Making up for this loss requires state action, including enabling adolescents to take ownership of their health rights and responsibilities. Ideally, this ownership would be matched by a guarantee of access across the region.

4 Despite major investments in education over the past few decades, major challenges remain, especially in the areas of tertiary education and vocational training. Removing the structural impediments to access to health and education is critical to harnessing the potential of AYAs.

As evidenced, adolescents are a distinct and yet communal cohort: still dependent, but not children; almost adult, but without full citizenship rights in their own countries or a claim in countries not their own. For citizen and non-citizen adolescents alike, they are supported by legal frameworks and mechanisms extended from the protections for children but which do not take fully into account the particular human and health security needs of adolescents (Grossman and Stangl, 2013; Pantelic et al., 2015). Adolescents must be given the tools, among them access to legal citizenship, to access their health security and thereby to contribute to that of their communities (International HIV/AIDS Alliance: Together to End AIDS, 2016; Li et al., 2013; Marten and Smith, 2018; Mburu et al., 2013; Gruskin et al., 2013; Christensen et al., 2013; Risher et al., 2013).

Such an approach could have positive reverberations for HIV prevention. It re-invigorates the debate for prevention that goes beyond individualized risk management approaches and current social determinants of health-based programming (e.g. combination HIV prevention) and brings human security into the heart of the debate.

A case for cross-border adolescent HIV and health access

Human and health security can influence the design of HIV interventions tailored to AYA against a backdrop of continual and intensifying population movements. Indeed, the case of HIV and AIDS illustrates that the question of the right to health and human security is less in dispute than before the eruption of that global epidemic. However, as treatment resistance and co-infections, notably of TB (including multi-drug-resistant and extremely drug-resistant TB strains, as well), and cross-border claims to access healthcare have increased,[8] the schism between the right and its realization has again widened. However, not meeting the demand for the right to health poses a risk to infection to both sedentary citizen as well as resident and migratory non-citizen populations (Šehović, 2018). This section focuses on answering the question: How might it be possible to protect the health of vulnerable adolescent populations across borders, including citizens and non-citizens?

That movements of disease as well as people are likely to increase reinforces the case for facilitated access to healthcare. Two scenarios, and three concrete options developed under the second scenario, present themselves as possible responses.

The first scenario would be to continue to allow migrants to cross territorial and political borders, while failing to formally recognize their human and health rights or to act on any corresponding citizenship responsibilities. This scenario would marginalize significant numbers of people, putting their own health (and the health of the populations with which they come into contact) at the mercy of NSAs that may or may not provide healthcare services for an uncertain amount of time, jeopardizing both access and continuity of care (Šehović, 2017). This would most certainly further marginalize already vulnerable populations, foremost among them adolescents with legal protections as minors. This would severely undercut the educational and economic and political potential of the individuals, communities and, ultimately, the nation states (Winter and Winter, 2018). The second scenario would be to issue identification documents (at the national or regional level) to document and enable access to state health and education as well as to facilitate participation in the formal economy and tax collection.[9]

The three concrete options are:

1 Regional protocols that focus on particular diseases could move beyond harmonization to treatment access. For instance, while the Harmonised Minimum Standards for the Prevention, Treatment and Management of Tuberculosis in the SADC Region (Directorate of Social & Human Development & Special Programs SADC Secretariat, 2010) and the HIV and AIDS Strategic Framework, 2010–2015 (SADC, 2010) seek to standardize treatments for those diseases in SADC, a further step would be for citizens, including those who migrate across borders, to access treatment in any of the participating countries. This would incentivize some to seek treatment and reduce the burden of treatment provision if additional providers are added to the cooperation.
2 The SADC Secretariat has expressed interest in the creation of cross-border initiatives for malaria and HIV (Janse van Rensburg and Fourie, 2016). Moving beyond particular disease treatment, cross-border initiatives could eventually could be applied to all health programs in the region.
3 The 2006–2015 Sexual and Reproductive Health Strategy for the SADC Region (2008), which included "vulnerable youth" as a unique target group slated for extra outreach and intervention, could be adapted and broadened. Its focus areas could also be integrated into a cross-border program.

Implementing such initiatives would go a long way towards providing for and protecting the health of vulnerable adolescent populations across borders.

Conclusion

This chapter analyzed the biological, social and legal "double vulnerability" of adolescents to HIV and EID infection in Eastern and Southern Africa. By looking through the lens of human security as it intersects with state security, the chapter made the conceptual case of including individuals, notably citizens and non-citizens, in any analysis of health security. First, it argued that a human-centric approach beyond citizenship would better capture the intermingled threats, risks and vulnerabilities that impact individual and population health security. Second, having made those identifications, the chapter delved into the particular conditions, biological and legal, that confront adolescents. In doing so, it paid particular attention to the added vulnerability of non-citizenship. Finally, it outlined two possible response scenarios and developed three operational ideas to address these vulnerabilities.

The chapter showed that citizenship status, whether existent, non-existent or compromised, constitutes a factor in adolescent access to health provisions and protections. In short, citizenship status is a contributing factor in adolescent marginalization. A "double vulnerability" follows from that, wherein biological vulnerability and legal vulnerability reinforce one another. Responding to this double vulnerability, as this chapter has shown, requires cross-border, regional concepts and operationalization of health interventions that expressly include citizen and non-citizen access to elevate health as a universal human right.

Health is increasingly accepted as a universal human right. More migrants than ever before are on the move. That means that health rights must move across borders. This reality reinforces the imperative to recognize universal health rights and to universally extend them beyond borders.

Notes

1 Quoted at the International Day of Democracy, 15 September 2014. Available at: www.way.org.my/press-release-menu/419-international-day-of-democracy.
2 Interview with M. Boddenberg, German Chamber of Commerce and Industry, Johannesburg, Republic of South Africa, April 2017.
3 The agency defines adolescents as persons between the ages of 10 and 19.
4 Interview with S. Timol, former educator in the Western Cape Province, Republic of South Africa, Cape Town, April 2017.
5 Interview with S. Timol, former educator in the Western Cape Province, Republic of South Africa, Cape Town, April 2017; also interview with Prof. Dr. Lynne Webber, University of Pretoria, April 2017.
6 Šehović, ethnographic notes taken in Pretoria, Republic of South Africa, April 2017.
7 Šehović, ethnographic notes taken in Pretoria, Republic of South Africa, April 2017.
8 Interview with K. Govender, HEARD, Durban, South Africa, 10 April 2017.
9 Tax collection in turn would help finance additional access to health and education services.

References

African Union. 2017. *State of Africa's Population 2017: Youth, Health and Development: Overcoming the Challenges towards Harnessing the Demographic Dividend.* STC-HPDC-2, Addis Ababa, 21–24 March.

Buzan, Barry, Ole Waever and Jaap de Wilde. 1998. *Security: A New Framework for Analysis*. Boulder, CO: Lynne Rienner.

Christensen, John L. Lynn Carol Miller, Paul Robert Appleby, Charisse Corsbie-Massay, Carlos Gustavo Godoy, Stacy C. Marsella and Stephen J. Read. 2013. Sexual stigma and discrimination as barriers to seeking appropriate healthcare among men who have sex with men in Eswatini, in *Global action to reduce HIV stigma and discrimination*, Anne L. Stangl and Cynthia I. Grossman, eds. *Journal of the International AIDS Society* Vol. 16, Suppl. 2, pp. 1–8 (121–129).

The Constitution of the Republic of South Africa. 1996. Available at: www.gov.za/documents/constitution/constitution-republic-south-africa-1996-1, last accessed 9 May 2018.

Directorate of Social & Human Development & Special Programs SADC Secretariat. 2010. Harmonised Minimum Standards for the Prevention, Treatment and Management of Tuberculosis in the SADC Region. Gaborone: SADC.

Elbe, Stefan. 2010. *Security and Global Health: Toward the Medicalization of Insecurity*. Cambridge: Blackwell Publishers.

Govender, K., W. Masebo, P. Nyamaruze, R. Cowden, B.T. Schunter and A. Bains. 2017. HIV prevention in adolescents and young people in the Eastern and Southern African Region: Key challenges impeding actions for an effective response. *HEARD Working Paper Series, N 2109/17* (submitted for publication)

Grossman, Cynthia I. and Anne L. Stangl. 2013. Impact of HIV-related stigma on treatment adherence: Systematic review and meta-synthesis, in *Global action to reduce HIV stigma and discrimination*, Anne L. Stangl and Cynthia I. Grossman, eds. *Journal of the International AIDS Society* Vol. 16, Suppl. 2, pp. 1–6 (8–13).

Gruskin, Sofia, Kelly Safreed-Harmon, Tamar Ezer, Anne Gathumbi, Jonathan Cohen and Patricia Kameri-Mbote. 2013. Assessment of HIV-related stigma in a US faith-based HIV education and testing: Reducing shame in a game that predicts HIV risk reduction for young adult men who have sex with men: A randomized trial delivered nationally over the web, in *Global action to reduce HIV stigma and discrimination*, Anne L. Stangl and Cynthia I. Grossman, eds. *Journal of the International AIDS Society* Vol. 16, Suppl. 2, pp. 1–7 (94–101).

Howell, Allison. 2014. The global politics of medicine: Beyond global health, against securitisation theory. *Review of International Studies* Vol. 40, Issue 5, pp. 961–987. doi:10.1017/S0260210514000369

Iliffe, J. 2006. *The African AIDS Epidemic: A History*. Oxford: James Currey.

International Health Regulations. 2005. Geneva: WHO.

International HIV/AIDS Alliance: Together to End AIDS. 2016. *Working with Young Key Populations in a Hostile Legal, Socio-cultural and Political Environment*. Experience of Alliance Burundaise Contre le SIDA implementing Link Up in Burundi, Case Study Burundi.

Janse van Rensburg, Andre and Pieter Fourie. 2016. Health policy and integrated mental health care in the SADC region: Strategic clarification using the Rainbow Model. International *Journal of Mental Health Systems* Vol. 10, p. 49. doi:10.1186/s13033-016-0081-7

Katz, Ingrid T., Annemarie E. Ryu, Afiachukwu G. Onuegbu, Christina Psaros, Sheri D. Weiser, David R. Bangsberg and Alexander C. Tsai. 2013. A systematic review of interventions to reduce HIV-related stigma and discrimination from 2002 to 2013: How far have we come? in *Global action to reduce HIV stigma and discrimination*, Anne L. Stangl and Cynthia I. Grossman, eds. *Journal of the International AIDS Society* Vol. 16, Suppl. 2, pp. 1–25 (14–37).

Kharsany, A., C. Cawood, D. Khanyile, L. Lewis, A. Grobler and A. Puren. 2018. Community-based HIV prevalence in KwaZulu-Natal, South Africa: Results of a cross-sectional household survey. *Lancet HIV* Vol. 5, Issue 8, pp. 427–437 (1 August).

Li, Chunqing Lin, Jihui Guan and Zunyou Wu. 2013. Access to justice: Evaluating law, health and human rights programmes in Kenya, in *Global action to reduce HIV stigma and discrimination*, Anne L. Stangl and Cynthia I. Grossman, eds. *Journal of the International AIDS Society* Vol. 16, Suppl. 2, pp. 1–7 (69–76).

Marten, Robert and Richard D. Smith. 2018. State support: A prerequisite for global health network effectiveness, comment on "four challenges that global health networks face". *International Journal of Health Policy Management* Vol. 7, Issue 3, pp. 275–277.

Mburu, Gitau, Mala Ram, Morten Skovdal, David Bitira, Ian Hodgson, Grace W. Mwai, Christine Stegling and Janet Seeley. 2013. Implementing a stigma reduction intervention in healthcare settings, in *Global action to reduce HIV stigma and discrimination*, Anne L. Stangl and Cynthia I. Grossman, eds. *Journal of the International AIDS Society* Vol. 16, Suppl. 2, pp. 1–7 (53–59).

Nef, Jorge. 1999. *Human Security and Mutual Vulnerability: The Global Policy Economy of Development and Underdevelopment*, 2nd edition. Ottawa: International Development Research Center.

Pantelic, Marija, Yulia Shenderovich, Lucie Cluver and Mark Boyes. 2015. Predictors of internalized HIV-related stigma: A systematic review of studies in sub-Saharan Africa. *Health Psychology Review* Vol. 9, Issue 4, pp. 469–490.

Paris, Roland. 2001. Human security: Paradigm shift of hot air? *International Security* Vol. 26, Issue 2, pp. 87–102 (Fall).

Risher, K. et al. 2013. Sexual stigma and discrimination as barriers to seeking appropriate healthcare among men who have sex with men in Swaziland. *Journal of the International AIDS Society*, Vol. 16, Issue Suppl 2, p. 18715. Available at: http://www.jiasociety.org/index.php/jias/article/view/18715.

SADC. 2008. *Sexual and Reproductive Health Strategy for the SADC Region 2006–2015*. Available at: www.sadc.int/files/7913/5293/3503/Sexual_And_Reproductive_Health_for_SADC_2006-2015.pdf.

SADC. 2010. *HIV and AIDS Strategic Framework, 2010–2015*. Available at: www.sadc.int/files/4213/5435/8109/SADCHIVandAIDSStrategyFramework2010-2015.pdf

Šehović, Annamarie Bindenagel. 2014. *HIV/AIDS and the South African State: The Responsibility to Respond*. Farnham: Ashgate.

Šehović, Annamarie Bindenagel. 2017. Identifying and addressing the governance accountability problem (GAP). *Global Public Health* (13 September). doi:10.1080/17441692.2017.1371203

Šehović, Annamarie Bindenagel. 2018. *Re-imagining Human Security Beyond Borders*. London: Palgrave Macmillan.

Sidibé, Michel and Eric P. Goosby. 2013. Editorial: Global action to reduce HIV stigma and discrimination, in *Global action to reduce HIV stigma and discrimination*, Anne L. Stangl and Cynthia I. Grossman, eds. *Journal of the International AIDS Society* Vol. 16, Suppl. 2.

Stangl, Anne L. and Cynthia I. Grossman., eds. 2013. Global action to reduce HIV stigma and discrimination. *Journal of the International AIDS Society* Vol. 16, Suppl. 2.

UNAIDS. 2008. *Uganda Country Progress Report*. Available at: http://data.unaids.org/pub/report/2008/uganda_2008_country_progress_report_en.pdf

UNDP. 1994. Human Development Report 1994: New Dimensions of Human Security. Available at: http://www.hdr.undp.org/en/content/human-development-report-1994

UNICEF. 2017a. *Adolescent Demographics*. Available at: https://data.unicef.org/topic/adolescents/adolescent-demographics/#

UNICEF. 2017b. *HIV/AIDS Adolescents and Young People*. Available at: https://data.unicef.org/topic/hivaids/adolescents-young-people/

US CDC. 2018. *Social Determinants of Health*. Available at: www.cdc.gov/socialdeterminants/, last accessed 8 May 2018.

Winter, Sebastian F. and Stefan F. Winter. 2018. Human dignity as leading principle in public health ethics: A multi-case analysis of 21st century German health policy decisions. *International Journal of Health Policy Management* Vol. 7, Issue 3, pp. 210–224.

World Health Organization. 2017. *Uganda Fact Sheet*. Available at: www.afro.who.int/sites/default/files/2017-08/UPHIA%20Uganda%20factsheet.pdf

World Health Organization. 2018. *Social Determinants of Heath*. Available at: www.who.int/social_determinants/sdh_definition/en/, last accessed 8 May 2018.

World Migration Report. 2015. *Migrants and Cities: New Partnerships to Manage Mobility*. Geneva: IOM.

Interviews

Blignaut, A. Teacher in Pretoria, 4 April 2017.

Boddenberg, Matthias. German Chamber of Commerce and Industry, Johannesburg, Republic of South Africa, April 2017.

Govender, Kaymarlin. HEARD, Durban, South Africa, 10 April 2017.

Kajee, Ayesha. Social science researcher, Johannesburg, Republic of South Africa, April 2017.

Panter, Clifford. Centurion/East London, Republic of South Africa, April 2017.

Timol, Suleiman. Former educator in the Western Cape Province, Republic of South Africa, Cape Town, April 2017.

Webber, Lynne. University of Pretoria Pathology, 4 April 2017.

Part II

7 Addressing structural drivers of HIV among young people in Eastern and Southern Africa

Evidence, challenges and recommendations for advancing the field

Mitzy Gafos, Tara Beattie, Kirsten Stoebenau, Deborah Baron, Renay Weiner, Joyce Wamoyi, Lebohang Letsela, James Hargreaves, Gerry Mshana, Saidi Kapiga, Anne Stangl, Michelle Remme, Lori Heise and Janet Seeley

Introduction

In 2016, of the 2.1 million adolescents (10–19 years) living with HIV globally, 84% were in sub-Saharan Africa. In this region, adolescent girls are twice as likely as boys to acquire HIV (UNAIDS, 2018b). This difference between adolescent girls and boys is greatest in Eastern and Southern Africa (ESA), where girls account for 78% of new infections in adolescents (UNICEF, 2018). In this chapter, we focus on the role of structural factors in exacerbating the risk of HIV among young people (10–24 years) in ESA and the structural interventions that aim to address them. Structural factors can be conceptualized as *drivers* of risk, which fundamentally shape and influence patterns of risk behaviour, and *mediators* of risk, which hinder or facilitate an individual's or group's ability to avoid HIV (Parkhurst, 2013).

Young people's primary proximal risk for HIV is sexual behaviour, including unprotected sex and partner selection (Figure 7.1). These risk factors are influenced by interpersonal and individual risks such as transactional sex, gender-based violence and harmful alcohol use. Structural factors function upstream of the individual, interpersonal and proximal determinants of HIV risk, increasing susceptibility to HIV and undermining both biomedical and behavioural prevention efforts (Blankenship et al., 2000; Kippax, 2008; Gupta et al., 2008; Hankins and de Zalduondo, 2010). As shown in Figure 7.1, gender inequality, stigma and discrimination, alcohol availability, lack of economic opportunity, lack of education and poor healthcare access are community-level structural drivers on the pathway to sexual risk behaviour and/or HIV infection. At the macro level, political, legal, cultural and religious, economic and corporate factors, as well as the social influence of the media,

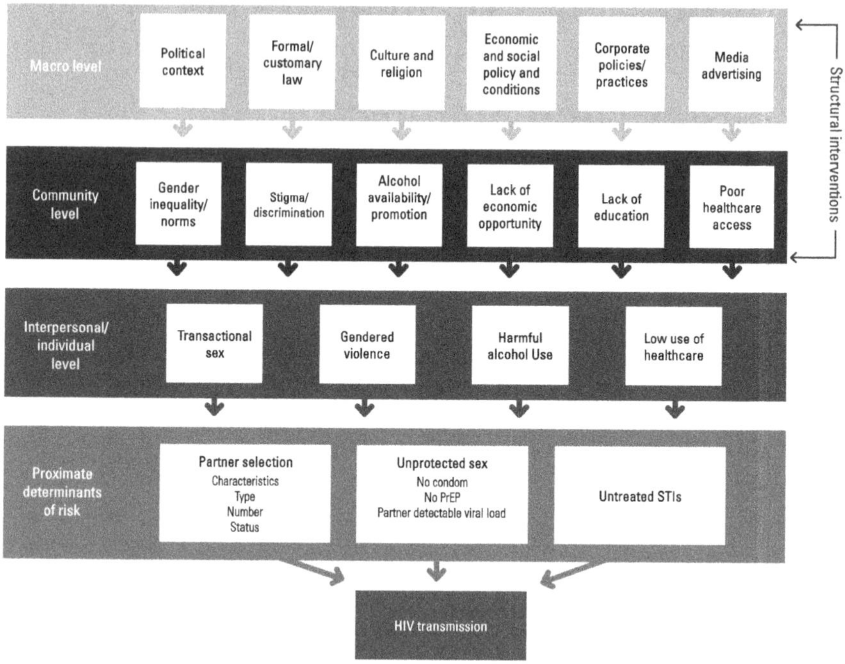

Figure 7.1 STRIVE conceptual framework mapping relationships between HIV, proximal determinants of risk and structural factors (http://strive.lshtm.ac.uk) Colour images available at: https://tinyurl.com/y5sbppxa

in turn impact on structural drivers of HIV. While these factors serve as drivers for all age groups, the impact on young people is exacerbated by their age and their relatively low social and economic position within society. Young people's experiences during adolescence lay the foundation for adulthood and define trajectories for future generations (Patton et al., 2016). It is therefore important to mitigate the risks posed by the structural drivers of HIV among this age group to improve prospects of future health and well-being.

Structural interventions aim to alter the social, economic and political contexts that influence the drivers or mediators of HIV (Blankenship et al., 2000). Structural interventions may tackle macro-level factors at an institutional level, such as addressing gender inequalities in the criminal justice system or changing the law to prevent child marriage. However, most structural interventions are intended to alter or mitigate drivers of HIV at the community level. As such, structural interventions can address factors such as socio-economic inequalities, harmful gender norms, gender-based violence, alcohol availability and promotion and HIV-related stigma. By targeting factors that increase young people's susceptibility to HIV, structural interventions have the potential to mitigate their risk of HIV. However, given that structural interventions function upstream of the proximal risk factors for HIV, they also have the potential to impact on other development outcomes and priorities. It has been argued that these interventions need to be integrated into both HIV prevention programmes and broader gender and development initiatives (Seeley et al., 2012). Addressing the structural drivers of HIV is an essential first step in creating enabling environments for young people to protect themselves from HIV and capitalize on the availability of development opportunities (Hardee et al., 2014). Only by addressing structural drivers will we be able to achieve the 'fast-track to end AIDS' strategic targets and the broader UN Sustainable Development Goals (SDGs) (UN, 2016; UNAIDS, 2015).

A previous literature review evaluated structural interventions among adolescents in sub-Saharan Africa that specifically aimed to change sexual risk behaviours (Wamoyi et al., 2014). The review included economic interventions such as income generation, cash transfer, support to start businesses or find work and support to attend school; gender empowerment interventions that focused on life skills and creating safe spaces for adolescent girls in the community; and behaviour change communication interventions that either provided mass-media information to support social change or to improve parent-child communication. Although a number of the interventions reviewed were then ongoing, there were several that demonstrated positive sexual and reproductive health outcomes especially from economic empowerment interventions. The review highlighted the need for interventions to be designed specifically to address the pathways that influence risk for young people, noting for example that in contrast to a microfinance trial that reduced risk for adult women, the pressures of repaying microcredit loans actually exacerbated risk among young women in one intervention.

In this chapter, we review interventions among young people aged 10–24 in ESA that are designed to impact more broadly on the upstream structural drivers of HIV. We review interventions that address limited livelihood options, including increasing school attendance and attainment, and reducing poverty and gender inequality, including gender norms and gender-based violence. At a time when the SDG agenda has re-focused people's attention on the potential of multi-sectoral action and synergistic developmental opportunities (Fritz and Heise, 2018), we aim to synthesize existing evidence of what works to alter the structural drivers of HIV for young people, identify the challenges of scaling up such interventions and achieving an impact on HIV incidence, and outline recommendations for policy-makers, implementers and researchers.

Causal pathways of risk

Structural interventions are designed to alter the mechanisms through which upstream structural drivers of HIV influence proximate risk behaviours within specific contexts and populations. These mechanisms of influence are delineated as causal pathways to HIV infection. In considering the causal pathways of interest in this review, we summarize evidence on the pathways through which education and poverty, and gender norms and violence, influence the risk of HIV.

Education

The relationship between education and HIV is thought to have reversed as the HIV epidemic has matured (Hargreaves and Glynn, 2002; Hargreaves et al., 2008). Current evidence suggests that each additional year of school attendance reduces the risk of HIV infection (Barnighausen et al., 2007), which in some studies is particularly pronounced for young women (De Neve et al., 2015; Pettifor et al., 2008). Similarly, evidence demonstrates that higher sexual risk behaviours are associated with being out of school among youth in ESA (Stroeken et al., 2012). Improving school attendance and educational attainment can impact on future socio-economic status; socio-cognitive factors including knowledge, attitudes, self-esteem and self-efficacy; social networks including sexual partnering; personal aspirations; and exposure to HIV prevention education (Jukes et al., 2008a). These factors are likely to play an important role in influencing sexual risk behaviours and adoption of HIV prevention options (Figure 7.2) (Prudden, 2017). There has been growing interest in structural interventions that aim to improve school enrolment, school attendance (as a predictor of school dropout), secondary school completion and educational attainment as a means to reduce the risk of HIV infection, with a particular interest in school-based interventions (Jukes et al., 2008b; Mason-Jones et al., 2016).

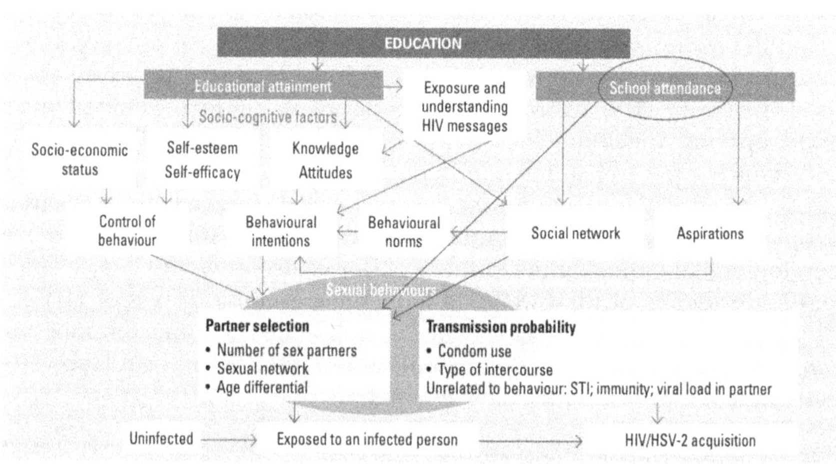

Figure 7.2 Potential pathways of change which may be influenced by greater attendance and greater attainment within schools

Poverty

Most reviews of the relationship between poverty and wealth with HIV infection find that macro-level economics, national wealth inequalities and gendered-wealth disparities have both positive and negative impacts on sexual risk behaviours and HIV risk (Wojcicki, 2005; Parkhurst, 2010; Fox, 2010). Certainly, HIV prevalence is highest in the wealthiest sub-Saharan African countries, although this can mask in-country disparities (Gupta et al., 2008). A number of studies suggest that relative poverty is not associated with HIV, with higher prevalence being observed in households with middle or higher quartile wealth indices (Barnighausen et al., 2007; Mishra et al., 2007). Other studies suggest that increasing socio-economic status either does not increase risk or can decrease sexual risk behaviours in countries with higher per capita income and in-country wealth inequalities (Wojcicki, 2005; Parkhurst, 2010). However, increasing access to resources for women also has the potential to increase risk-taking behaviours in some contexts (Wojcicki, 2005). The relative impact of poverty on HIV risk in different populations is further delineated by gender, marital status for women and urban or rural residency for both women and men (Wojcicki, 2005; Hallman, 2005b; Gillespie et al., 2007). As with education, there is a suggestion of a reversal in relationship between poverty and HIV risk in some countries, with declining prevalence in wealthy groups and increasing prevalence in poorer groups, especially among young women (Hargreaves, 2002; Hallman, 2005b; Parkhurst, 2010).

As shown in Figure 7.3, poverty can impact on HIV risk in terms of members of households being unable to meet the costs of food security, educational expenses and healthcare costs, which in turn influences young peoples' school attendance, health and well-being and engagement in gender-inequitable relationships (Parkhurst, 2013). There is currently increased attention to the role of youth poverty as an economic motivator of inequitable age-disparate and transactional sex relationships (Luke, 2003, 2005). A recent phylogenetic study in a hyperendemic area of South Africa highlighted the extent to which sexual partnering between young women and older men is driving new HIV infections among young women (de Oliveira et al., 2017). Transactional sexual relationships have been shown to be motivated by the desire for sexual relationships to meet basic financial needs and improve social status as well as sociocultural material expressions of love (Stoebenau et al., 2016). There has also been specific attention paid to the negative impact of household poverty on sexual risk behaviour for orphaned youth (Hallman, 2005a).

There is increasing interest in interventions that aim to alleviate poverty among groups for whom it has been shown to increase the risk of HIV. The UNAIDS fast-track target aims to strengthen HIV-sensitive national social

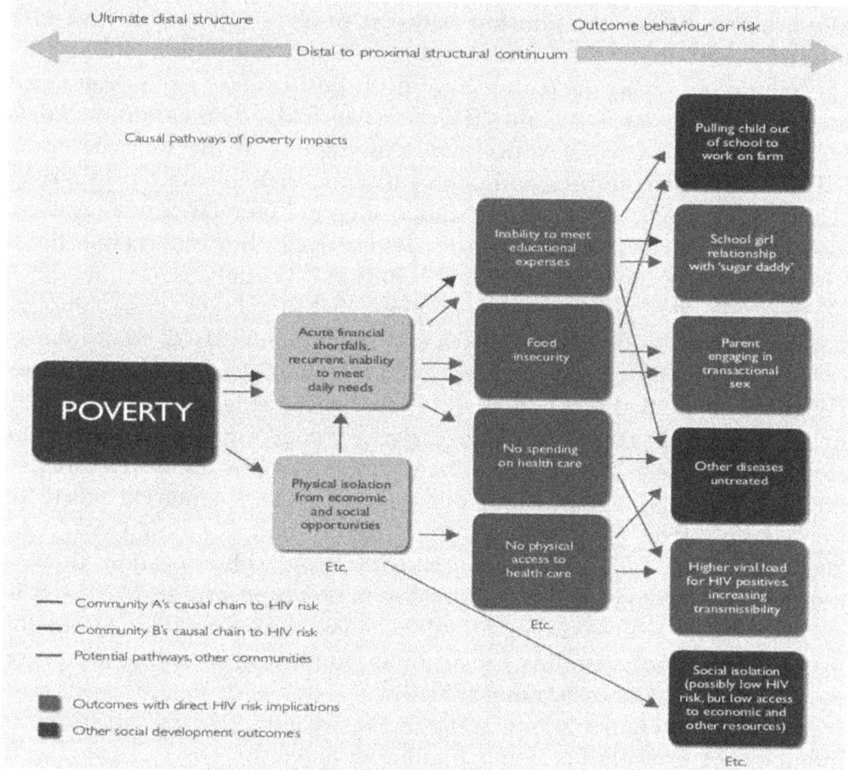

Figure 7.3 Potential pathways through which poverty impacts on HIV risk Figure available in colour at: https://tinyurl.com/y5sbppxa

and child protection systems to ensure 75% of people living with or at risk of HIV have access to social protection (UNAIDS, 2018a). Social protection interventions focus on ways to mitigate the impact of poverty, such as conditional and unconditional cash transfer programmes, income generation programmes such as vocational training and work generation, and microfinance programmes as standalone schemes or integrated in health programmes (Heise et al., 2013; Pega et al., 2017; Taaffe et al., 2016; Taaffe et al., 2017; Wilson, 2015; Kennedy et al., 2014; Lorenzetti et al., 2017).

Gender norms and gender-based violence

The causal pathways between gender-based violence and HIV are multifaceted and complex (Heise and McGrory, 2016). A number of studies have shown that young and adult women who experience physical and emotional intimate partner violence (IPV) are more likely to be HIV-positive than women who do not (Durevall and Lindskog, 2015a; Jewkes et al., 2010). However, a meta-analysis across ten countries in sub-Saharan Africa did not observe a link between sexual IPV and HIV among married women, suggesting that other indirect pathways are more influential (Durevall and Lindskog, 2015a). Similarly, studies have shown that men who are violent share a clustering of risk factors that increase their likelihood of being HIV-positive (Jewkes et al., 2011; Decker et al., 2009; Dunkle and Decker, 2013). The clustering of risk factors includes having multiple and concurrent partners; engagement in commercial sex, transactional sex, condomless sex and anal sex; and binge drinking (Dunkle et al., 2006; Dunkle and Decker, 2013; Gass et al., 2011; Gibbs et al., 2017; Durevall and Lindskog, 2015b). In addition, social norms of masculinity and femininity that reproduce the unequal position of women in society and associate masculinity with sexual risk-taking serve as upstream drivers of male IPV perpetration (Jewkes et al., 2010; Harrison et al., 2006).

Social norms are rules of behaviour shared by people in a given society that define what is 'normal' and appropriate behaviour. Social norms that discriminate against women, such as considering the education of boys more important than of girls, or norms which are harmful, such as norms supporting IPV, can exacerbate young women's risk of HIV. Social norms do not mandate behaviours such as IPV but by normalizing the practice can help maintain it, limiting women's ability to resist and community members' ability to intervene (Jewkes et al., 2015). Overall, young and adult women in relationships with violent men are at increased risk of being exposed to HIV and are least able to insist on safer sex practices (Durevall and Lindskog, 2015b; Kacanek et al., 2013).

Figure 7.4 illustrates how the causal pathways of IPV function through socio-economic insecurity, gender inequality and social norms condoning violence to influence sexual risk behaviours and HIV (Heise and McGrory, 2016). There has been increased interest in shifting harmful gender norms as a mechanism of effect on the pathway to the combined risks of gender-based violence and HIV (Cislaghi and Heise, 2016; Cislaghi et al., 2018). A number of reviews have evaluated the evidence of interventions to prevent violence, including for adolescents (De Koker et al., 2014; Lundgren and Amin, 2015; Maman et al., 2000; McCloskey et al., 2016; Shai and Sikweyiya, 2015). As mentioned earlier, there has been increasing interest in social protection interventions to address the upstream influences of poverty on gender-based violence. Gender transformative components such as gender equality training and gender empowerment programmes are increasingly being added to social protection interventions in order to change gender norms condoning violence; empower women socially, economically and politically in society; and address gender inequalities (Gibbs

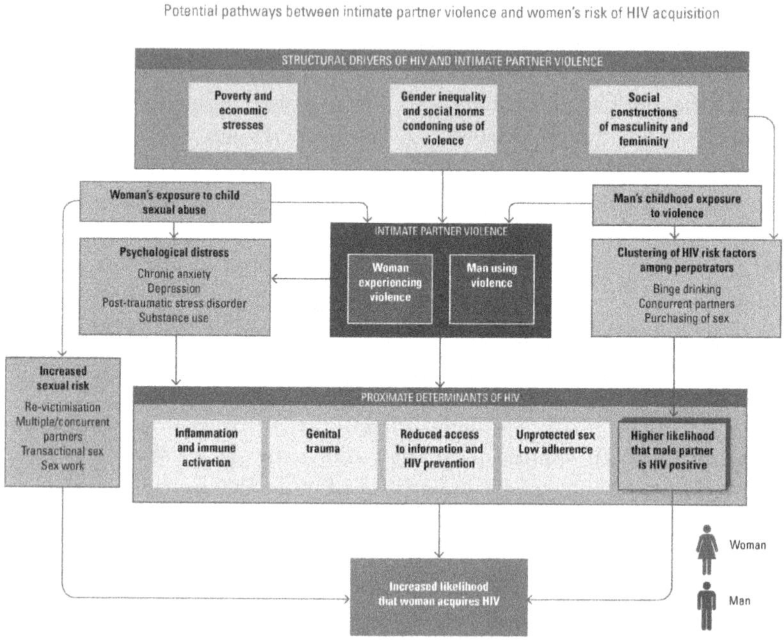

Figure 7.4 Potential pathways between intimate partner violence and women's risk of HIV acquisition Figure available in colour at: https://tinyurl.com/y5sbppxa

et al., 2012; Dworkin et al., 2013; Jewkes et al., 2015; Svanemyr et al., 2015; Buller et al., 2018).

Methods

In this study we review and synthesize findings from structural interventions among adolescents and young people in ESA. Between 8 and 16 January 2018 we conducted a systematic search of literature in Medline, Embase, Global Health, CINAHL Plus, Africa-Wide Information, PsycINFO, Web of Science Core Collection, Cochrane Library, and Scopus. The literature search was constructed using five concepts: young people (aged 10–24), structural drivers (livelihood, education, poverty, gender, social norms and gender-based violence), HIV prevention, ESA and intervention studies. The inclusion criteria were (1) English language publication; (2) interventions or evaluations of interventions addressing at least one structural driver of interest; (3) comparative evaluations or pre-post intervention evaluation; (4) publications from beginning of search engine records to January 2018; and (5) published literature only, based on the breadth of the review and the fact that we did not plan to do a systematic review of the literature or conduct a quality assessment. HIV endpoints were not part of the inclusion criteria. The search identified 2458 unique titles. After screening out 2386 references based on title and abstract, we reviewed 72 papers in full reporting on interventions. In total, 40 papers reporting on 27 interventions were included in the review. Interventions were identified from seven countries in ESA. A full description of the literature search methodology is available on request. This review and synthesis of the evidence was conducted by the STRIVE Research Programme Consortium, which aims to deliver new evidence, together with a synthesis of existing evidence, on individual and inter-related structural drivers of HIV, pathways of risk and infection, effective measurement tools of structural drivers and evaluation of structural interventions (http://strive.lshtm.ac.uk).

What we know about the effectiveness of interventions to address structural drivers of HIV

We now focus on the effectiveness of interventions to address (1) limited livelihood options including education and poverty and (2) gender inequalities including harmful gender norms and gender-based violence. We categorize the interventions based on their primary focus but cross-reference interventions that address multiple structural drivers. Tables 7.1 and 7.2 present an overview of the limited livelihood interventions, and Table 7.3 presents an overview of the gender inequalities interventions. Of the 27 interventions reviewed, 11 reported on improving school attendance, 7 on reducing poverty, 5 on reducing GBV and 4 on changing social norms. All interventions specifically aimed to intervene on the causal pathway between structural driver and HIV infection, yet most did not include HIV outcomes. Most interventions reported on multiple outcome measures. Figure 7.5 illustrates interventions that effectively impacted on structural drivers (education, poverty, social norms, GBV), sexual behaviour and clinical outcomes.

Addressing limited livelihood options to reduce HIV risk

We identified 11 interventions to improve school attendance, 5 to alleviate the impact of poverty more broadly and 2 that evaluated the impact of government cash transfer grants (Tables 7.1 and 7.2).

School attendance: OVC

Seven of the 11 education interventions focused on orphans and vulnerable children (OVC) aged 8–25 in Kenya, Zambia, Zimbabwe and Uganda.

Table 7.1 Structural interventions addressing education

Study name/ paper reference	*Aims of intervention*	*Intervention type and setting*	*Population (country, age group, if OVC, female [F] or male [M])*	*Evaluation design*	*Key findings*
Kenya-CT-OVC: Handa et al., 2014, 2015	The Kenya Cash Transfer for Orphans and Vulnerable Children (Kenya CT-OVC) project provided an unconditional cash transfer to caregivers of OVC.	Social protection, community-based	Kenya, <17, OVC, F/M	Cluster RCT (cRCT)	An evaluation of the government scheme in 2007 showed it had a significant impact on increasing school enrolment, whereby secondary school–aged youth were 8 percentage points more likely to be enrolled in school compared to the control group. A later evaluation in 2011 showed the intervention resulted in 31% reduced odds of sexual debut among recipients but had no impact on transactional sex, condom use or number of partners. An evaluation among young girls found a reduction in the likelihood of pregnancy but no impact on early marriage in the intervention group. The effects were partially explained as indirect impacts of keeping young people in school and reducing financial household instability.
Cho et al., 2011; Hallfors et al., 2012	A school-based invention that paid tuition and provided uniforms and community outreach workers to monitor and help avoid absenteeism for OVC.	Social protection, school-based	Kenya, 12–14, OVC, F/M	RCT	Results initially showed a reduction in school dropout, delayed sexual debut and attitudes supporting delaying sex, prosocial bonding and gender equity attitudes. However, an evaluation two years after the intervention demonstrated that most of these effects had dissipated.

Cho et al., 2017, 2018	A school-based invention that paid tuition and provided uniforms and community outreach workers to monitor and help avoid absenteeism for OVC.	Social protection, school-based	Kenya, 12–14, OVC, F/M	cRCT	Building on the Cho 2011 study, this intervention adapted on a larger scale had positive educational outcomes with reduced school dropout, more age-appropriate progression, higher average grades, higher matriculation into secondary school and increased expectations of completing college/university. However, there was no impact on primary and secondary school test scores. The intervention resulted in reduced transactional sex among sexually active participants, increased circumcision for male participants and improved quality of life indicators, including fewer reported problems with depression/anxiety and performance of usual activities. However, there was no impact on HIV or HSV-2 infection.
Hallfors et al., 2011, 2015; Iritani et al., 2016	A primary school intervention in which all schools received a universal daily feeding program; in addition, intervention participants received fees, uniforms and a school-based helper to monitor attendance and resolve problems.	Social protection, school-based	Zimbabwe, 10–16, OVC, F	cRC	At the three-year follow-up, OVC who received the intervention were less likely to drop out of school or get married, and they were more likely to endorse gender equity. At the five-year follow-up, the intervention group were more likely to still be in school and had achieved almost one additional year of schooling, and reported reduced sexual debut, marriage and pregnancy. The intervention still did not impact on HIV or HSV-2 acquisition. OVC in the intervention also reported eating more meals per day and better quality of life indicators (mobility, self-care, usual activities, pain/discomfort and anxiety/depression). An additional analysis found that the offer of school fees to girls during the transition from primary to secondary school likely has the most impact on school retention.

(Continued)

Table 7.1 (Continued)

Study name/ paper reference	*Aims of intervention*	*Intervention type and setting*	*Population (country, age group, if OVC, female [F] or male [M])*	*Evaluation design*	*Key findings*
Bwafwano: Chatterji et al., 2010	A community-based intervention that provided payment of school fees; school supplies; food, health and psychological services; and HIV prevention training.	Social protection, community-based	Zambia, 8–19, OVC, F/M	Cross sectional with control	The intervention was associated with reduced school dropout for 8–13-year-olds but not 14–19-year-olds. There is some suggestion that the intervention improved the proportion of young people in the correct grade for their age in the longer term.
Suubi: Curley et al., 2010; Ssewamala et al., 2009; Ssewamala 2010a, 2010b; Ssewamala et al., 2012; Ismayilova et al., 2012	This study compared usual school care for AIDS orphans in Uganda, which included school lunches, school materials, counselling, recreation activities and HIV education, to the Suubi intervention, which included a matched savings account for post-primary	Social protection, family-based	Uganda, 11–17, OVC, F/M	cRCT	The Suubi intervention was associated with improvements in self-rated health and mental health functioning, decreases in depression, higher levels of perceived caregiver support, willingness to discuss problems and sexual risk behaviours with caregivers, increased perceived support linked with improved attitudes to risk-taking behaviour, and reductions in sexual risk-taking intentions with higher impact among young girls than boys.

	schooling, 12 one-hour workshops on financial education, asset building and future planning, and monthly peer mentorship sessions.				
Suubi-Maka: Ssewamala et al., 2016; Jennings et al., 2016	This study compared usual school care for AIDS orphans in Uganda, which include school lunches, school materials, counselling, recreation activities and HIV education, to the Suubi-Maka intervention, which included a matched savings account for post-primary schooling, 12 one-hour workshops on financial education, asset-building, and future planning, and monthly peer mentorship sessions.	Social protection, family-based	Uganda, 12–16, OVC, F/M	cRCT	The Suubi-Maka intervention reduced the likelihood of orphans dropping out of school or repeating a year, and improved their grades, with girls faring better than boys. The intervention also resulted in lower levels of hopelessness, higher levels of self-concept (i.e. ability to achieve), increased cash savings and increases in HIV-prevention attitudinal scores.

(*Continued*)

Table 7.1 (Continued)

Study name/ paper reference	*Aims of intervention*	*Intervention type and setting*	*Population (country, age group, if OVC, female [F] or male [M])*	*Evaluation design*	*Key findings*
Zomba: Baird et al., 2012	The Zomba trial evaluated conditional (school attendance) and unconditional cash transfers to girls and their guardians, compared to no cash transfer in reducing the risk of STIs in young women.	Social protection, community-based	Malawi, 13–22, F	cRCT	The intervention observed a 64% reduction in HIV risk and a 76% reduction in HSV-2 risk. Young girls in the intervention were more likely to be enrolled in school and less likely to report sex at least once per week with at least one partner and having an age-disparate sexual partner aged 25 or older. There were no statistically significant differences between intervention and control group for marriage, pregnancy, sexual debut, condomless sex, syphilis or HIV testing. Approximately a quarter of sexually active participants reported transactional sex at baseline and although the trial did not measure intervention impact on transactional sex, reduction in HIV incidence was partially explained by a shift to younger partners with whom girls reported less frequent sex. Among students who had dropped out of school at baseline, girls in the intervention were less likely to be married or report sexual intercourse at least once in the last week, however prevalence of HIV and HSV-2 did not differ. There were few differences between the conditional and unconditional cash transfers expect for lower pregnancy in the unconditional arm.

Robertson et al., 2013; Fenton et al., 2016	A community cash-transfer programme that offered unconditional and conditional (school attendance) cash transfers.	Social protection, community-based	Zimbabwe, <18, F/M	cRCT	The programme found that receipt of unconditional and conditional (school attendance) cash transfers increased the likelihood of 6–12-year-olds and 13–17-year-olds attending school at least 80% of the time. Among 13–17-year-olds, the difference was greater in the conditional cash transfer group. An additional sub-analysis of associations by wealth differentials suggests that unconditional transfers had less effect than conditional transfers in the least poor quintile of the population. Conditional, but not unconditional, transfers reduced the likelihood of young people repeating a school grade. Both cash transfer options resulted in young people spending less time in paid employment.
HPTN068: Pettifor et al., 2016	The HPTN068 intervention provided a conditional cash transfer of ZAR 100 for girls (about USD 10 in 2012), and ZAR 200 (about USD 20 in 2012) for their parent or guardian every month, conditional on the young woman attending 80% of school days per month.	Social protection, community-based	South Africa, 13–20, F	RCT	The HPTN068 conditional (school attendance) cash transfer trial demonstrated that poor school attendance was associated with HIV acquisition. However, the intervention had no effect on school attendance (which was >95% in both the intervention and control groups), school dropout or HIV incidence. Young women who received cash transfers were less likely to report having a partner in the past 12 months, physical IPV in the past 12 months (relative risk 0.66) or condomless sex in the past three months. There were no differences in HSV-2 incidence, age-disparate relationships, transactional sex, pregnancy or age of sexual debut.

(*Continued*)

Table 7.1 (Continued)

Study name/ paper reference	*Aims of intervention*	*Intervention type and setting*	*Population (country, age group, if OVC, female [F] or male [M])*	*Evaluation design*	*Key findings*
Sherr et al., 2017	This study evaluated the impact of government grants in Malawi and South Africa on school attendance and performance.	Social protection, community-based	Malawi/South Africa, <10–15, F/M	Cross-sectional	The study found that grant receipt was associated with higher odds of attending school, lower absenteeism and being in the correct grade. However, it was not associated with school enrolment or performance. Grant receipt was associated with a reduced 'educational risk' (based on poor attendance, incorrect grade for age, slow learner, struggling in school, missing more than a week regularly) for girls but not for boys.

Table 7.2 Structural interventions addressing poverty

Study name/paper reference	*Aims of intervention*	*Intervention type and setting*	*Population (country, age group, if OVC, female (F) or male (M)*	*Evaluation design*	*Key findings*
SHAZ!: Dunbar et al., 2014	SHAZ! combination intervention compared life-skills and health education, vocational training, micro-grants and social support to life-skills and health education alone.	Social protection, community-based	Zimbabwe, 16–19, OVC, F	RCT	The intervention reduced food insecurity, increased independent income, lowered the risk of transactional sex and increased the likelihood of using a condom with a current partner. There was a borderline significant effect on reducing unintended pregnancies for young women.
Bantwana Program: Zuilkowski and Alon, 2015	The Bantwana Program provided training and materials to improve agricultural practices and product marketing, home visits for psychosocial support and referral to social services to families affected by HIV.	Social protection/ empowerment, community-based	Uganda, mean age 15.7, OVC, F/M	Pre-post intervention evaluation	The evaluation found positive trends over time in economic well-being and psychosocial functioning. In comparison to national data, completion of primary school and entry into secondary school was also higher in the intervention group.

(*Continued*)

Table 7.2 (Continued)

Study name/paper reference	*Aims of intervention*	*Intervention type and setting*	*Population (country, age group, if OVC, female (F) or male (M))*	*Evaluation design*	*Key findings*
Goodman et al., 2014	A combined cash transfer, income generation and empowerment programme that aimed to reduce poverty among orphans and vulnerable children in OVC headed-households.	Social protection/ empowerment, community-based	Kenya, 13–25, OVC, F/M	Cross-sectional comparison of year 1, 2, 3 of programme recipients	By comparing first-, second- and third-year recipients, the evaluation demonstrated that exposure to the programme improved financial status, access to essential medical care, food security, safe water access, literacy and completion of eight years in education. It also reduced the number of sexual partners in the last year and increased condom use at last sex for females but not for males.
StreetSmart: Rotheram-Borus et al., 2012	A vocational training programme consisting of apprenticeships with local artisans for training in hairdressing, catering, tailoring, mechanics, electronics, carpentry, cell phone repair and welding.	Social protection, youth centre based	Uganda, 13–23, F/M	Randomized, wait-listed pilot study	The intervention group were more likely to be employed and report better quality of life, greater increases in social support and fewer delinquent acts, although there were no significant differences in sexual risk behaviours.
Empowerment and Livelihood for Adolescents (ELA): Bandiera et al., 2012	ELA was designed to empower adolescent girls through the simultaneous provision of life skills to build knowledge and reduce	Social protection/ empowerment, youth centre based	Uganda, 14–20, F	RCT	Adolescent girls in the intervention were more likely to be engaged in income-generating activities, report safer sexual behaviour knowledge and practices, and

	sexual risk behaviours, and vocational training enabling girls to establish small-scale enterprises.				report higher indices of gender empowerment. In addition, among sexually active girls at baseline, there was a near elimination of reports of having sex unwillingly.
Cluver et al., 2013	Evaluation of child-focused state cash transfer grant.	Social protection, community-based	South Africa, 10–18, F/M	Case control	Receipt of a grant was associated with a reduction in transactional and age-disparate sexual relationships among girls but had no effect on other risk behaviours. The intervention had no effect on transactional sex or other risk behaviours among boys and did not reduce the likelihood of having sex after drinking for girls or boys.
Cluver et al., 2016	Evaluation of 14 different social protection grants.	Social protection, community-based	South Africa, 10–18, F/M	Prospective longitudinal	Child-focused grants, free schooling, school feeding, teacher support and parental monitoring were independently associated with reduced HIV-risk behaviour. Grant receipt was associated with lower reported economic sex (transactional and age disparate), higher-risk sex (condomless, multiple partners, sex while using alcohol or drugs) and pregnancy among girls, as well as economic and higher-risk sex among boys. The study also found cumulative risk-reduction benefits associated with combined social protection effects.

Table 7.3 Structural interventions addressing gender inequality

Study name/paper reference	*Aims of intervention*	*Intervention type and setting*	*Population (country, age group, female [F] or male [M])*	*Evaluation design*	*Key findings*
GBV					
Stepping Stones: Jewkes et al., 2008	Stepping Stones provides a series of single sex sessions of participatory learning that facilitates critical reflection, roleplay and drama and draws the everyday reality of participants' lives into the sessions. The sessions covered how we act and what shapes our actions; sex and love; conception and contraception; taking risks and sexual problems; unwanted pregnancy; sexually transmitted diseases and HIV; safer sex and condoms; gender-based violence; motivations for sexual behaviour; dealing with grief and loss; and communication skills. The intervention aimed to improve sexual health outcomes through building stronger, more gender-equitable relationships and improving communication between partners.	Gender transformative; community-based	South Africa; 15–26, F/M	cRCT	Stepping Stones demonstrated a 33% reduction in HSV-2 incidence in women and men but no difference in HIV incidence. Among men, the intervention reduced reported IPV perpetration, sexual risk behaviours, engagement in transaction sex, problem drinking, drug misuse initiation and depression. However, women initially reported increased engagement in transaction sex (at midpoint but not trial endpoint), and there were no reductions in reported IPV victimization or sexual risk behaviours.
Stepping Stones and Creating Futures: Jewkes et al., 2014	Stepping Stones was combined with the economic empowerment intervention, Creating Futures, and aimed to build stronger, more gender-equitable relationships, improve communication between partners and strengthen livelihoods by supporting participants to find work or set up a business, but did not provide cash or loans.	Gender transformative/ social protection; community-based	South Africa, 18–30 (83% <24), F/M	cRCT	The intervention resulted in a 38% reduction in women's experience of physical and sexual IPV combined, although the difference was only significant for sexual IPV when assessed individually. There were no differences in men's reports of IPV perpetration

					or transactional sex among women or men. The intervention resulted in increased earnings for women and men, improved gender attitudes among women and men, and reduced reported controlling behaviours by men in their relationships.
					There was also an increase in HIV testing behaviour and a reduction in reported symptoms of depression and suicidal ideation among men, and a reduction in alcohol and alcohol-related conflict among women.
PREPARE: Mathews et al., 2016	PREPARE was a multi-component, school-based HIV prevention intervention that provided an educational programme, a school health service and a school safety programme that aimed to reduce IPV (combined measure of emotional, physical and sexual IPV) and HIV risk behaviours.	Education/health services/safety programme; school-based	South Africa, 12–14, F/M	cRCT	The intervention reduced IPV victimization by 30% but had no impact on IPV perpetration or sexual risk behaviours.
Sarnquist et al., 2014	This school-based intervention aimed to evaluate the offer of life-skills education combined with empowerment, de-escalation and self-defence training compared to standard life-skills education to reduce the risk of sexual assault.	Empowerment/self-defence; school-based	Kenya, 13–20, F	Pre-post evaluation with control	In the intervention group, the reported incidence of sexual assault reduced by 60% from baseline to follow-up 10.5 months after the intervention. There were no decreases in the control group. Disclosure of sexual assault also increased significantly in the intervention but not in the control group.

(*Continued*)

Table 7.3 (Continued)

Study name/paper reference	*Aims of intervention*	*Intervention type and setting*	*Population (country, age group, female [F] or male [M])*	*Evaluation design*	*Key findings*
Women's Health CoOp: Wechsberg et al., 2013	The Women's Health CoOp (WHC) intervention is an empowerment-based, two-session HIV intervention designed to address alcohol and other drug use risks, IPV, sexual risk behaviours and gender inequality among underserved women using drugs.	Gender transformative/ alcohol reduction; community-based	South Africa, 18–33 (mean 23), F	RCT	The WHC intervention in Cape Town resulted in a 54% reduction in drug use but did not reduce physical IPV, alcohol use or sobriety at last sex (despite initial reductions at month six) or sexual risk behaviour.
Social Norms					
Regai Dzive Shiri: Cowan et al., 2010	The Regai Dzive Shiri intervention provided three programme components – a youth programme to improve knowledge and skills for in-school and out-of-school youth; a parents and community stakeholder to improve knowledge and communication skills; and a training programme for nurses and other staff working in rural clinics – and aimed to change social norms among adolescents.	Empowerment; community-based	Zimbabwe, 18–22, F/M	cRCT	The intervention positively impacted on women's attitudes to relationship control and gender empowerment. The intervention had limited impact on men's attitude to relationship control and gender empowerment. Women in the intervention were less likely to report ever being pregnant, but there were no other impacts on clinical outcomes (HIV, HSV-2 or current pregnancy), sexual behaviour or clinic attendance.

Moving the Goalposts (MTG): Woodcock et al., 2012	Moving the Goalposts (MTG) was a sports-based intervention aiming to empower young women by providing opportunities to develop 'important transferable life skills', including psychosocial and interpersonal skills, and psychological constructs such as confidence and self-efficacy, as well as knowledge and resources through participating in, developing and managing girls' football and associated health, educational and business initiatives.	Empowerment; sports-based	Kenya, 10–25, F	Cross-sectional	The evaluation found that duration in the intervention improved outcomes related to female empowerment, perceived life skills, social life, insights about HIV and leadership skills. Attendance at more established intervention sites was associated with greater benefits overall and with a positive outlook on life.
Mathare Youth Sport Association (MYSA): Delva et al., 2010	The MYSA HIV/AIDS Prevention and Awareness Project multi-component programme offered rotational facilitation, school outreach programmes, movement games and access to a resource centre facilitated by volunteer peer educators and peer counsellors. The study evaluated sexual behaviour and social norms of youth involved in the MYSA compared to a control group of non-MYSA members.	Skills building/peer support; sports-based	Kenya, 12–24, F/M	Cross-sectional	The intervention did not impact on subjective norms on virginity and gendered responsibility, risk-taking attitudes or behavioural intentions relating to condoms and fidelity. The intervention group were more likely to report condom use during their first and last sexual encounters and frequency of condom use, and score better on behavioural control of condoms (having condoms, knowing where to buy), but there were no other impacts on sexual behaviour.

(Continued)

Table 7.3 (Continued)

Study name/paper reference	*Aims of intervention*	*Intervention type and setting*	*Population (country, age group, female [F] or male [M])*	*Evaluation design*	*Key findings*
Fataki: Kaufman et al., 2013a	Fataki was a national multimedia campaign which aimed to shift social norms about cross-generational sex.	Mass media; community-based	Tanzania, >15 (mean 31.2), F/M	Post-intervention evaluation	While the campaign increased discussion about cross-generational sex and willingness to intervene to challenge such relationships, it did not shift social norms to oppose such relationships. Women who had been exposed to the campaign were less likely to be involved in cross-generational relationships with increasing exposure. However, there were no associations between intervention exposure and involvement in cross-generational relationships among men.

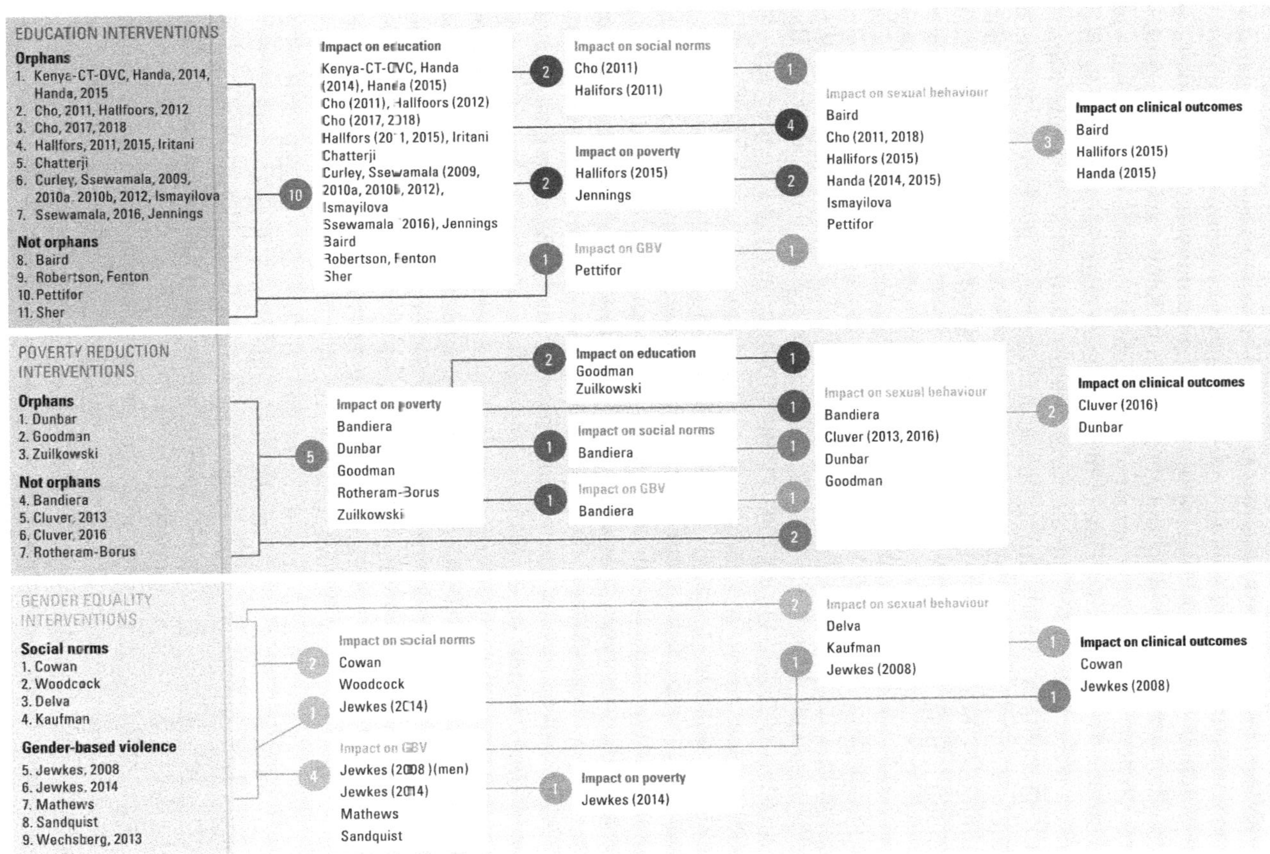

Figure 7.5 Structural HIV prevention interventions among adolescents in Eastern and Southern Africa and the impact on structural drivers (education, poverty, social norms, GBV), sexual behaviour and clinical outcomes Figure available in colour at: https://tinyurl.com/y5sbppxa

One intervention included young women only; the rest also included young men.

One study evaluated the impact of an unconditional cash transfer to caregivers of OVC in Kenya, and four evaluated broader social protection packages including paying tuition and exam fees, providing school uniforms and supplies, and providing support from community outreach workers to monitor and help avoid school absenteeism in Kenya, Zambia and Zimbabwe. The remaining two compared usual school care for AIDS orphans in Uganda, which includes school lunches, school materials, counselling, recreation activities and HIV education, with the Suubi (which means 'hope') or Suubi-Maka (which means 'hope for families') interventions, which included a matched savings account for post-primary schooling, 12 one-hour workshops on financial education, asset-building, future planning and monthly peer mentorship sessions.

All the interventions demonstrated positive impacts in terms of reducing school dropout. However, the intervention in Zambia reduced school dropout for 8–13-year-olds but not 14–19-year-olds (Chatterji et al., 2010). Analysis of an intervention among young girls in Zimbabwe found that the offer of school fees during the transition from primary to secondary school appeared to have the greatest impact on school retention (Iritani et al., 2016). Two studies reported on the maintenance of intervention effects. An evaluation of the Kenyan intervention two years after the programme ended demonstrated that the effect on school dropout had dissipated (Hallfors et al., 2012). However, an evaluation of the Zimbabwean pilot intervention at the five-year follow-up showed that the intervention group were more likely to still be in school and had achieved almost one additional year of schooling (Hallfors et al., 2015).

Only four interventions reported on educational attainment. One intervention resulted in more age-appropriate progression, higher average grade level in school, higher matriculation into secondary school and increased expectations of completing college/university, but no impact on primary and secondary school test scores (Cho et al., 2017). In the intervention that reduced school dropout only for 8–13-year-olds, there was some suggestion that the intervention improved the proportion of young people in the correct grade for their age in the longer term (Chatterji et al., 2010). The Suubi and Suubi-Maka interventions were both associated with improvements in academic grades, with girls faring better than boys in Suubi-Maka (Curley et al., 2010; Ssewamala et al., 2016).

Four of the seven interventions reported sexual behaviour outcomes. All four trials demonstrated an effect on reducing the probability of early age sexual debut (Handa et al., 2014; Cho et al., 2011; Hallfors et al., 2015), and one reduced transactional sex among sexually active participants (Cho et al., 2018). However, the Kenya unconditional cash transfer programme did not have an impact on transactional sex, condom use or number of partners (Handa et al., 2014). Two interventions measured early marriage as an outcome, with one showing no effect (Handa et al., 2015) and the other showing a reduction in the likelihood of early marriage (Hallfors et al., 2015).

Three interventions measured clinical outcomes. The unconditional cash transfer programme in Kenya and the broader social protection programme in Zimbabwe both reported reductions in the likelihood of pregnancy (Handa et al., 2015; Hallfors et al., 2015). However, neither of the two interventions that measured an impact on HIV or HSV-2 outcomes reduced infections within the timeline of the programme, with very few HIV cases observed (Hallfors et al., 2015; Cho et al., 2018). Only the broader social protection intervention in Kenya reported on uptake of voluntary medical male circumcision (VMMC), with young men in the intervention group being twice as likely than the control group to get circumcised (Cho et al., 2018).

Five studies suggest additional benefits of the interventions. These included improving attitudes towards delaying sex and more equal gender norms (Cho et al., 2011; Hallfors et al., 2011); improved quality of life indicators, including fewer reported problems with depression/anxiety/hopelessness; improved performance of usual activities and higher levels of confidence in the ability to achieve (Cho et al., 2018; Hallfors et al., 2015; Ssewamala et al., 2009; Ssewamala et al., 2012; Jennings et al., 2016); and improved support structures (Ismayilova et al., 2012; Cho et al., 2011), food security (Hallfors et al., 2015) and cash savings (Jennings et al., 2016).

School attendance: non-OVC

Of the remaining four interventions that aimed to improve school attendance beyond OVC, one evaluated conditional cash transfers and two evaluated conditional and unconditional cash transfer schemes in Malawi, Zimbabwe and South Africa. The conditional schemes were based on school attendance. The other study evaluated the impact of government grants in Malawi and South Africa. Two of the interventions included young women only, and the other two also included young men from younger than 10 to 22 years of age.

All but one of these interventions showed a positive impact on school attendance. Only the HPTN068 conditional cash transfer intervention in South Africa had no effect on school attendance, but attendance was >95% in both the intervention and control groups (Pettifor et al., 2016). Of the two trials that evaluated both conditional and unconditional cash transfers, one showed little difference between the schemes on school attendance (Baird et al., 2012). However, the other found that receipt of unconditional and conditional cash transfers increased the likelihood of 6–12-year-olds and 13–17-year-olds attending school at least 80% of the time, but the difference was greater in the conditional cash transfer group among

13–17-year-olds (Robertson et al., 2013). An additional sub-analysis of this intervention by wealth differentials suggests that unconditional transfers had less effect than conditional transfers in the least poor quintile of the population. In the same intervention, conditional (but not unconditional) transfers reduced the likelihood of young people repeating a school grade, and both cash transfer options resulted in young girls and boys spending less time in paid employment (Fenton et al., 2016). Evaluation of the impact of government grants in Malawi and South Africa found that grant receipt was associated with higher odds of attending school, lower absenteeism and being in the correct grade. However, it was not associated with school enrolment or performance. Grant receipt was associated with a reduced 'educational risk' (based on poor attendance, incorrect grade for age, slow learner, struggling in school, missing more than a week regularly) for girls but not for boys (Sherr et al., 2017).

Only two interventions reported an impact on sexual risk behaviours, both of which only included young women. Recipients of the Zomba intervention were less likely to report regular sex and having an age-disparate sexual partner aged 25 or older. However, there were no statistically significant differences between intervention and control group for sexual debut, condomless sex or early marriage. Among students who had dropped out of school at baseline, girls in the intervention were less likely to be married or report regular sex (Baird et al., 2012). In HPTN068, young women who received cash transfers were less likely to report having a partner in the last year or condomless sex in the last quarter. These impacts were likely due to the economic impact of the transfer given that there were no impacts on school attendance. There were no differences in age of sexual debut, age-disparate relationships or transactional sex (Pettifor et al., 2016).

The same two interventions measured clinical outcomes. The Zomba intervention resulted in a reduction in HIV, HSV-2 and pregnancy (Baird et al., 2012). The reduction in HIV incidence was partially explained by a shift to younger partners with whom girls reported less frequent sex. There were few differences between the conditional and unconditional cash transfers, expect for lower pregnancy in the unconditional arm (Baird et al., 2012). The HPTN068 trial demonstrated that poor school attendance was associated with HIV acquisition, but given that it did not influence school attendance, it is not surprising that it did not impact on HIV, HSV-2 or pregnancy (Pettifor et al., 2016). Few of these studies reported additional outcomes, but HPTN068 reported a 34% reduction in physical IPV (Pettifor et al., 2016).

Poverty reduction

We identified seven interventions that aimed to alleviate the impact of poverty: two on female and male OVC and one on only female OVC, aged 13–25 in Kenya, Zimbabwe and Uganda. The other four interventions were among 10–23-year-olds, one just with young women and the rest including young men, in South Africa and Uganda. Importantly, all interventions were community based and included young people out of school.

Among OVC, the SHAZ! intervention added vocational training, micro-grants and social support to the life-skills and health education curriculum in schools in Zimbabwe (Dunbar et al., 2014). The Bantwana Program in Uganda provided OVC households with training and materials to improve agricultural practices and product marketing, home visits for psychosocial support and referrals to social services (Zuilkowski and Alon, 2015). The Kenyan intervention combined cash transfers, income generation and empowerment training (Goodman et al., 2014). Among non-OVC groups, the StreetSmart intervention provided vocational training to young women and men living in slums in Kampala in a wait-listed trial design (Rotheram-Borus et al., 2012). The Empowerment and Livelihood for Adolescents (ELA) programme in Uganda offered young girls life-skills and vocational training to support the establishment of small-scale enterprises (Bandiera et al., 2012). The final two studies evaluated the impact of state grants, both conditional and unconditional, among young women and men in South Africa on sexual risk behaviours, but did not report socio-economic outcomes (Cluver et al., 2013; Cluver et al., 2016).

All five interventions that aimed to improve socio-economic outcomes had a positive effect. Among OVC, this included reduced food insecurity, improved financial status and economic well-being, increased independent income and improved access to essential medical care and safe water (Dunbar et al., 2014; Zuilkowski and Alon, 2015; Goodman et al., 2014). Among non-OVC, there was increased likelihood of being employed (Rotheram-Borus et al., 2012) and of young girls being engaged in income-generating activities (Bandiera et al., 2012).

All but one of the seven interventions reported sexual behaviour outcomes. Among OVC, this included a reduction in risk of transactional sex and increased likelihood of using a condom with a current partner among young women in Zimbabwe (Dunbar et al., 2014) and a reduction in number of sexual partners in the last year and increased condom use at last sex for young women but not for young men in Kenya (Goodman et al., 2014). Among non-OVC, there were reports of safer sexual behaviour among young women in the ELA intervention in Uganda (Bandiera et al., 2012) but no difference in sexual risk behaviours among young women and men in the StreetSmart intervention, also in Uganda (Rotheram-Borus et al., 2012). Evaluation of the impact of child grants on young people in South Africa found the receipt of a grant was associated with a reduction in transactional and age-disparate sexual relationships among girls but had no effect on other risk behaviours for girls or on any risk behaviours among boys (Cluver et al., 2013). Evaluation of 14 different social protection grants in South Africa found that child-focused grants, free schooling, school feeding, teacher support and parental monitoring were independently associated with reduced HIV-risk behaviours, including reductions in economic sex (transactional and age disparate) and higher risk sex (condomless, multiple partners, sex while using alcohol or drugs) in young girls and boys. The study also found cumulative risk-reduction benefits associated with combined social protection grants (Cluver et al., 2016).

Only two studies reported on clinical outcomes. The SHAZ! intervention observed a borderline significant effect on reducing unintended pregnancies among young women (Dunbar et al., 2014), and grant receipt reduced pregnancy among girls in South Africa (Cluver et al., 2016). Other reported benefits among OVC included improvements in psychosocial functioning and higher completion of primary school and entry into secondary school (when compared to national data) (Zuilkowski and Alon, 2015), and higher literacy and completion of eight years in education (Goodman et al., 2014). Among non-OVC, other benefits included better quality of life, increased social support and fewer delinquent acts among StreetSmart participants (Rotheram-Borus et al., 2012), and higher indices of gender empowerment and near elimination of reports of having sex unwillingly among sexually active young women (Bandiera et al., 2012).

Addressing gender inequality to reduce the risk of HIV

We identified nine interventions that aimed to address gender inequalities (Table 7.3). Five aimed to address gender-based violence, although only three exclusively included young people aged 12–26 in Kenya and South Africa. Two additional interventions in South Africa included cohorts of women aged 18–30, but with 83% below 24 years of age, and aged 18–33 but with a mean age of 23, so we are including them here. In addition, four interventions aimed to shift social norms: one was exclusively for young women and two included young women and men, ranging in age from 10 to 25 years old in Kenya and Zimbabwe. A mass media campaign in Tanzania included young people and adults, and although the evaluation included respondents of a median age of 31, we report it here as a rare example of an intervention that aimed to shift national social norms regarding young peoples' sexual partnerships.

Gender-based violence

Four interventions that aimed to address gender-based violence focus on IPV and one on sexual assault. Three of the interventions were community based and two were school based. Four included gender-transformative components, one in combination with social protection components. The other was a skills-based training intervention.

Stepping Stones is an HIV prevention intervention in South Africa among young women and men that aims to improve sexual health outcomes through building stronger, more gender-equitable relationships and improving communication between partners (Jewkes et al., 2008). In a subsequent community-based intervention also in South Africa, Stepping Stones was combined with Creating Futures, an economic empowerment programme to strengthen livelihoods by supporting participants to find work or set up a business, but did not provide cash or loans (Jewkes et al., 2014). A school-based intervention in Kenya offered empowerment, de-escalation and self-defence training to adolescent girls in addition to standard life-skills education to reduce the risk of sexual assault (Sarnquist et al., 2014). PREPARE was a multi-component, school-based HIV prevention intervention including after-school educational sessions, school health services and a school-based safety programme designed to reduce IPV and HIV risk behaviours (Mathews et al., 2016). Finally, the Women's Health CoOp (WHC) intervention in Cape Town enrolled women reporting drug or alcohol use in an empowerment and skills-building programme (Wechsberg et al., 2013).

Four of the five interventions demonstrated positive impacts on IPV victimization, perpetration or sexual assault. Stepping Stones and Creating Futures resulted in a 38% reduction in women's experience of physical and sexual IPV combined, although the difference was only significant for sexual IPV when assessed individually. There were no differences in men's reports of IPV perpetration (Jewkes et al., 2014). PREPARE reduced IPV victimization (composite of emotional, physical, sexual) by 30% but had no impact on IPV perpetration (Mathews et al., 2016). Stepping Stones did not reduce IPV victimization (physical and sexual) among young women but did reduce reported IPV perpetration (physical and sexual) among men (Jewkes et al., 2008). The one intervention among substance-using women in Cape Town showed no impact on physical IPV (Wechsberg et al., 2013). In the Kenya study, there was a 60% reduction in the reported incidence of sexual assault between baseline and follow-up, 10.5 months after the intervention. There were no decreases in the control group. Disclosure of sexual assault also increased significantly in the intervention but not in the control group (Sarnquist et al., 2014).

Four studies reported sexual behaviour outcomes. Among men, Stepping Stones reduced sexual risk behaviours, including engagement in transactional sex. However, women initially reported increased engagement in transactional sex (at midpoint but not trial endpoint) and no reductions in other sexual risk behaviours (Jewkes et al., 2008). There were no impacts on sexual risk behaviours including transactional sex in the other interventions (Jewkes et al., 2014; Mathews et al., 2016; Wechsberg et al., 2013). Only Stepping Stones reported a clinical outcome, demonstrating a 33% reduction in HSV-2 incidence in women and men but no difference in HIV incidence (Jewkes et al., 2008).

Additional benefits included increased earnings for women and men, improved gender norms in terms of attitudes among women and men and reduced reported controlling behaviours by men in their relationships, an increase in HIV testing behaviour and a reduction in reported symptoms of depression and suicidal ideation among men, and a reduction in alcohol and alcohol-related conflict among women in Stepping Stones and Creating Futures (Jewkes et al., 2014). Stepping Stones resulted in a reduction in problem drinking (AUDIT score), drug misuse initiation and depression among men (Jewkes et al., 2008). The WHC intervention in Cape Town reduced drug use but did not reduce alcohol use or sobriety at last sex (despite initial reductions at month six) (Wechsberg et al., 2013).

Social norms

In addition to the GBV intervention that influenced social norms, mentioned earlier (Jewkes et al., 2014), four community-based interventions primarily aimed to address social norms. The Regai Dzive Shiri programme in Zimbabwe for in-school and out-of-school youth included peer education and participatory learning, community-based sessions for parents and community stakeholders, and training for nurses and other staff in rural clinics. It aimed to change social norms about sex among adolescents to support individual behaviour change (Cowan et al., 2010). There were two sports-based interventions in Kenya: the Moving the Goalposts (MTG) football programme aiming to empower young women (Woodcock et al., 2012) and the Mathare Youth Sport Association (MYSA) with adolescent girls and boys, which evaluated the impact of participation on social norms around gender and sexual behaviour (Delva et al., 2010). Finally, Fataki was a national multimedia campaign in Tanzania to address social norms relating to cross-generational sex (CGS) by mobilizing communities to intervene in CGS relationships. The evaluation was conducted with young people and adults age 15 or older, with a mean participant age of 31 (Kaufman et al., 2013a).

Two of the interventions demonstrated shifts in social norms. Regai Dzive Shiri positively affected young women's attitudes to relationship control and gender empowerment but had limited impact among young men (Cowan et al., 2010). The MTG evaluation found that duration in the intervention improved outcomes related to female empowerment (equal educational opportunities and playing sport during menses), perceived life skills, social life, insights about HIV, and leadership skills. Attendance at more established intervention sites was associated with greater benefits overall and with a positive outlook on life (Woodcock et al., 2012). Youth involved in the MYSA, compared to youth from youth clubs, schools and social organizations in the same areas, did not differ in terms of gendered subjective norms on virginity, responsibility or fidelity; behavioural attitudes towards risk-avoiding behaviour; or behavioural intentions concerning condom use (Delva et al., 2010). The Fataki campaign increased discussion about cross-generational sex and willingness to intervene to challenge such relationships but did not shift social norms to oppose such relationships, although the evaluation did not report results for participants under age 24 (Kaufman et al., 2013a).

Three of the interventions reported sexual behaviour outcomes. MYSA youth were more likely to report condom use during their first and last sexual encounters, but there were no other impacts on sexual behaviour in this study (Delva et al., 2010) or in Regai Dzive Shiri (Cowan et al., 2010). Women who had been exposed to the Fataki campaign were less likely to be involved in cross-generational relationships, although there was no association between intervention exposure and involvement in cross-generational relationships among men (Kaufman et al., 2013a). Only the Regai Dzive Shiri intervention measured clinical outcomes and found that young women in the intervention were less likely to report ever being pregnant, but there were no other impacts on HIV, HSV-2 or current pregnancy (Cowan et al., 2010).

Lessons and challenges for the future

Within the scope of this review, all but one of the structural interventions designed to improve school attendance had a positive impact on schooling. All structural interventions designed to reduce poverty had a positive impact on socio-economic outcomes. When evaluating educational attainment in the context of age-appropriate grades, the outcomes were generally positive, although there is clearly a need for additional evaluation of the impact on educational achievement, such as exam scores. While all of the seven poverty alleviation interventions included young people out of school, only one of the educational interventions included them (Baird et al., 2012). There is need for further interventions to re-engage out-of-school youth in education, including those who have dropped out of school due to an adverse outcome such as unintended pregnancy, both to improve their educational outcomes as well as their sexual and reproductive health outcomes, including HIV risk.

The evidence for structural interventions to address gender inequalities is less consistent, with two out of four social norm interventions and one out of five GBV interventions that measured norms demonstrating a shift in norms. Given the importance of social norms in shaping perceptions of violence, it is striking that most of the GBV interventions did not measure changes in social norms. There is a need for the inclusion of social norms outcomes in more multi-component structural interventions in the future. Of five GBV interventions, there were three reported reductions in physical and/or sexual victimization, although sometimes one and not the other, and one in physical and sexual perpetration. These findings support the argument that the mechanisms of effect differ for emotional, physical, and sexual IPV victimization, and between victimization and perpetration. However, differences in studies are also likely to be due to the lack of standardized implementation methods and inconsistent measurement tools.

There have been important developments in the establishment of standardized measurement tools of IPV which should be used in future evaluations (Heise and Hossain, 2017). There is a growing body of evidence on the use of qualitative vignettes to measure social norms, but there are still substantial challenges in designing effective quantitative measures (Cislaghi, 2017).

During screening, we identified a further five GBV interventions that included young people age 14 and older. All five reduced the risk of IPV victimization or IPV perpetration or sexual assault. However, they did not stratify results by age, so we excluded them from the review (Pronyk et al., 2006; Wagman et al., 2015; Abramsky et al., 2014; Parcesepe et al., 2016; Wechsberg et al., 2011). SASA! was a highly effective community-based intervention, and the authors confirmed that there were no differences in intervention impacts on IPV among 18–24-year-olds, although these results were not published (personal communication with Tanya Abramsky; Abramsky et al., 2014). Approximately a third of the cohorts in four of these trials were under age 24, and stratifying the results by age could have contributed further to our understanding of how to intervene to reduce the risk of violence among young people.

In considering the breadth of the evidence on effect, there is a strong possibility of publication bias, as we did not include unpublished and other grey literature in our search and are aware of a number of relevant studies with flat or partially flat results that have thus far only been presented at conferences (Kaufman et al., 2013b; Abdool-Karim et al., 2015).

The evidence suggests that the timing of educational interventions is critical, potentially having a larger impact when intervening early to keep young people in school (Bruce, 2015). Overall, there appear to be few differences between conditional and unconditional social protection schemes, although there is a suggestion from one trial that conditional transfers may be more important for older youth from less impoverished households and have a more marked impact on educational attainment. A previous meta-analysis suggested that it is the intensity of the stipulations and monitoring of the conditionality rather than the conditionality itself that has the largest effect on school attendance (Baird et al., 2013). The relative benefit of conditional versus unconditional transfers, weighed against the complexity of large-scale implementation, is an important issue for ongoing debate. Stepping Stones and Creating Futures was the only GBV intervention to include an economic empowerment component, and resulted in positive impacts on social norms, IPV and poverty. There is increasing interest in combined gender and economic empowerment approaches.

From the available evidence, there were few differences for young women and men in terms of both education and poverty alleviation. Only two educational interventions among non-OVC youth included both young women and men, one of which suggested that the impact of unconditional grants was more pronounced for young women. However, the gender inequality interventions appear to have a more pronounced effect among young women, and potentially require a broader and more intensive engagement at a societal level to achieve a shift in gender norms and violence as seen in SASA! The need to engage both women and men across the generations to shift gendered perceptions remains a priority, as this also impacts on young women's access to education and economic opportunity. Certainly, a previous review of studies to prevent violence against women found greatest promise from studies that included group training for women and men, community mobilization, and combining livelihood and training interventions for women (Ellsberg et al., 2015).

There are cross-over benefits of structural interventions among youth, with two of the education interventions demonstrating positive impacts on socio-economic outcomes, one on IPV, and two on social norms; two poverty interventions impacting on educational outcomes and one on GBV and social norms; and one GBV intervention impacting on poverty (Figure 7.5). Given that singular structural drivers, such as poverty, influence the causal pathway to HIV through multiple routes, combining interventions to tackle multiple influencers of risk is vital. However, there are financial challenges to implementing multi-sectoral interventions. Zomba was the only structural intervention in this review to reduce HIV risk for young women, yet it was unlikely to be cost-effective from an HIV perspective (Baird et al., 2012). Indeed, a cost-effectiveness assessment showed that if each sector (education and health) adopted a siloed approach and assessed the value of the intervention in its sectoral silo, the intervention would not have been funded (Remme et al., 2014). By contrast, if sectors pooled their resources through a co-financing mechanism to jointly achieve their outcomes, they would be able to cover the full cost of the intervention and even spend less for the same outcomes than they would have each spent in their own sectors (Remme et al., 2012; Remme and McGuire, 2018). A pilot study in sub-Saharan Africa is currently assessing the practicalities of operationalizing the co-financing approach in governmental planning and budgeting (Vassall, 2018).

A few of the interventions suggest the importance of assessing the impact at multiple time points, ensuring sufficient time for the upstream changes to take effect, and assessing the duration of the impact. This has been highlighted in other GBV interventions as well (Wagman et al., 2015). We did not extract details on the duration of intervention or time points of evaluation from the papers reviewed. Building a body of evidence on the optimal intensity and duration for effect and timelines for evaluation will be useful going forward.

The measure of proximal risk factors and HIV infection were not inclusion criteria for this review. The self-reported nature of sexual behaviour data makes it sensitive to social desirability bias, but it still provides a useful indicator of risk behaviour change (Krumpal, 2013). Eleven out of 12 education and poverty interventions that measured sexual behaviour outcomes reported some positive effects. Of the five gender inequality interventions, only one had a positive impact on sexual behaviour. However, the two social norm interventions that did not impact on norms did impact on sexual behaviour, suggesting additional mechanisms of effect. The sexual behaviour results were not consistent, with some showing impact on measures such as sexual debut, transactional sex and condomless sex, but others not, and with differences by gender. The HPTN068 trial results highlight the point that cash transfers have the potential to function through multiple routes; despite having no impact on education, the intervention still resulted in positive impacts on sexual behaviour outcomes. Only three interventions assessed early marriage as an outcome, with split results. The measure of early marriage is important, as it can be a trigger for school dropout, limit young women's ability to negotiate safer sex or indicate forced child marriage, which is a risk factor for partner violence (Lloyd and Mensch, 2008; Durevall and Lindskog, 2015a).

Six of the seven educational and poverty interventions that measured clinical outcomes showed a positive effect predominantly in terms of pregnancy, while two of the gender inequality interventions showed clinical impacts on HSV-2 and ever being pregnant. Only one trial, Zomba, demonstrated a positive impact on HIV as well as HSV-2, with no impact in the other three interventions that measured HIV. Overall, there was stronger evidence for sexual behaviour and clinical impact among young women than among men. This may well reflect the differential risk for young women and men in this age group and the differential reporting bias on sexual behaviour due to social desirability (Krumpal, 2013). Although all the evidence suggests that keeping young girls in school, alleviating poverty and addressing gender inequalities will help mitigate the risk of acquiring HIV, a key challenge is establishing whether these interventions have an effect on HIV incidence. Limited evidence on the direct impact on HIV incidence is a major challenge to financing and scaling up such interventions. We need to find better ways to estimate impact over the longer term.

We conducted a comprehensive and expansive review of structural interventions among young people in ESA designed to intervene on the causal pathways to HIV infection. However, in summarizing this evidence we need to consider a number of limitations of the review. The majority of the structural interventions designed to address school attendance and poverty focused on OVC. We aimed to identify structural interventions with educational and socio-economic outcomes but which were designed to intervene on the pathway to HIV. It is possible that this search strategy emphasized the identification of interventions with OVC from households affected by HIV and failed to identify other educational and socio-economic structural interventions that may also have been relevant. There were surprisingly few interventions among young people addressing gender inequalities and, although expert review by authors supports the findings, there is a chance that their absence is a manifestation of our search strategy, especially our reliance only on the published literature. It is also noteworthy that the studies included in the review were all concentrated in only seven countries in ESA: Kenya, Malawi, South Africa, Tanzania, Uganda, Zambia and Zimbabwe. From experience, we know that the majority of HIV prevention research is taking place in these countries, although it is also likely that our focus on English language literature restricted evidence from other countries in the region.

Recommendations and next steps

A growing body of evidence points to the benefits of structural interventions to improve livelihood and gender equality for young people in ESA. To build on this evidence base, it will be useful to have consistent and multi-sectoral measures of effect. School attendance is a clear outcome measure, but it would be helpful to also assess a broader range of educational achievement and socio-economic indices consistently. Measures for IPV are now well defined, but there is a need for reliable tools to measure social norm change. Similarly, using consistent measures of proximal determinants would aid comparison. Recent clarifications have been made to the definition and validation of measurement tools for transactional sex (Stoebenau et al., 2016; Wamoyi et al., 2016; Wamoyi et al., 2017; UNAIDS/STRIVE, 2018). Looking forward, we have to consider the best way to capture measures of 'protected' versus 'unprotected' sex beyond just condom use, as the availability of oral pre-exposure prophylaxis increases and the benefits of universal test and treat and VMMC are realized. In the context of expanded prevention options, it is also critical to pay attention to structural drivers that serve as barriers to prevention services, such as stigma restricting access to comprehensive sexual and reproductive health services for young people (Krishnaratne et al., 2016; Stangl, in press; Stangl et al., 2017; Stangl and Sievwright, 2016; Stangl et al., 2013; Delany-Moretlwe, 2018). The challenges of measuring an impact on HIV incidence within short time frames are clear; it would therefore be useful to collect other indices of exposure including pregnancy, HSV-2 and other relevant sexually transmitted infections (STIs) such as syphilis and chlamydia (Pinkerton et al., 2002).

While the evidence base for structural interventions is strong, the pathways of impact are not consistent. Few papers included the theory of change that underpinned the design of the intervention. It would be useful to define clearly the underlying theory of change in each intervention in order to evaluate the mechanisms of effect for individual and combined interventional components. Similarly, definitions and comparisons of intervention duration, time to impact and measures of maintenance of impact would all enhance our understanding of the value, cost-effectiveness and scalability of interventions. Differences in age groups should also be investigated (Kinghorn et al., 2018). This is as true of educational interventions, where the age of intervention appears to be important, as it is for IPV interventions that tend to enrol predominantly adult cohorts. All interventions should ensure sufficient statistical power to stratify results by gender. A further noteworthy challenge of structural interventions with adolescents is the need for parental consent to participate, and the potential for the most vulnerable young people to be excluded from either the intervention or the evaluation process, because they cannot gain parental consent, thereby impacting the generalizability of the findings.

The evaluation of interventions in a more diverse set of countries would further contribute to our understanding of the contextual sensitivities of some of these interventions. Evidence on livelihood interventions, particularly in East Africa, derives substantially from OVC households; applying lessons from OVC interventions to other vulnerable groups of young people, including out-of-school youth and young married women, could yield additional valuable evidence. Evaluations of government social protection programmes were particularly valuable in this review. As governments in sub-Saharan Africa expand social protection programming, there is the potential to evaluate the impact on structural drivers of HIV and on HIV infection among young people.

Finally, the most important challenge for the future is to move evidence into practice. Improving educational attainment, reducing poverty, challenging restricting and harmful gender norms and mitigating the risk of gender-based violence are important steps to interrupt the causal pathway towards HIV infection. The evidence supports a multi-sectoral approach for multiple outcomes. Such approaches need to be integrated into HIV prevention, gender empowerment and broader development initiatives in line with the SDG priorities. To achieve this, we need further evidence on the best mechanisms to achieve scale, integration into existing programmes and sustained effectiveness. We also need more information on the implementation of cross-sectoral co-financing as an innovative strategy to support upstream interventions that yield multiple benefits, thus increasing efficiency in the allocation of government, donor and other budget holders' resources. The priority must be the implementation of high-impact interventions that can achieve multiple health and social impacts for young people in the process of mitigating the risk of HIV and achieving cost-efficiencies across the interconnected SDGs.

References

Abdool-Karim, Q., Leask, K., Kharsany, A., Humphries, H., Ntombela, F., Samsunder, N., Baxter, C., Frohlich, J., Van Der Elst, L. & Abdool-Karim, S. 2015. Impact of conditional cash incentives on HSV-2 and HIV prevention in rural South African high school students: Results of the CAPRISA 007 cluster randomized controlled trial. *Journal of the International AIDS Society*, 18.

Abramsky, T., Devries, K., Kiss, L., Nakuti, J., Kyegombe, N., Starmann, E., Cundill, B., Francisco, L., Kaye, D., Musuya, T., Michau, L. & Watts, C. 2014. Findings from the SASA! Study: A cluster randomized controlled trial to assess the impact of a community mobilization intervention to prevent violence against women and reduce HIV risk in Kampala, Uganda. *BMC Medicine*, 12, 122.

Baird, S.J., Ferreira, H.G., Özler, B. & Woolcock, M. 2013. Relative effectiveness of conditional and unconditional cash transfers for schooling outcomes in developing countries: A systematic review. *Campbell Systematic Reviews*, 8.

Baird, S.J., Garfein, R.S., Mcintosh, C.T. & Özler, B. 2012. Effect of a cash transfer programme for schooling on prevalence of HIV and herpes simplex type 2 in Malawi: A cluster randomised trial. *Lancet*, 379, 1320–1329.

Bandiera, O., Buehren, N., Burgess, R., Goldstein, M., Gulesci, S., Rasul, I. & Sulaiman, M. 2012. *Empowering adolescent girls: Evidence from a randomized control trial in Uganda*. Semantics Scholar. [Online] Available: http://econ.lse.ac.uk/staff/rburgess/wp/ELA.pdf

Barnighausen, T., Hosegood, V., Timaeus, I.M. & Newell, M.L. 2007. The socioeconomic determinants of HIV incidence: Evidence from a longitudinal, population-based study in rural South Africa. *AIDS*, 21 Suppl 7, S29–S38.

Blankenship, K.M., Bray, S.J. & Merson, M.H. 2000. Structural interventions in public health. *AIDS*, 14 Suppl 1, S11–S21.

Bruce, J. 2015. Commentary: Investing in the poorest girls in the poorest communities early enough to make a difference. *Global Public Health*, 10, 225–227.

Buller, A.M., Peterman, A., Ranganathan, M., Bleile, A., Hidrobo, M. & Heise, L. 2018. *A mixed-method review of cash transfers and intimate partner violence in low and middle-income countries*. London: STRIVE, London School of Hygiene and Tropical Medicine.

Chatterji, M., Hutchinson, P., Buek, K., Murray, N., Mulenga, Y. & Ventimiglia, T. 2010. Evaluating the impact of community-based interventions on schooling outcomes among orphans and vulnerable children in Lusaka, Zambia. *Vulnerable Children and Youth Studies*, 5, 130–141.

Cho, H., Hallfors, D.D., Mbai, II, Itindi, J., Milimo, B.W., Halpern, C.T. & Iritani, B.J. 2011. Keeping adolescent orphans in school to prevent human immunodeficiency virus infection: Evidence from a randomized controlled trial in Kenya. *Journal of Adolescent Health*, 48, 523–526.

Cho, H., Mbai, I., Luseno, W.K., Hobbs, M., Halpern, C. & Hallfors, D.D. 2018. School support as structural HIV prevention for adolescent orphans in Western Kenya. *Journal of Adolescent Health*, 62, 44–51.

Cho, H., Ryberg, R.C., Hwang, K., Pearce, L.D. & Iritani, B.J. 2017. A school support intervention and educational outcomes among orphaned adolescents: Results of a cluster randomized controlled trial in Kenya. *Prevention Science*, 18, 943–954.

Cislaghi, B. & Heise, L. 2016. *Measuring gender-related social norms, learning report 1. Learning group on social norms and gender-related harmful practices*. London: STRIVE, London School of Hygiene and Tropical Medicine.

Cislaghi, B., Heise, L., 2017. *STRIVE technical brief: Measuring social norms*. London: STRIVE, London School of Hygiene and Tropical Medicine.

Cislaghi, B., Manji, K. & Heise, L. 2018. *Social norms and gender-related harmful practices. Learning report 2: Theory in support of better practice*. Learning Group on Social Norms and Gender- related Harmful Practices. London: STRIVE, London School of Hygiene and Tropical Medicine.

Cluver, L.D., Boyes, M., Orkin, M., Pantelic, M., Molwena, T. & Sherr, L. 2013. Child-focused state cash transfers and adolescent risk of HIV infection in South Africa: A propensity-score-matched case-control study. *Lancet Global Health*, 1, e362–e370.

Cluver, L.D., Orkin, F.M., Yakubovich, A.R. & Sherr, L. 2016. Combination social protection for reducing HIV-risk behavior among adolescents in South Africa. *Journal of Acquired Immune Deficiency Syndromes: JAIDS*, 72, 96–104.

Cowan, F.M., Pascoe, S.J., Langhaug, L.F., Mavhu, W., Chidiya, S., Jaffar, S., Mbizvo, M.T., Stephenson, J.M., Johnson, A.M., Power, R.M., Woelk, G., Hayes, R.J. & Regai Dzive Shiri Trial, T. 2010. The Regai Dzive Shiri project: Results of a randomized trial of an HIV prevention intervention for youth. *AIDS*, 24, 2541–2552.

Curley, J., Ssewamala, F. & Han, C.K. 2010. Assets and educational outcomes: Child development accounts (CDAs) for orphaned children in Uganda. *Children and Youth Services Review*, 32, 1585–1590.

De Koker, P., Mathews, C., Zuch, M., Bastien, S. & Mason-Jones, A.J. 2014. A systematic review of interventions for preventing adolescent intimate partner violence. *Journal of Adolescent Health*, 54, 3–13.

De Neve, J.W., Fink, G., Subramanian, S.V., Moyo, S. & Bor, J. 2015. Length of secondary schooling and risk of HIV infection in Botswana: Evidence from a natural experiment. *Lancet Global Health*, 3, e470–e477.

De Oliveira, T., Kharsany, A., Gräf, T., Cawood, C., Khanyile, D., Grobler, A., Puren, A., Madurai, S., Baxter, C., Karim, Q. & Karim, S. 2017. Transmission networks and risk of HIV infection in KwaZulu-Natal, South Africa: A community-wide phylogenetic study. *Lancet HIV*, 4, e41–e50.

Decker, M.R., Seage, G.R., 3rd, Hemenway, D., Raj, A., Saggurti, N., Balaiah, D. & Silverman, J.G. 2009. Intimate partner violence functions as both a risk marker and risk factor for women's HIV infection: Findings from Indian husband-wife dyads. *Journal of Acquired Immune Deficiency Syndrome*, 51, 593–600.

Delany-Moretlwe, S., Hargreaves, J., Stangl, A., Gafos, M. 2018. *STRIVE technical brief: Biomedical and structural prevention: STRIVE in the era of 'cascades'*. London: STRIVE, London School of Hygiene and Tropical Medicine.

Delva, W., Michielsen, K., Meulders, B., Groeninck, S., Wasonga, E., Ajwang, P., Temmerman, M. & Vanreusel, B. 2010. HIV prevention through sport: The case of the Mathare Youth Sport Association in Kenya. *Aids Care-Psychological and Socio-Medical Aspects of AIDS/HIV*, 22, 1012–1020.

Dunbar, M.S., Kang Dufour, M.S., Lambdin, B., Mudekunye-Mahaka, I., Nhamo, D. & Padian, N.S. 2014. The SHAZ! project: Results from a pilot randomized trial of a structural intervention to prevent HIV among adolescent women in Zimbabwe. *PLoS One [Electronic Resource]*, 9, e113621.

Dunkle, K.L. & Decker, M.R. 2013. Gender-based violence and HIV: Reviewing the evidence for links and causal pathways in the general population and high-risk groups. *American Journal of Reproductive Immunology*, 69 Suppl 1, 20–26.

Dunkle, K.L., Jewkes, R.K., Nduna, M., Levin, J., Jama, N., Khuzwayo, N., Koss, M.P. & Duvvury, N. 2006. Perpetration of partner violence and HIV risk behaviour among young men in the rural Eastern Cape, South Africa. *AIDS*, 20, 2107–2114.

Durevall, D. & Lindskog, A. 2015a. Intimate partner violence and HIV in ten sub-Saharan African countries: What do the demographic and health surveys tell us? *Lancet Global Health*, 3, e34–e43.

Durevall, D. & Lindskog, A. 2015b. Intimate partner violence and HIV infection in sub-Saharan Africa. *World Development*, 72, 27–42.

Dworkin, S.L., Treves-Kagan, S. & Lippman, S.A. 2013. Gender-transformative interventions to reduce HIV risks and violence with heterosexually-active men: A review of the global evidence. *AIDS and Behavior*, 17, 2845–2863.

Ellsberg, M., Arango, D.J., Morton, M., Gennari, F., Kiplesund, S., Contreras, M. & Watts, C. 2015. Prevention of violence against women and girls: What does the evidence say? *Lancet*, 385, 1555–1566.

Fenton, R., Nyamukapa, C., Gregson, S., Robertson, L., Mushati, P., Thomas, R. & Eaton, J.W. 2016. Wealth differentials in the impact of conditional and unconditional cash transfers on education: Findings from a community-randomised controlled trial in Zimbabwe. *Psychology, Health & Medicine*, 21, 909–917.

Fox, A.M. 2010. The social determinants of HIV serostatus in sub-Saharan Africa: An inverse relationship between poverty and HIV? *Public Health Reports*, 125 Suppl 4, 16–24.

Fritz, K. & Heise, L. 2018. *STRIVE technical brief: A moment of convergence: STRIVE and the sustainable development goals*. London: STRIVE, London School of Hygiene and Tropical Medicine.

Gass, J.D., Stein, D.J., Williams, D.R. & Seedat, S. 2011. Gender differences in risk for intimate partner violence among South African adults. *Journal of Interpersonal Violence*, 26, 2764–2789.

Gibbs, A., Jacobson, J. & Kerr Wilson, A. 2017. A global comprehensive review of economic interventions to prevent intimate partner violence and HIV risk behaviours. *Global Health Action*, 10, 1290427.

Gibbs, A., Willan, S., Misselhorn, A. & Mangoma, J. 2012. Combined structural interventions for gender equality and livelihood security: A critical review of the evidence from southern and eastern Africa and the implications for young people. *Journal of the International Aids Society*, 15.

Gillespie, S., Kadiyala, S. & Greener, R. 2007. Is poverty or wealth driving HIV transmission? *AIDS*, 21 Suppl 7, S5–S16.

Goodman, M.L., Kaberia, R., Morgan, R.O. & Keiser, P.H. 2014. Health and livelihood outcomes associated with participation in a community-based empowerment program for orphan families in semirural Kenya: A cross-sectional study. *Vulnerable Children and Youth Studies*, 9, 365–376.

Gupta, G.R., Parkhurst, J.O., Ogden, J.A., Aggleton, P. & Mahal, A. 2008. Structural approaches to HIV prevention. *Lancet*, 372, 764–775.

Hallfors, D., Cho, H., Mbai, I., Milimo, B. & Itindi, J. 2012. Process and outcome evaluation of a community intervention for orphan adolescents in western Kenya. *Journal of Community Health*, 37, 1101–1109.

Hallfors, D., Cho, H., Rusakaniko, S., Iritani, B., Mapfumo, J. & Halpern, C. 2011. Supporting adolescent orphan girls to stay in school as HIV risk prevention: Evidence from a randomized controlled trial in Zimbabwe. *American Journal of Public Health*, 101, 1082–1088.

Hallfors, D., Cho, H., Rusakaniko, S., Mapfumo, J., Iritani, B., Zhang, L., Luseno, W. & Miller, T. 2015. The impact of school subsidies on HIV-related outcomes among adolescent female orphans. *Journal of Adolescent Health*, 56, 79–84.

Hallman, K. 2005a. The effects of orphaning and poverty on sexual debut in KwaZulu-Natal, South Arica. *IUSSP Seminar on "Poverty and HIV/ AIDS"*. Cape Town, South Africa: University of Cape Town.

Hallman, K. 2005b. Gendered socioeconomic conditions and HIV risk behaviours among young people in South Africa. *African Journal of AIDS Research*, 4, 37–50.

Handa, S., Halpern, C.T., Pettifor, A. & Thirumurthy, H. 2014. The government of Kenya's cash transfer program reduces the risk of sexual debut among young people age 15–25. *PLoS One [Electronic Resource]*, 9, e85473.

Handa, S., Peterman, A., Huang, C., Halpern, C., Pettifor, A. & Thirumurthy, H. 2015. Impact of the Kenya cash transfer for orphans and vulnerable children on early pregnancy and marriage of adolescent girls. *Social Science & Medicine*, 141, 36–45.

Hankins, C.A. & De Zalduondo, B.O. 2010. Combination prevention: A deeper understanding of effective HIV prevention. *AIDS*, 24 Suppl 4, S70–S80.

Hardee, K., Gay, J., Croce-Galis, M. & Peltz, A. 2014. Strengthening the enabling environment for women and girls: What is the evidence in social and structural approaches in the HIV response? *Journal of the International AIDS Society*, 17, 18619.

Hargreaves, J.R. 2002. Socioeconomic status and risk of HIV infection in an urban population in Kenya. *Tropical Medicine & International Health*, 7, 793–802.

Hargreaves, J.R., Bonell, C.P., Boler, T., Boccia, D., Birdthistle, I., Fletcher, A., Pronyk, P.M. & Glynn, J.R. 2008. Systematic review exploring time trends in the association between educational attainment and risk of HIV infection in sub-Saharan Africa. *AIDS*, 22, 403–414.

Hargreaves, J.R. & Glynn, J.R. 2002. Educational attainment and HIV-1 infection in developing countries: A systematic review. *Tropical Medicine & International Health*, 7, 489–498.

Harrison, A., O'Sullivan, L.F., Hoffman, S., Dolezal, C. & Morrell, R. 2006. Gender role and relationship norms among young adults in South Africa: Measuring the context of masculinity and HIV risk. *Journal of Urban Health*, 83, 709–722.

Heise, L. & Hossain, M. 2017. *STRIVE technical brief: Measuring intimate partner violence.* London: STRIVE, London School of Hygiene and Tropical Medicine.

Heise, L., Lutz, B., Ranganathan, M. & Watts, C. 2013. Cash transfers for HIV prevention: Considering their potential. *Journal of the International Aids Society*, 16.

Heise, L. & McGrory, E. 2016. *Violence against women and girls and HIV: Report on a high level consultation on the evidence and its implications, 12–14 May, 2015.* Greentree Estate. London: STRIVE Research Consortium.

Iritani, B.J., Cho, H., Rusakaniko, S., Mapfumo, J., Hartman, S. & Hallfors, D.D. 2016. Educational outcomes for orphan girls in rural Zimbabwe: Effects of a school support intervention. *Health Care for Women International*, 37, 301–322.

Ismayilova, L., Ssewamala, F.M. & Karimli, L. 2012. Family support as a mediator of change in sexual risk-taking attitudes among orphaned adolescents in rural Uganda. *Journal of Adolescent Health*, 50, 228–235.

Jennings, L., Ssewamala, F.M. & Nabunya, P. 2016. Effect of savings-led economic empowerment on HIV preventive practices among orphaned adolescents in rural Uganda: Results from the Suubi-Maka randomized experiment. *AIDS Care*, 28, 273–282.

Jewkes, R., Dunkle, K., Nduna, M. & Shai, N. 2010. Intimate partner violence, relationship power inequity, and incidence of HIV infection in young women in South Africa: A cohort study. *Lancet*, 376, 41–48.

Jewkes, R., Flood, M. & Lang, J. 2015. From work with men and boys to changes of social norms and reduction of inequities in gender relations: A conceptual shift in prevention of violence against women and girls. *Lancet*, 385, 1580–1589.

Jewkes, R., Gibbs, A., Jama-Shai, N., Willan, S., Misselhorn, A., Mushinga, M., Washington, L., Mbatha, N. & Sikweyiya, Y. 2014. Stepping Stones and Creating Futures intervention: Shortened interrupted time series evaluation of a behavioural and structural health promotion and violence prevention intervention for young people in informal settlements in Durban, South Africa. *BMC Public Health*, 14.

Jewkes, R., Nduna, M., Levin, J., Jama, N., Dunkle, K., Puren, A. & Duvvury, N. 2008. Impact of stepping stones on incidence of HIV and HSV-2 and sexual behaviour in rural South Africa: Cluster randomised controlled trial. *British Medical Journal*, 337, a506.

Jewkes, R., Sikweyiya, Y., Morrell, R. & Dunkle, K. 2011. The relationship between intimate partner violence, rape and HIV amongst South African men: A cross-sectional study. *PLoS One*, 6, e24256.

Jukes, M., Simmons, S. & Bundy, D. 2008a. Education and vulnerability: The role of schools in protecting young women and girls from HIV in southern Africa. *AIDS*, 22 Suppl 4, S41–S56.

Jukes, M., Simmons, S. & Bundy, D. 2008b. Education and vulnerability: The role of schools in protecting young women and girls from HIV in southern Africa (Vulnerability of young women and girls to HIV infection in the hyperendemic countries of southern Africa.). *AIDS*, 22, S41–S56.

Kacanek, D., Bostrom, A., Montgomery, E. T., Ramjee, G., De Bruyn, G., Blanchard, K., Rock, A., Mtetwa, S., Van Der Straten, A. & Team, M. 2013. Intimate partner violence and condom and diaphragm nonadherence among women in an HIV prevention trial in southern Africa. *Journal of Acquired Immune Deficiency Syndrome*, 64, 400–408.

Kaufman, M. R., Mooney, A., Kamala, B., Modarres, N., Karam, R. & Ng'wanansabi, D. 2013a. Effects of the Fataki campaign: Addressing cross-generational sex in Tanzania by mobilizing communities to intervene. *AIDS Behaviour*, 17, 2053–2062.

Kaufman, Z. A., E B Kaufman, E. B., Dringus, S., Weiss, H. A., Delany-Moretlwe, S. & Ross, D. A. 2013b. Baseline results: Of a cluster-randomised trial assessing the effectiveness of sport-based HIV prevention in South African schools. *Sexually Transmitted Infections*, 89, A1–A428.

Kennedy, C. E., Fonner, V. A., O'Reilly, K. R. & Sweat, M. D. 2014. A systematic review of income generation interventions, including microfinance and vocational skills training, for HIV prevention. *AIDS Care*, 26, 659–673.

Kinghorn, A., Shanaube, K., Toska, E., Cluver, C. & Bekker, L. 2018. Defining adolescence: Priorities from a global health perspective. *Lancet: Child and Adolescent Health*, 2(5), e10.

Kippax, S. 2008. Understanding and integrating the structural and biomedical determinants of HIV infection: A way forward for prevention. *Current Opinion in HIV & AIDS*, 3, 489–494.

Krishnaratne, S., Hensen, B., Cordes, J., Enstone, J. & Hargreaves, J. R. 2016. Interventions to strengthen the HIV prevention cascade: A systematic review of reviews. *Lancet HIV*, 3, e307–e317.

Krumpal, I. 2013. Determinants of social desirability bias in sensitive surveys: A literature review. *Quality & Quantity*, 47.

Lloyd, C. B. & Mensch, B. S. 2008. Marriage and childbirth as factors in dropping out from school: An analysis of DHS data from sub-Saharan Africa. *Population Studies (Camb)*, 62, 1–13.

Lorenzetti, L. M. J., Leatherman, S. & Flax, V. L. 2017. Evaluating the effect of integrated microfinance and health interventions: An updated review of the evidence. *Health Policy and Planning*, 32, 732–756.

Luke, N. 2003. Age and economic asymmetries in the sexual relationships of adolescent girls in sub-Saharan Africa. *Studies in Family Planning*, 34, 67–86.

Luke, N. 2005. Confronting the 'sugar daddy' stereotype: Age and economic asymmetries and risky sexual behavior in urban Kenya. *International Family Planning Perspective*, 31, 6–14.

Lundgren, R. & Amin, A. 2015. Addressing intimate partner violence and sexual violence among adolescents: Emerging evidence of effectiveness. *Journal of Adolescent Health*, 56, S42–S50.

Maman, S., Campbell, J., Sweat, M. D. & Gielen, A. C. 2000. The intersections of HIV and violence: Directions for future research and interventions. *Social Science & Medicine*, 50, 459–78.

Mason-Jones, A. J., Sinclair, D., Mathews, C., Kagee, A., Hillman, A. & Lombard, C. 2016. School-based interventions for preventing HIV, sexually transmitted infections, and pregnancy in adolescents. *Cochrane Database of Systematic Reviews*, 11, CD006417.

Mathews, C., Eggers, S., Townsend, L., Aarø, L., Vries, P., Mason-Jones, A., Koker, P., McClinton Appollis, T., Mtshizana, Y., Koech, J., Wubs, A. & Vries, H. 2016. Effects of prepare, a multi-component, school-based HIV and intimate partner violence (IPV) prevention programme on adolescent sexual risk behaviour and IPV: Cluster randomised controlled trial. *AIDS & Behavior*, 20, 1821–1840.

McCloskey, L. A., Boonzaier, F., Steinbrenner, S. Y. & Hunter, T. 2016. Determinants of intimate partner violence in sub-Saharan Africa: A review of prevention and intervention programs. *Partner Abuse*, 7, 277–315.

Mishra, V., Assche, S. B., Greener, R., Vaessen, M., Hong, R., Ghys, P. D., Boerma, J. T., Van Assche, A., Khan, S. & Rutstein, S. 2007. HIV infection does not disproportionately affect the poorer in sub-Saharan Africa. *AIDS*, 21 Suppl 7, S17–S28.

Parcesepe, A. M., Engle, K. L. L., Martin, S. L., Green, S., Sinkele, W., Suchindran, C., Speizer, I. S., Mwarogo, P. & Kingola, N. 2016. The impact of an alcohol harm reduction intervention on interpersonal violence and engagement in sex work among female sex workers in Mombasa, Kenya: Results from a randomized controlled trial. *Drug & Alcohol Dependence*, 161, 21–28.

Parkhurst, J. O. 2010. Understanding the correlations between wealth, poverty and human immunodeficiency virus infection in African countries. *Bulletin of the World Health Organization*, 88, 519–526.

Parkhurst, J. O. 2013. Structural drivers, interventions, and approaches for prevention of sexually transmitted HIV in general populations: Definitions and an operational approach. *Structural Approaches to HIV Prevention Position Paper Series.* London: STRIVE, London School of Hygiene and Tropical Medicine.

Patton, G. C., Sawyer, S. M., Santelli, J. S., Ross, D. A., Afifi, R., Allen, N. B., Arora, M., Azzopardi, P., Baldwin, W., Bonell, C., Kakuma, R., Kennedy, E., Mahon, J., McGovern, T., Mokdad, A. H., Patel, V., Petroni, S., Reavley, N., Taiwo, K., Waldfogel, J., Wickremarathne, D., Barroso, C., Bhutta, Z., Fatusi, A. O., Mattoo, A., Diers, J., Fang, J., Ferguson, J., Ssewamala, F. & Viner, R. M. 2016. Our future: A *Lancet* commission on adolescent health and wellbeing. *Lancet*, 387, 2423–2478.

Pega, F., Liu, S. Y., Walter, S., Pabayo, R., Saith, R. & Lhachimi, S. K. 2017. Unconditional cash transfers for reducing poverty and vulnerabilities: Effect on use of health services and health outcomes in low- and middle-income countries. *Cochrane Database of Systematic Reviews*, (11), Art. No.: CD011135.

Pettifor, A., Levandowski, B. A., Macphail, C., Padian, N. S., Cohen, M. S. & Rees, H. V. 2008. Keep them in school: The importance of education as a protective factor against HIV infection among young South African women. *International Journal of Epidemiology*, 37, 1266–1273.

Pettifor, A., Macphail, C., Hughes, J. P., Selin, A., Wang, J., Gomez-Olive, F. X., Eshleman, S. H., Wagner, R. G., Mabuza, W., Khoza, N., Suchindran, C., Mokoena, I., Twine, R., Andrew, P., Townley, E., Laeyendecker, O., Agyei, Y., Tollman, S. &

Kahn, K. 2016. The effect of a conditional cash transfer on HIV incidence in young women in rural South Africa (HPTN 068): A phase 3, randomised controlled trial. *Lancet Global Health*, 4, e978–e988.

Pinkerton, S. D., Layde, P. M. & NIMH Multisite HIV Prevention Trial Group. 2002. Using sexually transmitted disease incidence as a surrogate marker for HIV incidence in prevention trials: A modeling study. *Sexually Transmitted Diseases*, 29, 298–307.

Pronyk, P. M., Hargreaves, J. R., Kim, J. C., Morison, L. A., Phetla, G., Watts, C., Busza, J. & Porter, J. D. 2006. Effect of a structural intervention for the prevention of intimate-partner violence and HIV in rural South Africa: A cluster randomised trial. *Lancet*, 368, 1973–1983.

Prudden, H. 2017. *Incorporating structural interventions in country HIV programme planning and resource allocation: Report from an expert consultation convened by STRIVE and the HIV modelling consortium with support from the global fund to fight AIDS, Tuberculosis and Malaria.* London: STRIVE, London School of Hygiene and Tropical Medicine.

Remme, M. & McGuire, F. 2018. *STRIVE technical brief: Development synergies and co-financing.* London: STRIVE, London School of Hygiene and Tropical Medicine.

Remme, M., Vassall, A., Lutz, B., Luna, J. & Watts, C. 2014. Financing structural interventions: Going beyond HIV-only value for money assessments. *AIDS*, 28, 425–434.

Remme, M., Vassall, A., Lutz, B. & Watts, C. 2012. Paying girls to stay in school: A good return on HIV investment? *Lancet*, 379, 2150.

Robertson, L., Mushati, P., Eaton, J. W., Dumba, L., Mavise, G., Makoni, J., Schumacher, C., Crea, T., Monasch, R., Sherr, L., Garnett, G. P., Nyamukapa, C. & Gregson, S. 2013. Effects of unconditional and conditional cash transfers on child health and development in Zimbabwe: A cluster-randomised trial. *Lancet*, 381, 1283–1292.

Rotheram-Borus, M. J., Lightfoot, M., Kasirye, R. & Desmond, K. 2012. Vocational training with HIV prevention for Ugandan youth. *AIDS & Behavior*, 16, 1133–1137.

Sarnquist, C., Omondi, B., Sinclair, J., Gitau, C., Paiva, L., Mulinge, M., Cornfield, D. N. & Maldonado, Y. 2014. Rape prevention through empowerment of adolescent girls. *Pediatrics*, 133, e1226–e1232.

Seeley, J., Watts, C. H., Kippax, S., Russell, S., Heise, L. & Whiteside, A. 2012. Addressing the structural drivers of HIV: A luxury or necessity for programmes? *Journal of International AIDS Society*, 15 Suppl 1, 1–4.

Shai, N. J. & Sikweyiya, Y. 2015. Programmes for change addressing sexual and intimate partner violence in South Africa. *South African Crime Quarterly*, 31–41.

Sherr, L., Tomlinson, M., Macedo, A., Skeen, S., Hensels, I. S. & Cluver, L. D. 2017. Can cash break the cycle of educational risks for young children in high HIV-affected communities? A cross-sectional study in South Africa and Malawi. *Journal of Global Health*, 7.

Ssewamala, F. M., Han, C. K. & Neilands, T. B. 2009. Asset ownership and health and mental health functioning among AIDS-orphaned adolescents: Findings from a randomized clinical trial in rural Uganda. *Social Science & Medicine*, 69, 191–198.

Ssewamala, F. M., Karimli, L., Torsten, N., Wang, J. S., Han, C. K., Ilic, V. & Nabunya, P. 2016. Applying a family-level economic strengthening intervention to improve education and health-related outcomes of school-going AIDS-orphaned children: Lessons from a randomized experiment in Southern Uganda. *Prevention Science*, 17, 134–143.

Ssewamala, F. M., Han, C. K., Neilands, T. B., Ismayilova, L. & Sperber, E. 2010a. Effect of economic assets on sexual risk-taking intentions among orphaned adolescents in Uganda. *American Journal of Public Health*, 100(3), 483–488. doi:10.2105/AJPH.2008.158840

Ssewamala, F. M., Ismayilova, L., McKay, M., Sperber, E., Bannon, W. Jr. & Alicea, S. 2010b. Gender and the effects of an economic empowerment program on attitudes toward sexual risk-taking among AIDS-orphaned adolescent youth in Uganda. *Journal of Adolescent Health*, 46(4), 372–378.

Ssewamala, F.M., Neilands, T.B., Waldfogel, J. & Ismayilova, L. 2012. The impact of a comprehensive microfinance intervention on depression levels of AIDS-orphaned children in Uganda. *Journal of Adolescent Health*, 50, 346–352.

Stangl, A., Brady, L. & Fritz, K. 2017. *STRIVE technical brief: Measuring HIV stigma and discrimination*. Washington, DC: International Center for Research on Women.

Stangl, A., Lloyd, J.K., Brady, L.M., Holland, C.E. & Baral, S. 2013. A systematic review of interventions to reduce HIV-related stigma and discrimination from 2002 to 2013: How far have we come? *Journal of International AIDS Society*, 16, 18734.

Stangl, A. & Sievwright, K. 2016. HIV-related stigma and children. *In:* Chenneville, T. (ed.) *A clinical guide to pediatric HIV: Bridging the gaps between research and practice*. New York: Springer.

Stangl, A., Singh, D., Windle, M., Sievwright, K., Footer, K., Iovita, A., Mukasa, S., Baral, S. in press. A systematic review of human rights programs to improve HIV-related outcomes from 2003 to 2015: What do we know? *BMC Infectious Diseases*.

Stoebenau, K., Heise, L., Wamoyi, J. & Bobrova, N. 2016. Revisiting the understanding of "transactional sex" in sub-Saharan Africa: A review and synthesis of the literature. *Social Science & Medicine*, 168, 186–197.

Stroeken, K., Remes, P., De Koker, P., Michielsen, K., Van Vossole, A. & Temmerman, M. 2012. HIV among out-of-school youth in Eastern and Southern Africa: A review. *AIDS Care*, 24, 186–194.

Svanemyr, J., Amin, A., Robles, O.J. & Greene, M.E. 2015. Creating an enabling environment for adolescent sexual and reproductive health: A framework and promising approaches. *Journal of Adolescent Health*, 56, S7–S14.

Taaffe, J.E., Cheikh, N. & Wilson, D. 2016. The use of cash transfers for HIV prevention – are we there yet? *African Journal of AIDS Research*, 15, 17–25.

Taaffe, J.E., Longosz, A.F. & Wilson, D. 2017. The impact of cash transfers on livelihoods, education, health and HIV – what's the evidence? *Development Policy Review*, 35, 601–619.

UN. 2016. *Sustainable development goals*. [Online] Available: https://sustainabledevelopment.un.org

UNAIDS. 2015. *On the fast-track to end AIDS: 2016–2021 strategy*. Geneva: UNAIDS.

UNAIDS. 2018a. *Social protection: A fast-track commitment to end AIDS. Guidance for policy-makers, and people living with, at risk of or affected by HIV*. Geneva: UNAIDS.

UNAIDS. 2018b. *Women and girls and HIV*. Geneva: UNAIDS.

UNAIDS/STRIVE. 2018. *Transactional sex and HIV risk: From analysis to action*. Geneva: Joint United Nations Programme on HIV/AIDS and STRIVE.

UNICEF. 2018. *Turning the tide against AIDS will require more concentrated focus on adolescents and young people*. [Online] Available: https://data.unicef.org/topic/hivaids/adolescents-young-people/

Vassall, A. & Remme, M., 2018. *STRIVE impact case study: Cross-sectoral co-financing for HIV and development synergies*. London: STRIVE, London School of Hygiene and Tropical Medicine.

Wagman, J.A., Gray, R.H., Campbell, J.C., Thoma, M., Ndyanabo, A., Ssekasanvu, J., Nalugoda, F., Kagaayi, J., Nakigozi, G., Serwadda, D. & Brahmbhatt, H. 2015. Effectiveness of an integrated intimate partner violence and HIV prevention intervention in Rakai, Uganda: Analysis of an intervention in an existing cluster randomised cohort. *Lancet Global Health*, 3, e23–e33.

Wamoyi, J., Mshana, G., Mongi, A., Neke, N., Kapiga, S. & Changalucha, J. 2014. A review of interventions addressing structural drivers of adolescents' sexual and reproductive health vulnerability in sub-Saharan Africa: Implications for sexual health programming. *Reproductive Health*, 11.

Wamoyi, J., Stobeanau, K., Bobrova, N., Abramsky, T. & Watts, C. 2016. Transactional sex and risk for HIV infection in sub-Saharan Africa: A systematic review and meta-analysis. *Journal of International AIDS Society*, 19, 20992.

Wamoyi, J., Stoebenau, K., Kyegombe, N., Heise, L. & Ranganathan, M. 2017. *STRIVE Technical brief: Measuring transactional sex and HIV risk*. Tanzania: National Institute of Medical Research, Mwanza; Washington, DC: International Center for Research on Women; London: London School of Hygiene and Tropical Medicine.

Wechsberg, W., Jewkes, R., Novak, S.P., Kline, T., Myers, B., Browne, F.A., Carney, T., Morgan Lopez, A.A. & Parry, C. 2013. A brief intervention for drug use, sexual risk behaviours and violence prevention with vulnerable women in South Africa: A randomised trial of the women's health CoOp. *BMJ Open*, 3.

Wechsberg, W., Zule, W., Luseno, W., Kline, T., Browne, F., Novak, S. & Middlesteadt-Ellerson, R. 2011. Effectiveness of an adapted evidence-based woman-focused intervention for sex workers and non-sex workers: The women's health CoOp in South Africa. *Journal of Drug Issues*, 41, 233–252.

Wilson, D. 2015. Social protection, financial incentives, and prevention of HIV. *Topics in Antiviral Medicine*, 23, 30–31.

Wojcicki, J.M. 2005. Socioeconomic status as a risk factor for HIV infection in women in East, Central and Southern Africa: A systematic review. *Journal of Biosocial Science*, 37, 1–36.

Woodcock, A., Cronin, O. & Forde, S. 2012. Quantitative evidence for the benefits of moving the goalposts, a sport for development project in rural Kenya. *Evaluation & Program Planning*, 35, 370–381.

Zuilkowski, S.S. & Alon, I. 2015. Promoting education for vulnerable children by supporting families: A holistic intervention in Uganda. *Journal of Social Service Research*, 41, 454–465.

8 Young key populations in Southern Africa

An analysis of the social determinants of HIV risk and barriers to sexual and reproductive health services

Jane Freedman, Tamaryn L. Crankshaw, Carolien Aantjes, Russell Armstrong and Nana K. Poku

Introduction

The health and well-being of young people (10–24 years) is vital to the social and economic development goals of the Africa continent, which is home to a youthful and growing population.[1] Protecting the sexual and reproductive health and rights (SRHR)[2] of these young people is clearly a fundamental requisite. However, there remain substantial barriers to young people accessing quality health services, and they face a range of serious health challenges, particularly with regard to their sexual and reproductive health (SRH) (Kabiru, 2013; Fatusi, 2016). In sub-Saharan Africa, HIV prevention remains a persistent challenge among young people, where 37% of all new infections are among youth aged 15–24 and where females are disproportionately affected (UNAIDS, 2019). Likewise, there exist high rates of teenage pregnancy, unsafe abortion and maternal mortality and morbidity in the region, all underpinned by pervasive sexual and gender-based violence (SGBV) and harmful cultural and gendered practices (Juma and Klot, 2011; Anderson, 2015).

Adolescence is a life phase in which rapid physical maturation and psychological and cognitive change takes place, with adolescent development fundamentally impacted by their structural and social environments. Differential exposure to these environments has the potential to positively or negatively shape adolescent health and psychological well-being, with strong associations between socio-economic status and health behaviours and concomitant long-term outcomes (Fatusi and Hindin, 2010; Sawyer et al., 2012). Young people who are also members of key populations (KP)[3] are one example of young people facing compounded vulnerabilities since they share a number of specific barriers and challenges concerning their SRHR, linked to legal, social and political structures, which undermine their ability to access healthcare (Cornell and Dovel, 2018), and this is reflected in the poor SRH indicators for this group. Given these overlapping and intersectional challenges, there is need to apply a comprehensive framework of analysis which draws on all aspects of their lifestyles and choices, peer groups and networks as well as broader social, economic and political structures. This comprehensive approach is indispensable to efforts to fully understand the challenges these young people face, and to plan and take action on appropriate policy and programmatic interventions to improve their overall health and well-being.

This chapter presents an overview of what is known about the SRHR of young key populations (YKP) in Southern Africa, using specific examples from five countries, namely Angola, Madagascar, Mozambique, Zambia and Zimbabwe, to anchor the discussion. The discussion draws on the social determinants of health framework to structure an analysis of what is known about the determinants and drivers of sexual and reproductive health (SRH) risk and to highlight the gaps in evidence and understanding of specific vulnerabilities of these groups of youth. The social determinants of health framework allows for an analysis that goes beyond some current approaches which are over-reliant on psychosocial or behavioural factors of risk and vulnerability and which fail to adequately consider the underlying structural and social factors which shape and limit these behaviours and psychological predispositions (Ross, 2010). The discussion is based on a review of academic and grey literature concerning the SRH of YKPs in Southern Africa, together with a series of interviews with key informants from relevant government ministries, international organisations and international and national non-governmental organisations (NGOs) working with key populations in each country. Our initial findings point to the importance of understanding the vulnerabilities and risks faced by young people in these key populations in the context of a wider consideration of the social determinants of health of all young people, as well as in the context of the full range of SRH needs and priorities which include but go beyond HIV alone. Moreover, looking more broadly at the economic situation of young people, educational and employment opportunities, health systems, and peer and family networks will give us a more complete picture that will help us to understand how and why certain young people are more at risk for negative SRH outcomes than others. This more comprehensive approach creates the foundations for the development of equally comprehensive and more inclusive policies and programmes to protect and promote the SRHR of all young people in the region in all of their diversity.

The research informing this chapter is part of an ongoing study being carried out by the Health Economics and HIV and AIDS Research Division (HEARD) as part of a joint four-year project in collaboration with United Nations Development Programme (UNDP) and African Men for Sexual Health and Rights (AMSHeR), supported by funding from the government of the Netherlands. The overall project aims to strengthen HIV/SRH-related rights of young key populations in law, policy and strategy in five

Southern African countries (Angola, Madagascar, Mozambique, Zambia and Zimbabwe) and at the SADC regional level. The long-term objective of the project is to improve the SRH outcomes for young key populations in SADC countries.

Why a focus on young key populations?

In the context of the HIV and AIDS response, key populations have been defined as groups who are at increased risk of HIV infection and who are often faced with legal and social barriers and discrimination which increase their vulnerability to HIV and prevent them from accessing the concomitant SRH services.[4] Young members of key populations are located at a critical juncture of overlapping vulnerability for poor SRH, facing both the challenges associated with adolescence and the stigma and discriminations experienced by key population groups. Despite growing attention to the health of key populations in the Southern African region, there is a paucity of research on SRHR (including HIV) of YKPs, in part because of the methodological difficulties in identifying and reaching these young people, who in most cases have good reason to remain "hidden" because of the discrimination, stigmatisation and possible criminalisation that they may face. There are also important ethical challenges in carrying out research among young people under the age of 18, and while the 15–18-year-old segment of the young key populations is more under-researched than their older counterparts, the reality is that many of these 15–18-year-olds are also sexually active and in need of quality SRH services. Given the above, there are few studies which specifically explore how and why young people from these key populations may face specific challenges regarding their SRHR.

The paucity of reliable data and the lack of in-depth knowledge are sufficient reason for pursuing further research into the situations of YKPs. But what we do know makes this even more urgent, as available data suggest a range of negative SRH indicators for young people in general, and in particular for young people in key populations. An analysis conducted by UNICEF estimates that 9.6 million young people aged 15–24 will be newly infected with HIV in sub-Saharan Africa between 2017 and 2050 (UNICEF, 2018). Other estimates suggest that 50% of new HIV infections worldwide occur among members of young key populations (WHO, 2014). Young people in key populations also experience heightened risk of other STIs, unintended pregnancy, violence and other negative health outcomes. This is indicative of the vulnerable situation in which these young people find themselves, a vulnerability which is heightened in many cases by punitive legal contexts, stigma and discrimination. Restrictive legal contexts which criminalise same-sex activity, sex work or drug use – and the social stigma attached to these – affect all key populations, but for young people there are additional barriers. In some cases, health service providers face legal restrictions in providing SRH services such as HIV testing or provision of contraception to young people under the age of 18 without parental consent (Mbeba et al., 2012; Chandra-Mouli et al., 2015; Delany-Moretlwe et al., 2015). NGOs and associations working with key populations may also be reluctant to engage with young people for fear of being accused of promoting homosexuality or sex work, for example (Muller et al., 2018). Like other adolescents and young people, YKPs are at a crucial age of social and sexual development where they face pressure from families, peers and community and require support and access to services to ensure positive health for their present and future lives. The combination of being young and being a member of a key population means that many of these YKPs find themselves in a situation of high vulnerability with little or no access to SRH services or to social support groups or networks. Improving the SRHR of these young people is thus a major challenge, and one which requires understanding of the very specific situations in which they find themselves in order to design programmes and interventions which can really make a difference to their health outcomes.

Deconstructing the categories of key populations

For over a decade, key populations have been central in policies and interventions on HIV and AIDS at international levels.[5] The focus on key populations is justified by these groups' vulnerability and risks of HIV infection as mentioned earlier. However, without detracting from the importance of the attention to key populations – a focus which has been necessary in the more targeted responses to HIV and AIDS – it is important to deconstruct and analyse these categories and to acknowledge that both between and within different key populations there is a wide variety of different situations of risk and vulnerability, and also possibilities for action and resilience. Research studies have shown the diversity within each of the so-called key population groups (Paiva et al., 2015; Parker et al., 2016; Garcia et al., 2016), but the continuing usage of the term in policy and programming masks this diversity and thus erases the impacts of varying social, economic and political inequalities on individual members of the groups. The category of men who have sex with men (MSM), for instance, encompasses men in a wide range of social and economic situations, from those who are living in poverty and engaging in transactional sex for economic survival to others who are in an economically and socially privileged position but who may in turn be marginalised by legal restrictions or stigmatisation by peers. The ways in which MSM identify and experience their sexual orientations and gender identities also varies from one person to another (Alcala-Alezones et al., 2018; Sandfort and Reddy, 2013; Sheehy et al., 2014). Creating generalised categories such as MSM can risk excluding and marginalising those who feel that they cannot or should not be categorised as such (Kaplan et al., 2016). Similarly, the category of "sex workers" will encompass both more professional and visible women who sell sex who may be organised in associations to defend their interests, and young men and women engaging in transactional sexual relations in a more informal way, who may not even acknowledge or recognise that they are involved in selling sex. Young women and men engage in transactional sex for a variety of often interconnected reasons including economic necessity, gender norms or cultural practices. Reducing this range of meanings and motivations to one categorisation may lead to misrepresenting or misunderstanding the complex nature of transactional sex (Stoebenau et al., 2016; Wamoyi et al., 2016). Moreover, labelling any member of a key population primarily by function of this identity runs the risk of classifying their risks and vulnerability in unidimensional terms and ignoring other intersectional forms of discrimination and domination which they may face. Women who sell sex have argued that this identification as a "sex worker" ignores their experiences as women affected by norms related to gender and sexuality, and also their social and economic positioning and experiences (Weitzer, 2009). Further, the use of the notion of YKPs to indicate those young people most at risk of HIV infection may risk further stigmatising these young people by casting them in a negative framework which does not create space for the positive and pleasurable aspects of their sexual and gender identities and behaviours.

This diversity of situations is true for all the key populations as currently defined, making any research or policy recommendations complicated. Moreover, there is a lack of research and data on some of the key populations, leading to them being hidden or invisible in policy-related or programmatic discussions. In all of the five countries studied, there is comparatively little data on young transgender people, young people in prison or other forms of detention and young people who inject drugs. In many cases, what evidence does exist seems to indicate a "crossover" between these young people in a situation of complex and intersectional identities with cross-established categorisations. For example, many young transgender people may also be involved in transactional sex or inject drugs. These crossovers render even more problematic any forms of analysis or interventions which attempt to consider YKPs as discrete categories separate from one another.

In order to be able to develop more effective policy and interventions to respond to the needs of all members of key populations, we need to better understand these variations and the multiplicity and complexity of the SRH situations and outcomes that exist in particular social contexts. In order to do this, we need to move beyond unidimensional analyses which focus on only one factor affecting the SRHR of key populations. Whilst any individual factor may be important, examining it in isolation from a wider range of determinants of health will give only a partial picture. Detailing legislative frameworks on sex work, homosexuality or drug use, for example, may help to provide some elements of the context in which members of key populations SRHR are determined, but it will not be able to explain why certain members of these groups have better outcomes than others.

Evidence shows that de-criminalisation of homosexuality, for example, does not necessarily improve the SRHR of MSM or transgender people in these countries (Beyrer et al., 2013). Thus a multi-dimensional approach is vital in understanding the SRHR of young people who are designated as members of key populations. This multi-dimensional approach will also allow us to question the definitions and boundaries of key populations and to unpack the a priori categorisations which might limit the impacts of policies and interventions aimed at improving SRHR for young people.

Using a social determinants of health framework to understand the vulnerability of young key populations

To better understand the HIV and SRHR situation of young people who are designated as members of key populations, we have thus chosen to use a social determinants of health (SDH) framework (Solar and Irwin, 2010; Viner et al., 2012). This framework analyses the complex interactions between different levels of factors in determining the health of individuals within varying groups in a general population. Wider structural and systemic determinants, such as economic inequalities, political or legal systems (e.g. punitive laws) and health systems, interact with more proximate determinants such as family, peer or community networks and micro-level individual and behavioural-level determinants (e.g. substance abuse). This interaction will be mediated by factors related to social constructions of gender identity and sexual orientation. There is thus a complex interplay of factors which shapes risks and vulnerability, with intersecting social, physical, economic and policy factors at both macro and micro levels. Thus each individual, situated at a different point within this matrix, has their own unique situation of risk, vulnerability or possibility in terms of health outcomes. Using this framework will help us to understand how and why certain individuals are more at risk or vulnerable in terms of SRHR, and how policies and interventions could be better designed to target specific determinants and effect a real shift in health outcomes. Whilst the SDH framework has been in use for some time, there are still few empirically based studies which fully consider determinants at all levels of the framework and their interactions. Further, the framework may need to be adapted for considering young people, for whom various determinants, such as peer networks, may be found to play a larger role than for adults.

The research on young people who are members of key populations is central here because of the youthful "demographic bulge" of the countries of the SADC region and also because of the specific sets of determinants which affect young people's health outcomes particularly. In all five countries studied here, as in the region more generally, the majority of the population is under 25 years old. The health of these young people is thus central for the future health of the country and the region. A focus on young people is also necessary and justified by a life-course approach to health, which makes it evident that poor sexual and reproductive health during this period of life will have severe ongoing consequences for the whole of an individual's lifespan. The complex physical, psychological, emotional and social changes that take place during adolescence have immediate and long-term implications for individuals. For example, the onset of puberty is linked to the initiation of sexual activity and subsequent exposure to the risk of pregnancy and STIs, including HIV. Awareness of sexual orientation and gender identity may emerge or become clearer during this period. Social determinants of health are also very specific to the period of adolescence and early adulthood, with an increased influence of family and peer networks (Viner et al., 2012).

Researching SRHR of young key populations also necessitates widening the focus beyond the exclusive concentration on HIV and AIDS. Whilst HIV remains a critical issue for most of the countries in the region, the young people with whom we are concerned also face multiple other and often linked SRH challenges which must be considered and which, in fact, can impact the HIV prevention agenda (Crankshaw et al., 2016; Patton et al., 2016). For young women who sell sex, for example, our initial research highlights a predominantly HIV-dominated intervention response with very little attention paid to these young people's reproductive health, including access to contraception, the problem of unintended pregnancy or unsafe abortion. These challenges are inextricably linked with HIV prevention efforts (e.g. elimination of mother-to-child transmission of HIV or safer conception strategies) and share cross-cutting systemic challenges (e.g. SGBV) which render some more vulnerable to poor health outcomes than others.

Applying the social determinants framework to our baseline findings

Global research has shown that the strongest determinants of adolescent health in general are structural factors such as national wealth, income inequality and access to education (Viner et al., 2012). Our findings point to the major impacts of low levels of national wealth and of economic inequalities on the young people in the five countries studied. Poverty and low levels of national wealth affect spending and availability of public services such as health and education. In many of the project countries there is a basic lack of health infrastructure, and populations, particularly in rural areas, have little access to basic health services (Marks et al., 2016; Ray and Masuka, 2017). For young people, and particularly those in key populations who may experience additional discrimination and stigma, finding appropriate and suitable health advice and care for issues related to SRH issues is often an unsurmountable challenge. The lack of educational opportunities for young people is also a component in creating situations of risk and vulnerability for young people and is linked to worse sexual and reproductive health outcomes (Van Stam et al., 2014).

Young people are particularly affected by income inequality. In all five countries, our baseline research showed particularly high levels of poverty among young people and high levels of youth unemployment. In Madagascar, for example, where recent estimates indicate that extreme poverty impacts 56.5% of the population (IMF, 2017), poverty has a "predominantly young face" (World Bank, 2014). There, young aged 15–24 face immense difficulties in entering the labour market and 75% of the unemployed in the country are under 30 years old (ILO Instat, 2014). Similar situations are found in the other countries studied. In Mozambique, the majority of young people have no access to formal employment (ADB, 2012), and the high youth unemployment levels have been described as leaving young people in a "state of waithood . . . a situation of waiting to become full adults" (p. 16). Poverty and economic inequality impact on young people's SRHR in various ways, including in their abilities to pay for health services and in their survival strategies, which may in the absence of alternatives lead them to sex work, for example. In Madagascar, increasing rates of transactional sex and sex tourism have been noted in recent years (PSI, 2017; Freedman et al., forthcoming). Although reasons for transactional sex and routes into sex work are not by any means straightforward or unidimensional, there is strong evidence that for many girls and young women transactional sex is primarily a means to be able to buy basic necessities for themselves or their families (PSI, 2017). Evidence from our research, particularly in the south of the country, showed the ways in which traditional and customary gender norms have become imbricated with current structural conditions of poverty and lack of employment, to create situations where transactional sex is a "way of life" for young women. Similar patterns are in evidence in Zimbabwe, where increasing poverty has led to sex work becoming less formalised with the emergence of different forms of transactional sex, and interactions between women who sell sex and clients becoming riskier (Elmes et al., 2017). Young women engaged in this less formalised sex work may not view themselves as "commercial sex workers" and so may risk being missed by targeted health interventions yet struggle to access necessary healthcare elsewhere given conservative community norms around youth and sexuality, and barriers posed by age of consent laws in Zimbabwe and the region more broadly. In Zambia, research has shown that the influence of poverty and inequality as "pathways" to sex work is greater for young women than for other members of the population (Butts et al., 2017). Engaging in transactional sex renders young people vulnerable to infection with HIV and other STIs, unwanted pregnancies and SGBV (Stobeanau et al., 2016). This vulnerability is heightened by legal and policy contexts in which sex work is criminalised, as is the case in Zambia and Zimbabwe, where young people selling sex work may fear reporting SGBV and receiving the necessary care for fear of being arrested themselves. These contexts will interact with economic factors (e.g. out-of-pocket costs to access healthcare) to render young women who sell sex even more vulnerable to poor HIV and other SRH outcomes.

As suggested above, legal and political structures also act as determinants on the SRH of young key populations. In Zambia and Zimbabwe, homosexuality is criminalised, meaning that young people are often scared to reveal their sexual orientations or gender identities for fear of arrest, detention or physical abuse (Hachoonda, 2017; Meer et al., 2017). But even in Madagascar and Mozambique, where homosexuality is legal, norms which strongly favour heterosexuality may mean that young people choose to hide or deny their homosexuality for fear of negative reactions, stigmatisation or violence. Gay or transgender people may thus become "invisible," a status which can prevent them from accessing health services and push them into marginalised positions within society. In Mozambique, for example, while the decriminalisation of homosexuality has been an important structural change for the legal position of young gays and lesbians, the strongly normative stance on gender relations and identities of key opinion leaders has not shifted much, leading to a continuing marginalisation of young MSM and pressure on them to raise a family (Macia et al., 2011). Marginalisation and stigmatisation of young lesbian, gay, bisexual, transgender and intersex (LGBTI) people, sex workers and injecting drug users (IDUs) are often a fundamental barrier to these YKPs accessing health services where attitudes towards them are discriminatory and where the care provided is inappropriate or unresponsive to these young people's specific SRH needs. Young women who sell sex, for example, have been found not to disclose their work to health professionals or to misrepresent their health problems or even to avoid care entirely because of their fears of discrimination (Scorgie et al., 2011; Lafort et al., 2016; Mwashita, 2017).

Health systems themselves are an intermediate determinant of health through which differences in health vulnerabilities and risks are exacerbated or mitigated. The five country case studies have different organisations of health systems, but a common factor seems to be health systems which suffer from lack of resources and which may be fragmented in their delivery of services, with vertical delivery of services, for example, separating structures dealing with HIV/AIDS from those addressing other SRH needs. In Mozambique, for example, there is only one methadone treatment site in the country, which is situated in the psychiatric hospital in Maputo. Key informants revealed that people who inject drugs who sign up for this programme often leave prematurely, as they are hospitalised together with psychiatric patients and alcoholics and find it difficult to cope in such an environment. Cost of services and distance from health facilities remain major barriers for many people in accessing care (Marks et al., 2016; Garchitorena et al., 2017). For YKPs these problems may be intensified in country contexts where their health needs are marginalised. For example, despite provision for treatment for AIDS, TB and hepatitis in Mozambique's Prison Policy (2002), the Integrated Biological and Behavioural Survey found that prisoners often faced interruptions and discontinuation of their treatment regimens

(INS, 2013). A serious lack of health provision for prisoners or for IDUs in many countries reinforces the vulnerabilities of these young people to poor SRH outcomes.

Structures of gender inequality and the persistence of traditional attitudes and norms towards gender and sexuality in conjunction with the existing socio-economic and political systems in each country may thus impact on the SRHR and the general health and well-being of persons belonging to gender or sexual minorities. Similarly, traditional gender norms which place an important prime on heterosexuality and "traditional" family structures create a context within which young women have little control over their sexuality and face particular risks to their sexual and reproductive health. Proximal determinants such as family and peer networks mediate the effects of these structural determinants and have a strong impact on young people's SRHR. Globally research has shown how social networks including family and peers shape sexual behaviour (Marston and King, 2006). Again, our research shows the potential negative impacts on SRH of young people in communities where there is strong peer pressure on young people to have sexual relations at an early age, or where young men feel peer pressure to engage in multiple sexual partnerships. In Madagascar, the research has shown that strong pressure both from family and peers to engage in sexual relations at an early age, in combination with a lack of access to contraception and to SRH services, has led to high rates of pregnancy among young women and also to high rates of illegal abortion (Focus Development, 2007). Young people with weak sex-work peer networks, as our research suggests may be the case for adolescents who sell sex in Zimbabwe, may not benefit from targeted interventions accessed via these referral pathways.

A final piece in the social determinants framework is the individual behavioural-level determinants, which means that two young people who are seemingly in near identical socio-economic conditions, with similar family and peer networks, gender identities and sexual orientations, may still have very different SRH outcomes. These issues are not explored in the baseline literature review and key informant interviews, and thus need further in-depth research and analysis. One of the objectives of our ongoing research will be to aim to capture these individual-level determinants by in-depth biographical interview techniques to understand better young people's choice and pathways to vulnerability or resilience. This understanding should lead to recommendations on how better to engage young people from key populations to promote behaviours and choices which will improve their SRH.

Conclusion: moving forward

The initial baseline analysis of the sexual and reproductive health of young key populations in these five countries using a social determinants of health framework has shown the multiple interlocking factors that may lead to poor HIV and SRH outcomes, including infection with HIV and other STIs, unwanted pregnancies, sexual and gender-based violence. This acknowledgement of the multiplicity of pathways into vulnerability for these young people and the intersectional nature of the barriers and risks they face points to the need for more in-depth research to fully understand how policy and programming could address these determinants to improve SRH for young people in key populations. Questions for further research emerge directly from a lack of data on certain young key populations – especially young prisoners, young transgender people and young IDUs – and others push to explore further the ways in which varying constellations of social determinants will lead to individual outcomes of risk or vulnerability for young people's SRHR and how these may be better addressed in the future.

Further, our baseline studies point to more serious issues with the categorisation of young key populations and the ways in which these categorisations have been employed. Thus issues which need to be considered in future research concern the ways in which a social determinants of health framework might lead to re-consideration of the categories of key populations in the SADC region as applied to young people. We need to better understand who these populations are and how exactly they are rendered vulnerable. Given a certain set of systemic and structural determinants, how and why do certain individuals and groups have more negative health outcomes than others? And which policy interventions would be most effective in transforming the social determinants for YKPs, thus ensuring better sexual and reproductive health outcomes?

Notes

1 Approximately two-fifths of Africa's population are 14 years or younger, and nearly one-fifth (19%) are between the ages of 15 and 24 (African Union, 2015, 2017; UNECA, 2017).

2 Sexual and reproductive health and rights (SRHR) is broadly defined as "a state of physical, emotional, mental, and social wellbeing in relation to all aspects of sexuality and reproduction, not merely the absence of disease, dysfunction, or infirmity. Therefore, a positive approach to sexuality and reproduction should recognise the part played by pleasurable sexual relationships, trust, and communication in the promotion of self-esteem and overall wellbeing. All individuals have a right to make decisions governing their bodies and to access services that support that right" (Guttmacher-Lancet Commission, 2018).

3 Key populations are generally defined as men who have sex with men (MSM), people who inject drugs, people in prisons and forms of detention, sex workers and transgender people (UNAIDS, 2014).

4 www.unaids.org/en/topic/key-populations.

5 It should be noted that the introduction of KP programmes has been varied across this time, with a somewhat later adoption in Africa due to the focus on more generalised epidemics in many countries on the continent and in some cases political resistance to programmes targeting criminalised or otherwise marginalised groups.

References

ADB. (2012), *African Economic Outlook: Mozambique*, Abidjan: African Development Bank.

African Union. (2015), *Agenda 2063: The Africa We Want*, Addis Ababa: African Union.

African Union. (2017), *AU Roadmap on Harnessing the Demographic Dividend Through Investments in Youth: In Response to AU Assembly Decision (Assembly/AU/Dec.601 (XXVI) on the 2017 Theme of the Year*, Addis Ababa: African Union.

Alcala-Alezones, C. et al. (2018), 'South African Men Who Have Sex with Both Men and Women and How They Differ from Men Who Have Sex with Men Exclusively', *The Journal of Sex Research*, 55(8): 1048–1055.

Anderson, E. L. (2015), *Gender, HIV and Risk*, Basingstoke: Palgrave Macmillan.

Beyrer, C. et al. (2013), 'The Increase in Global HIV Epidemics in MSM', *AIDS*, 27(17): 2665–2678.

Butts, S. et al. (2017), 'Let Us Fight and Support One Another: Adolescent Girls and Young Women on Contributors and Solutions for HIV Risks in Zambia', *International Journal of Women's Health*, 9: 727–737.

Chandra-Mouli, V. et al. (2015), 'Twenty Years After International Conference on Population and Development: Where Are We with Adolescent Sexual and Reproductive Health and Rights?' *Journal of Adolescent Health*, 56(1): S1–S6.

Cornell, M., & Dovel, K. (2018), 'Reaching Key Adolescent Populations', *Current Opinion HIV and AIDS*, 13(3): 274–280. Medline:29432229. Doi:10.1097/COH.0000000000000457.

Crankshaw, T. L., Smit, J. A., & Beksinska, M. E. (2016), 'Placing Contraception at the Centre of the HIV Prevention Agenda', *African Journal of AIDS Research*, 15(2): 157–162.

Delany-Moretlwe, S. et al. (2015), 'Providing Comprehensive Health Services for Young Key Populations: Needs, Barriers and Gaps', *Journal of the International AIDS Society*, 18(1): 29–41.

Elmes, J. et al. (2017), 'A Reconfiguration of the Sex Trade: How Social and Structural Changes in Eastern Zimbabwe Left Women Involved in Sex Work and Transactional Sex More Vulnerable', *PLoS One*, 12: e0171916.

Fatusi, A. O. (2016), 'Young People's Sexual and Reproductive Health Interventions in Developing Countries: Making the Investments Count', *Journal of Adolescent Health*, 59: S1–S3.

Fatusi, A. O., & Hindin, M. J. (2010), 'Adolescents and Youth in Developing Countries: Health and Development Issues in Context', *Journal of Adolescence*, 33(4): 499–508.

Focus Development. (2007), *Etude sur l'avortement clandestine à Madagascar*, Antananarivo: FISA-IPPF.

Freedman, J. et al. (forthcoming), 'Economies of Transactional Sex in Madagascar', *World Development*.

Garchitorena, A. et al. (2017), 'In Madagascar, Use of Health Care Services Increased When Fees Were Removed: Lessons For Universal Health Coverage', *Health Affairs*, 36(8): 1443–1451.

Garcia, J., Parker, R. G., Parker, C., Wilson, P. A., Philbin, M., & Hirsch, J. S. (2016), 'The Limitations of "Black MSM" as a Category: Why Gender, Sexuality, and Desire Still Matter for Social and Biomedical HIV Prevention Methods', *Global Public Health*, 11(7–8): 1026–1048.

Guttmacher-Lancet Commission. (2018), *Accelerate Progress—Sexual and Reproductive Health and Rights for All: Report of the Guttmacher–Lancet Commission.* https://www.thelancet.com/commissions/sexual-and-reproductive-health-and-rights.

Hachoonda, H. (2017), *Final Report of the Desk Review and Stakeholder Consultations on Human Rights Status of People of Diverse Sexual Orientation and Gender Identity in Zambia,* Lusaka: UNDP and OHCHR.

ILO Instat. (2014), *Transition relativement rapide des jeunes vers des emplois précaires et vulnérables. Enquête sur la transition des jeunes vers la vie active.* Madagascar: ETVA.

IMF. (2017), *Republic of Madagascar: Economic Development Document,* IMF Country Report, No. 17/25. https://www.imf.org/en/Publications/CR/Issues/2017/07/18/Republic-of-Madagascar-Economic-Development-Document-45099.

INS. (2013), *Assessment of the Situation of HIV, STIs, TB and Health Needs in Prisons in Mozambique,* Maputo: Instituto Nacional de Saude, United Nations Office on Drugs and Crime.

Juma, M.K., & Klot, J. (2011), *HIV/AIDS, Gender, Human Security and Violence in Southern Africa,* Pretoria: Africa Institute of South Africa.

Kabiru, C.W. (2013), 'The Health and Wellbeing of Young People in sub-Saharan Africa: An Under-Researched Area?', *BMC International Health and Human Rights,* 13(11): 1–7.

Kaplan, R.L., Sevelius, J., & Ribeiro, K. (2016), 'In the Name of Brevity: The Problem with Binary HIV Risk Categories', *Global Public Health,* 11(7–8): 824–834.

Lafort, Y. et al. (2016), 'Barriers to HIV and Sexual and Reproductive Health Care for Female Sex Workers in Tete, Mozambique: Results from a Cross-Sectional Survey and Focus Group Discussions', *BMC Public Health,* 16(1): 608.

Macia, M. et al. (2011), 'Masculinity and Male Sexual Behaviour in Mozambique', *Culture, Health and Sexuality,* 13(10): 1181–1192.

Marks, F. et al. (2016), 'A Way Forward for Healthcare in Madagascar?', *Clinical Infectious Diseases,* 62(15): 76–79.

Marston, C., & King, E. (2006), 'Factors That Shape Young People's Sexual Behaviour: A Systematic Review', *Lancet,* 368(9547): 1581–1586.

Mbeba, Rita M. et al. (2012), 'Barriers to Sexual Reproductive Health Services and Rights Among Young People in Mtwara District, Tanzania: A Qualitative Study', *Pan African Medical Journal,* 13(Suppl 1): 13.

Meer, T. et al. (2017), *Lesbian, Gay, Bisexual, Transgender and Intersex Human Rights in Southern Africa: A Contemporary Literature Review 2012–2016,* Johannesburg: HIVOS.

Muller, A. et al. (2018), 'The No-Go Zone: A Qualitative Study of Access to Sexual and Reproductive Health Services for Sexual and Gender Minority Adolescents in Southern Africa', *Reproductive Health,* 15(12).

Mwashita, F. (2017), *Young Women in Commercial Sexual Exploitation Along Two Transport Corridors in Zimbabwe,* Harare: Zimbabwe National Council for the Welfare of Children.

Paiva, V. et al. (2015), 'The Current State of Play of Research on the Social, Political and Legal Dimensions of HIV', *Cadernos de Saúde Pública,* 31(3): 477–486. doi:10.1590/0102-311X00172514. Accessed 4 February 2019.

Parker, R., Aggleton, P., & Perez-Brumer, A.G. (2016), 'The Trouble with "Categories": Rethinking Men Who Have Sex with Men, Transgender and Their Equivalents in HIV Prevention and Health Promotion', *Global Public Health,* 11(7–8): 819–823.

Patton, G.C. et al. (2016), 'Our Future: A *Lancet* Commission on Adolescent Health and Well-Being', *Lancet*, 387(10036): 2423–2478.

PSI (2017), *Étude Formative pour comprendre les archétypes des professionnelles de sexe*, Antananarivo: PSI.

Ray, S., & Masuka, N. (2017), 'Facilitators and Barriers to Effective Primary Health Care in Zimbabwe', *African Journal of Primary Healthcare and Family Medicine*, 9(1): 1639.

Ross, D.A. (2010), 'Behavioural Interventions to Reduce HIV Risk: What Works?', *AIDS*, 24: S4–S14.

Sandfort, T., & Reddy, V. (2013), 'African Same-Sex Sexualities and Gender-Diversity: An Introduction', *Culture, Health & Sexuality*, 15(Supp 1): 1–6.

Sawyer, S. et al. (2012), 'Adolescence: A Foundation for Future Health', *Lancet*, 379(9826): 1630–1640.

Scorgie, F. et al. (2011), ' "I Expected to Be Abused and I Have Fear": Sex Workers' Experiences of Human Rights Violations and Barriers to Accessing Health Care in Four African Countries', *Culture, Health and Sexuality*, 15(4): 450–465.

Sheehy, M. et al. (2014), 'High Levels of Bisexual Behavior and Factors Associated with Bisexual Behavior Among Men Having Sex with Men (MSM) in Nigeria', *Journal of AIDS Care*, 26(1): 116–122.

Solar, O., & Irwin, A. (2010), *A Conceptual Framework for Action on the Social Determinants of Health*, Social Determinants of Health Discussion Paper 2 (Policy and Practice), Geneva: World Health Organization.

Stoebenau, K. et al. (2016), 'Revisiting the Understanding of "Transactional Sex" in sub-Saharan Africa: A Review and Synthesis of the Literature', *Social Science and Medicine*, 168: 186–197.

UNECA. (2017), *Demographic Datasets for Africa*, Addis Ababa: United Nations Economic Commission for Africa.

UNAIDS (2014), *UNAIDS Interagency Working Group on Key Populations*. https://www.who.int/hiv/pub/guidelines/briefs_ykp_2014.pdf

UNAIDS (2019), *UNAIDS Data 2019*. https://www.unaids.org/sites/default/files/media_asset/2019-UNAIDS-data_en.pdf

UNICEF. (2018), *Opportunity in Crisis: Preventing HIV from Early Adolescence to Young Adulthood*, New York: UNICEF.

Van Stam, M. et al. (2014), 'The Impact of Education and Globalization on Sexual and Reproductive Health: Retrospective Evidence from Eastern and Southern Africa', *AIDS Care*, 26(3): 379–386.

Viner, R. et al. (2012), 'Adolescence and the Social Determinants of Health', *Lancet*, 379(9826): 1641–1652.

Wamoyi, J. et al. (2016), 'Transactional Sex and Risk for HIV Infection in Sub-Saharan Africa: A Systematic Review and Meta-Analysis', *Journal of the International AIDS Society*, 19(1): 20992.

Weitzer, R. (2009), 'The Sociology of Sex Work', *Annual Review of Sociology*, 35: 213–234.

WHO (2014), *Working Briefs on Key Populations*, https://www.who.int/hiv/pub/guidelines/briefs_ykp_2014.pdf.

World Bank. (2014), *Face of Poverty in Madagascar: Poverty, Gender and Inequality Assessment*, Washington, DC: World Bank.

9 Are adolescent boys and young men being left behind? missing discourse and missed opportunities for engagement in HIV prevention in Eastern and Southern Africa

Joanne E. Mantell, Susie Hoffman, Andrea Low, Elizabeth A. Kelvin and Philip Kreniske

Introduction

Worldwide, HIV incidence among young females aged 15–24 is 44% higher than it is among their male counterparts (UNAIDS (Joint United Nations Programme on HIV/AIDS), 2017). This gender divide is especially pronounced in Eastern and Southern Africa (ESA), where young women accounted for 26% of new HIV infections in 2016 despite comprising about 10% of the population (UNAIDS, 2017). Adolescent girls and young women (AGYW) have therefore been the focal point for HIV prevention initiatives, whereas adolescent boys and young men (ABYM) have been relatively overlooked. Although HIV prevalence peaks among men in sub-Saharan Africa (SSA) at a much later age than it does among women, ABYM are not at zero risk. Moreover, behavioural patterns formed during early adolescence become ingrained in adulthood (Woog and Kagesten, 2017), setting the stage for adolescent boys' increasing risk of HIV acquisition as they age. Early adolescence provides an opportunity for instilling positive sexual and reproductive health attitudes and behaviours.

Pronounced gender disparities occur across the HIV care continuum (DiCarlo et al., 2014; Gari et al., 2014; Staveteig et al., 2017). ABYM, especially those who have sex with other boys or men (Cornell and Dovel, 2018), continue to be left behind in efforts to achieve the 90–90–90 goals (UNAIDS, 2017a). Studies in many ESA countries have shown that HIV testing rates are sub-optimal among 15–24-year-old ABYM (9% ever tested vs 13% of girls the same age) (United Nations Children's Fund (UNICEF), 2018), as are initiation of and adherence to antiretroviral therapy (Ochieng-Ooko et al., 2010), retention in HIV care (Koole et al., 2014; Dovel et al., 2015, 2016), and viral suppression.

For these reasons, ABYM have been described as the "forgotten fifty per cent" (Varga, 2001). Funding support for HIV prevention for ABYM has been limited compared to that for AGYW, resulting in insufficient data on the intersecting multi-level factors that contribute to HIV risk among them, and to the dearth of risk-reduction programmes. Despite this, we are unaware of any synthesis of HIV prevention research regarding ABYM in SSA. In response to this gap, we conducted a focused review in ESA countries to identify the HIV prevention research findings among ABYM aged 10–24 and to address three issues:

1 What factors create contexts of risk for HIV acquisition and promote or limit adoption of HIV prevention behaviours among ABYM in ESA?
2 What types of evidence-based HIV prevention interventions have been conducted with ABYM in ESA and what are their results?
3 What are key gaps in research on HIV prevention among ABYM in ESA?

We used a social-ecological framework (Bronfenbrenner and Ceci, 1994) to map and synthesize the multi-level factors that drive risk of HIV acquisition and to describe types of interventions for ABYM. Five researchers conducted a focused literature search to identify relevant studies, including studies on sexual risk behaviours and substance use as well as interventions – structural (e.g. cash transfers), biomedical (e.g. HIV testing and counselling, voluntary medical male circumcision [VMMC] and pre-exposure prophylaxis [PrEP]) and behavioural (e.g. condom promotion, school-based risk-reduction and interpersonal violence). Searches were limited to English articles and to the 24 countries in eastern (Burundi, Comoros, Djibouti, Eritrea, Ethiopia, Kenya, Mauritius, Rwanda, Seychelles, Somalia, South Sudan, Tanzania and Uganda) and southern Africa (Angola, Botswana, Eswatini [Swaziland], Lesotho, Madagascar, Malawi, Mozambique, Namibia, South Africa, Zambia and Zimbabwe) between 2005 and March 2018 (to capture data after ART roll-out). Quantitative and qualitative studies that included data on ABYM aged 10–24 were included. We excluded studies that did not have male-specific data within our specified age range as well as studies on preventing onward HIV transmission among people living with HIV.

Factors associated with HIV acquisition among ABYM

Transitioning from adolescence to young adulthood is a period of key biological and developmental life-course changes including completion of school, marriage, and childbearing, all of which may influence the risk of HIV acquisition (Lloyd, 2005). These life transitions differ for men and women and are largely shaped by culturally based social norms, especially those related to gender. In the context of this developmental period, young men's risk of HIV acquisition is driven by a constellation of intersecting social-structural, interpersonal and individual-level risk factors, as described in the following.

Social-structural risk factors. Education, marital status, employment and income have been studied as potential risk factors for HIV acquisition among adolescents in SSA. For example, whether higher educational attainment has any relationship to the risk of HIV in ESA has been investigated since early in the epidemic. A systematic review conducted in 2002 (Hargreaves and Glynn, 2002) concluded that higher educational attainment was more often associated with greater risk of HIV than was lower educational attainment. Two subsequent systematic reviews – one of studies published between 2001 and 2006 (not restricted to youth) (Hargreaves et al., 2008) and the other of studies published between 2007 and 2017 (restricted to youth) (Pace, 2018) – indicated that the pattern of association appears to be changing over time, despite considerable heterogeneity (Hargreaves et al., 2015). Higher educational attainment was protective against HIV infection more often in studies conducted after 1996 (Hargreaves et al., 2008). This trend continued in studies included in the 2007–2017 review (Pace, 2018); more studies showed a protective effect of education, with higher educational attainment associated with decreased HIV risk.

Evidence is limited concerning whether educational attainment has a differential impact on boys than girls. In the most recent review, covering 17 studies conducted in ESA, only two reported differences by gender (Pace, 2018). One study of HIV incidence in rural South Africa reported a statistically significant protective association between secondary education and HIV infection for women but not for men (Hargreaves et al., 2008). In a study of HIV incidence in Uganda, being enrolled in school was protective for both women and men but completing secondary school (relative to completing only primary school) was protective only for men (Santelli et al., 2013).

Marriage has been associated with protection against HIV acquisition in some studies and systematic reviews, and divorce or separation has been associated with increased risk. For example, data from 6741 sexually experienced youth aged 15–24 in the Ugandan Rakai Community Cohort Study between 1999 and 2008 found that formerly married ABYM and AGYW had higher risk of new HIV infections than married and never married youth (Santelli et al., 2013), perhaps because formerly married youth had more sexual partnerships than the other groups.

The search for work is one of the main drivers of youth mobility across ESA (Boerma et al., 2002; Camlin et al., 2014; Schuyler et al., 2017; Olawore et al., 2018), and people involved in certain occupations appear to be at higher risk for HIV infection (Serwadda et al., 1992; Kagaayi et al., 2014). Occupations such as motorcycle taxi drivers, truck drivers, traders, police and security officers and those in hospitality service industries (bar, restaurant and hotel workers) place people at greater risk for HIV infection. In contrast, low-risk occupations include jobs in engineering and mechanics, subsistence farming and government (such as health workers or educators). For youth, these high-risk occupations are frequently the only wage-earning jobs available, and these structural forces place youth at increased risk for HIV infection (Kreniske et al., 2019). There are a number of reasons why mobility is associated with higher risk of HIV among migrants and the partners they leave behind, including demographic factors, separation from partners, family and friends, multiple concurrent sexual partners, frequent partner change and disparities in access to prevention services (Weine and Kashuba, 2012; Magadi, 2013; Olawore et al., 2018). Additionally, structural factors may place migrants in situations where uneven power dynamics force them to make decisions that increase risk for HIV infection (Kreniske et al., 2019). There are significant gender disparities in HIV risk among 15–24-year-old migrants in SSA. AGYW are 2.5 times more likely to be HIV-positive than ABYM, even when demographic and sexual behaviour factors are taken into account (Magadi, 2013).

Peer and family norms. During early adolescence, young people become cognizant of peer norms. A wealth of research has focused on how social constructions of gender that privilege men and dominant ideas about masculinity are detrimental to AGYW by condoning male control over sex and condom use, and violence against women (Barker and Ricardo, 2005). However, social constructions of manhood also increase men's risk for HIV by valorising multiple sexual partnerships, transactional sex and condomless sex. These norms also constrain ABYM usage of health services and adoption of HIV prevention behaviours such as HIV testing, safer sex communications with partners, and avoidance of alcohol and drug use (UNAIDS, 2017a).

The importance of these norms was demonstrated in a study of 14–17-year-old youth in South Africa. Boys' perceptions of whether their male and female peers were sexually active, a stronger belief that it is "ok for a girl to propose love to a boy" and stronger support for the idea that it is "ok for a girl to refuse sex when her boyfriend refuses to use a condom" were statistically significant predictors of ever having had sexual intercourse (Harrison et al., 2012). Older boys, boys who strongly endorsed the idea that "using condoms is a way to show love and respect for your partner," and boys who perceived that male peers were using condoms had significantly higher odds of condom use at last sex. These findings indicate that peer norms can have a positive impact on adolescent boys' use of condoms, and they point to a strategy of targeting peer norms in risk-reduction interventions for adolescent boys.

A study in South Africa's Eastern Cape also showed a relationship between holding more gender-equitable norms and condom use among ABYM aged 15–26 (Shai et al., 2012). Consistent condom users held less conservative gender attitudes, were less violent, and engaged in less risky sexual behaviour than inconsistent condom users, highlighting the need for focusing on healthy masculinities in HIV prevention interventions.

A recent systematic review also pointed to the salient role of family in influencing young adolescents' construction of gender norms (Kågesten et al., 2016). For example, adolescent boys in Botswana recruited from secondary schools and after-school and sports programmes were more likely than adolescent girls to report positive relationships with parents. Additionally, boys perceived greater community normative beliefs that condoned sexual risk behaviour. However, both boys and girls reported low levels of parental monitoring, parental reinforcement, and parental communication and comfort in addressing questions about sexuality and sexual development (Sun et al., 2018).

Health services. Access to sexual and reproductive health services has often been challenging to adolescents because services are not attuned to the developmental needs of youth. These challenges include inconvenient clinic hours for in-school youth, limited transportation to clinics (Wood and Jewkes, 2006; Lightfoot et al., 2017), pervasive stigma around sexual and reproductive health reflected in verbal harassment, name-calling, social isolation and punishment by providers, peers, family and community members, and in some cases, need for parental consent (Nyblade et al., 2017). This issue is intensified for ABYM because public-sector health facilities in many ESA countries are not typically oriented to male needs. Due to limited research, we know little about the experience of ABYM seeking healthcare services (Fortenberry, 2017). Some studies suggest that youth-friendly services that do not interfere with school attendance or work can increase access to HIV testing for both adolescent boys and girls (Francis, 2010). For sexual and gender minority youth, barriers to accessing sexual and reproductive health services may be even more acute than for heterosexual and cisgender youth due to social stigma, assumptions of heterosexuality, healthcare providers' moral values and criminalisation of consensual sexual activities with same-sex partners (Müller et al., 2018).

Interpersonal-level/social risk factors

Partnership and sexual networks

Characteristics of partnerships and social networks may contribute to the risk of HIV acquisition, but studies of age-disparate partnerships and HIV risk have been examined among young women and have produced mixed findings (Harling et al., 2014; Schaefer et al., 2017). Less is known about the sexual partnerships of ABYM, although we know that concurrent sexual partnerships are common. Multiple sexual partnerships were more common among 15–19-year-old ABYM in SSA than their female counterparts based on 2000–2010 DHS and AIDS Indicator Survey data (Doyle et al., 2012). Data also indicate that some ABYM have sex with older women ("sugar mommies") for economic gain (Onoya et al., 2015). Little is known about which of these behaviours and in what contexts are most risky. However, one study from Uganda found that the number of sexual partners in the last 12 months was not associated with incident HIV infection in young men, although it was among young women (Santelli et al., 2013).

Communication with sexual partners

There is a dearth of studies on communication between ABYM and their sexual partners in ESA. However, one cross-sectional survey of potential HIV risk factors in 983 boys and girls aged 14–17 in rural South Africa found that discussion of condom use with a partner was the strongest predictor of condom use at last sex, with a sevenfold increase for boys compared to a fivefold increase for girls (Harrison et al., 2012).

Parental influence on ABYM prevention practices

Parents/guardians can be an influence in shaping cultural and gender norms in adolescents, and this may in turn affect their risk of HIV. However, parents may play a limited role in supporting their sons to adopt HIV preventive behaviours. This conclusion emerged from a study of parental role in supporting voluntary medical male circumcision (VMMC). In interviews in 2015–2016 with 1293 ABYM aged 10–19 who intended to or who were recently circumcised and focus groups with 192 of their parents/guardians in South Africa, Tanzania and Zimbabwe, parents/guardians noted challenges in talking to their sons about VMMC, especially if they did not accompany their sons to the clinic (Dam et al., 2018). Parents in all countries reported they had discussed the benefits and risks of VMMC with their sons prior to the procedure, and that their son's age influenced the level of information they shared. Most parents/guardians believed that the decision to undergo VMMC was their son's or a joint parent-son decision. Parents/guardians of youth aged 10–14 were more likely than those of 15–19-year-olds to accompany their son to pre-VMMC procedure counselling (56.5% vs 12.5%; $p < .001$), and older adolescents were more resistant to a parent being present during the procedure and post-procedure wound care.

Parents reported that they rarely talked about sex, HIV, and condoms with older ABYM and not at all with those aged 10–12, and that they did not want HIV risk and sexual health information to be discussed in their son's VMMC counselling sessions. Although this study demonstrates the important role that parents/guardians can play in supporting uptake of HIV prevention strategies such as VMMC by younger ABYM, it also reveals the discomfort that parents/guardians have about candid sexual discussions with their children.

Intimate partner violence

The epidemics of intimate partner violence (IPV) and HIV overlap in ESA. Nearly 40% of women in eastern Africa and 30% in southern Africa have experienced IPV (Devries et al., 2013; UNAIDS, 2016b), and there is a large body of research linking women's IPV victimization with increased risk of

HIV infection (Maman et al., 2002; Fonck et al., 2005; Dude, 2011; Kayibanda et al., 2012; Kouyoumdjian et al., 2013). Some studies have shown that young men who perpetrate IPV are more likely to engage in HIV risk behaviours (Dunkle et al., 2006; Jewkes et al., 2011; Mullinax et al., 2017) including abusing alcohol, having multiple sexual partners, and engaging in condomless sex (Dunkle and Decker, 2013). These risk behaviours have been linked to commonly accepted ideas about masculinity, as discussed above, and they are reinforced by social-structural inequalities (Jewkes et al., 2011). For example, focus group and in-depth interview data from the Stepping Stones and Creating Futures Interventions in South Africa found that young men in two urban informal settlements manifested their masculinity through IPV, control of female sexual partners, and having multiple sexual partners in response to their high levels of unemployment and poverty and their concomitant inability to achieve economic security (Gibbs et al., 2014).

Despite strong evidence associating men's IPV perpetration and their engagement in HIV risk behaviours, only one study to our knowledge has shown a significant relationship between IPV perpetration and HIV prevalence in young men (Jewkes et al., 2011). In that study, 18–24-year-old ABYM who stated they were physically violent towards an intimate partner were more likely to be HIV-positive than those who did not report such violence, but no association was found between reporting rape perpetration and HIV prevalence.

Few studies in ESA have examined IPV perpetration against men, that is, whether men report being a victim of IPV and/or women report they perpetrated violence against male partners. A review of IPV research in high-income countries found that men and women were equally likely to perpetrate IPV (Capaldi et al., 2012), and two ESA studies that examined this question found similar proportions of women and men reported having perpetuated IPV and having been victimized (Gass et al., 2011; Mulawa et al., 2018). Both experiences (IPV victimization and perpetration) could contribute to the increased risk of acquiring HIV among ABYM.

Individual-level risk factors

Substance use

Alcohol and drug use may affect risk of HIV acquisition due to the disinhibitory effects of these substances on decision-making about sexual behaviours such as condom use (Kalichman et al., 2007). A number of studies in ESA have shown greater alcohol use among school-age males than females. A review of national prevalence and sentinel surveillance studies in South Africa found significant gender differences in alcohol use, with adolescent males more likely to have ever consumed alcohol, engaged in binge drinking, and driven or walked under the influence of alcohol than their female counterparts (Ramsoomar and Morojele, 2012). For example, in one such study, the percentage of adolescent boys aged 14–17 who reported alcohol use more than once a month was twice as high as it was among their female counterparts (30.3% vs 14.2%; $p < 0.01$) (Miller et al., 2017). Another study, in peri-urban areas of South Africa, found that adolescent males aged 16–18 who had been exposed to violence and those who were sexually active were four times as likely to have used alcohol in the past six months than those not having these experiences. In comparison, adolescent females who had been exposed to violence and who were sexually active each were 2.5 times more likely to have used alcohol in this period. Regarding drug use, being older (17 or 18 vs 16 years) and sexually active were associated with drug use among male adolescents (Magidson et al., 2017), whereas depressive symptomatology was a correlate of drug use among female adolescents. These findings suggest that targeted interventions to reduce alcohol and drug use may be important for reducing HIV risk among ABYM. One such intervention showing promise for reducing drug and alcohol use was conducted among unemployed men aged 18–25 in two Cape Town neighbourhoods that were randomized to an immediate intervention condition with access to a soccer program, random rapid diagnostic tests for alcohol and drug use, and an opportunity to enter a vocational training program, or a delayed control condition. Between the pre and post assessments, the frequency of substance use decreased, and employment and income increased in the immediate condition compared to the delayed condition (Rotheram-Borus et al., 2016).

Mental health

Few studies have examined associations between mental health and sexual risk behaviour among HIV-negative youth in ESA, but several have shown that mental health status is associated with sexual risk behaviour among ABYM, and that indicators of social, political and economic marginalisation of young people may be a contributory factor to their depressive symptomology (Gibbs et al., 2016). For example, in Tanzania, among 1113 sexually active young men, 43.4% of whom were aged 15–24, higher anxiety and depression scores were significantly associated with both decreased condom use and increased partnership concurrency (Hill et al., 2017). Additionally, baseline data from a cluster randomized controlled trial of the Stepping Stones HIV prevention intervention in South Africa with 1002 female and 976 male volunteers aged 15 to 26 found that ABYM with depressive symptoms were significantly more likely to report ever having had transactional sex and ever having perpetrated IPV and rape, and were less likely to report correct condom use at last sex; at 12 months follow-up, baseline depressive symptomology was significantly associated with failure to use a condom at last sex among ABYM. A cross-sectional survey among 1495 Zimbabwean youth aged 15–23 from 12 rural communities found that being at risk for affective disorders was associated with having multiple sexual partners, younger age of sexual debut, and alcohol and drug use among both ABYM and AGYW (Langhaug et al., 2010).

Key social-cognitive factors

Accurate knowledge of HIV prevention among young people aged 15–24 was similar between ABYM and AGYW, based on household survey data from 23 priority focus countries (the majority in SSA) between 2011 and 2016 (UNAIDS, 2017b). A recent review of 63 HIV prevention studies that addressed the effects of sexual self-efficacy (one's perceived control of or confidence in the ability to perform a given sexual behaviour) on condom use and sexual refusal among male and female adolescents aged 10–25 in SSA indicated that ABYM generally had higher condom use self-efficacy than AGYW, and promotion of condom self-efficacy was reported to increase condom use among ABYM only (Closson et al., 2018).

Risk perception is an important cognition, as individuals who perceive themselves to be at risk may engage in avoidant behaviours to reduce acquisition of HIV (Brewer et al., 2004). Most studies have focused on individual-level factors that influence young people's perceived risk of HIV, but school/community-level factors can also be determinants of risk perception (Anderson et al., 2007; Maticka-Tyndale and Tenkorang, 2010). A cross-sectional study of sexually experienced primary school youth in Kenya included measures at the individual and community levels; it found that among adolescent boys, individual-level correlates of higher risk perception included higher knowledge about HIV/AIDS, rejection of myths surrounding HIV transmission and higher condom self-efficacy (Tenkorang and Maticka-Tyndale, 2014a). At the community level, boys living in communities with higher AIDS-related mortality had higher risk perceptions, indicating that community-level factors are also important.

Sexual practices

Sexual debut. Delaying sexual debut is a key prevention strategy among youth. Early sexual debut, often defined having had first sexual intercourse at age 14 or younger (Doyle et al., 2012; Richter et al., 2015; Durowade et al., 2017) (though there are variations by country and researcher), is more prevalent in girls than boys in many SSA countries (Idele et al., 2014) and has been associated with increased risk of HIV/STI acquisition (Singh et al., 2000). For example, a cross-sectional household survey in rural South Africa found that among ABYM aged 15–24 who reported sexual debut before age 15 (13.1%), 19% did not use condoms compared to 9% among those initiating sex after age 15, and in multivariable analysis, early sexual debut was a strong and statistically significant predictor of having three or more partners in the past three years (Harrison et al., 2010).

A study in Kenya among students aged 11–17 found that a greater proportion of boys reported having engaged in sex by age 12 (36%) compared to girls (16%) (Tenkorang and Maticka-Tyndale, 2014b). In multivariable analysis, after controlling for individual and school/community-level factors, perceiving a small or moderate risk of HIV, experiencing high levels of sexual pressure, knowing someone who died of AIDS, or endorsing a greater number of myths about HIV transmission were associated with early sexual debut among both male and female youth. Among males, sexual debut was delayed in communities where abstinence was the predominant message communicated to youth but sexual debut was positively associated with the number of male relatives talked to about AIDS. In terms of school- and community-level factors, for both male and female youth, living in communities where AIDS deaths were publicly acknowledged and attendance at schools where a Primary School Action for Better Health Programme had been present were associated with delayed sexual debut. Among males, living in communities in which promotion of abstinence was the predominant HIV prevention message communicated to youth was associated with delayed sexual debut, whereas living in communities where festivals incorporated HIV programming was associated with earlier sexual debut relative to youth in other communities.

Anal sex. Anal intercourse is often underreported or not acknowledged as a risk factor for HIV among young people in ESA. A growing body of research (Kalichman et al., 2009, 2011; Ybarra et al., 2018), including a systematic review (Baggaley et al., 2010; Owen et al., 2017), indicates that this practice is prevalent among adolescents and young people (Kalichman et al., 2009, 2011; Maswanya et al., 2012; Ybarra et al., 2018). Youth may engage in anal intercourse as a form of birth control (Roye et al., 2013; Duby and Colvin, 2014), as a means to preserve virginity and to provide male pleasure, and as an HIV risk-reduction strategy (on the basis of belief that there is a lower risk of HIV infection from anal than vaginal intercourse) (Harrison et al., 2006). A representative campus-wide survey in a South African tertiary institution found that 10.7% of young men and 3.4% of young women reported ever having engaged in anal sex (Hoffman et al., 2017). In a 2012 cross-sectional survey of 937 secondary school students aged 16–24 in South Africa, nearly three times the number of ABYM than AGYW reported ever having had anal sex (31% vs 11%), with only 5 of 349 ABYM reporting anal sex exclusively (Ybarra et al., 2018). The percentage of males who reported ever having anal sex increased with age: 55% among those aged 20–24 compared with 16% of those aged 16–17. The proportion of females who reported anal sex also increased with age, but to a lesser extent (10% among those aged 16–17 and 16% among those aged 20–24). This study did not distinguish between opposite-sex and same-sex partners, nor whether (for men) the anal sex was insertive or receptive. A population-based South African youth survey reported that young, presumably heterosexual men aged 15–24 who engaged in anal intercourse were twice as likely to be infected compared to those reporting vaginal intercourse only (Lane et al., 2006), with those aged 15–19 being about four times as likely to be infected if they engaged in anal intercourse, even accounting for associated risk behaviours. Of the studies of men who have sex with men, few include adolescent boys. Those that do are primarily bio-behavioural surveys to estimate HIV prevalence, viral load and HIV-related risk behaviours, and these studies generally do not provide age-disaggregated data on correlates of HIV infection (Hladik et al., 2017).

Transactional sex. Transactional sex – non-marital, non-commercial sex in exchange for material goods including money, gifts, as well as favours, in non-commercial relationships (Choudhry et al., 2015; Stoebenau et al., 2016) – has been associated with HIV risk. Some studies have shown high rates of transactional sex among AGYW, whereas others have shown transactional sex to be more common among ABYM. A recent review reported that several studies found a positive association between transactional sex and HIV infection among men, whereas other studies have found a weak and statistically non-significant inverse association (Wamoyi et al., 2016). Childhood exposure to abuse has been found to be a predictor of transactional sex among young rural men aged 15–26 in South Africa (Dunkle et al., 2007). In a community-based study of 15–24-year-old AIDS-orphaned and AIDS-affected adolescents and young adults in South Africa, living in an AIDS-affected family, being abused, and experiencing food insecurity were associated with heightened risk of transactional sex among both ABYM and AGYW.

Analysis of sexually active young people (1516 ABYM and 2824 AGYW) aged 15–24 from a nationally representative population-based survey in Uganda found that transactional sex increased the risk of HIV infection (Choudhry et al., 2015). Among ABYM, 5.2% reported paying for sex, and their HIV prevalence was eight times higher than that of ABYM who did not report paying for sex, even after adjusting for socio-demographic characteristics and other risky sexual behaviours. Lower educational level, ever having been forced to have sex against their will, and having multiple concurrent sexual relationships were significantly associated with having paid for sex in the 12 months prior to the survey; paying for sex was also associated with increased odds of testing HIV-positive, even after adjusting for socio-demographics and other risky sexual behaviours. Similarly, another study in Uganda found that providing or seeking gifts, money, or compensation in exchange for sex was common among both male and female university students (23% of males; 38% of females) (Choudhry et al., 2014). Survey data from a 2012 nationally representative sample of 1574 adolescents aged 10–19 in Nigeria reported that significantly fewer male (11.6%) than female (29.1%) adolescents had engaged in transactional sex ($p < 0.001$) and had sex with partners who were ten or more years older (4.6% of males; 18.2% of females among those who knew age of their sexual partners) ($p<0.001$) (Folayan et al., 2014).

Group sex. Group sex and partner swapping associated with experimentation and pleasing partners and peers have been reported as an emerging sexual risk behaviour, increasing the likelihood of condomless sex, by both adolescent boys and girls in South Africa (Dietrich et al., 2011). The prevalence of this practice is unknown in ESA.

HIV testing

HIV testing is an important component of various prevention strategies and a key component of the WHO 90–90–90 targets, with the first goal being that 90% of those infected with HIV know that they are infected by 2020.

Prevalence of undiagnosed HIV is higher among adolescents than adults (UNAIDS, 2017; WHO et al., 2013). Between 2005 and 2010, fewer than 1 in 5 women and men aged 15–24 were estimated to be aware of their HIV status. Additionally, between 2005 and 2012, AIDS-related deaths among adolescents increased by about 50% (from 71,000 in 2005 to 110,000 in 2012) compared to a 32% decrease in all other age groups during the same period. One study has suggested that this high mortality rate may be due to the low HIV testing rates, which contribute to late initiation of care (Idele et al., 2014).

In ESA, there have been long-standing concerns about the low HIV testing rates among adult men compared to women (WHO et al., 2013). Adolescents have less access to HIV testing and counselling services than adults, but many studies have documented similar gender patterns in testing (Pettifor et al., 2005; MacPhail et al., 2009; Ramirez-Avila et al., 2012; Peltzer and Matseke, 2013; Idele et al., 2014). Based on data from 2006 to 2012, HIV testing rates among boys aged 15–19 in ESA were estimated at 20% compared to 29% among girls of the same age (Idele et al., 2014). In SSA between 2005 and 2009, only about 4% of boys and 6% of girls aged 15–19 (ratio of 1:1.5) tested for HIV and received the test results in the prior 12 months, and while the proportion tested increased in both age groups between 2010 and 2015, the gender disparities also increased (9% of boys and 14% of girls; ratio of 1:1.6) (UNICEF, 2016b). A similar trend of increasing testing rates among adolescents coupled with increasing gender disparities was seen in South Africa's national surveys, with 17.7% of male and 32.7% of female sexually experienced youth aged 15–24 ever having been tested for HIV in 2003 (ratio of 1:1.9) compared with 36.3% and 75.5% in 2008, respectively (ratio of 1:2.1) (Peltzer and Matseke, 2013). The lower testing rates among ABYM is an important gap to address, given that HIV testing is the gateway to treatment access. The gap may be due to several factors, including masculine norms which dissuade men from using health services (Skovdal et al., 2011; Wyrod, 2011), women's greater use of health services because of pregnancy, and insufficiently targeted male prevention programmes.

As with adults, gender differences in HIV testing among adolescents may be related to early pregnancy, as pregnant women of all ages are tested as part of antenatal care (Idele et al., 2014). An analysis from South Africa's 2003 national survey data of predictors of ever having tested for HIV among sexually active 15–24-year-olds found that ever having talked to a parent about HIV/AIDS, having participated in loveLife (an HIV education and prevention program), and higher frequency of health clinic visits were significantly associated with having been tested among both ABYM and AGYW. Ever having been pregnant, urban residence, and ever having initiated a conversation about HIV/AIDS were predictors of having been tested among AGYW only. Knowing someone who died of AIDS, older age, and having completed high school were predictors of having been tested for ABYM only (MacPhail et al., 2009; Peltzer and Matseke, 2013). In a 2006–2007 household serosurvey in Tanzania in which voluntary testing and counselling was offered, 15–24-year-old ABYM were significantly less likely to accept testing than men aged 25–34, but this was not the case for AGYW in relation to older women. An intervention in Zambia that offered door-to-door HIV testing to 15–19-year-old adolescents found that the most common reason for refusing among younger adolescents was that they did not feel they were at risk for HIV (37% of males and 32% of females age 15), and among 19-year-old adolescents, the most common reason for refusing was having tested recently (35% males and 44% females) (Shanaube et al., 2017). A study in Mozambique among 16–20-year-old adolescents recruited from two schools found that boys were less likely to have ever been tested (19.1% vs 46.7% of girls), although they were more likely to perceive themselves as being at risk for HIV infection (46% vs 28.6% of girls) (Hector et al., 2018).

Restrictions related to the age of consent for testing can hinder access to HIV testing and other health services for both ABYM and AGYW (Fox et al., 2013; WHO et al., 2013). Depending on the ESA country, the age of consent for HIV testing ranges from 12 to 18, with three countries having no law or policy and two countries not defining an age of consent (Armstrong et al., 2018). However, a number of countries include conditions under which minors can provide consent despite not being of legal age. Pregnancy is one such exception in a number of countries (Fox et al., 2013). In a qualitative study among 13–18-year-olds and their caregivers who were recruited from healthcare clinics in Kenya, both boys and girls wanted the power to consent to HIV testing without needing a guardian's permission. However, their caregivers felt that they should be notified of the HIV test results even if the adolescent under their care did not want to share them (Wilson et al., 2017). Other studies in Kenya among healthcare providers found that many were uncomfortable providing HIV testing and counselling services to adolescents. Their concerns included doubts about younger adolescents' autonomy to consent and fear they would inappropriately disclose their HIV-positive test results and be stigmatized, uncertainty that adolescents would adhere to providers' advice given during counselling and testing, and the providers' own lack of confidence in counselling and communication with adolescents in general (Godia et al., 2013; Wagner et al., 2018).

The intervention landscape

Biomedical prevention strategies

Pre-exposure prophylaxis (PrEP)

In 2018 the US Food and Drug Administration (FDA) and World Health Organization (WHO) expanded approval of Truvada (emtricitabine/tenofovir disoproxil fumarate) as pre-exposure prophylaxis (PrEP) against HIV to include its use by adolescents at risk (Gilead Sciences, 2018). Nevertheless, PrEP data relevant to adolescents are lacking (World Health Organization, 2016), including guidelines around episodic use (Elsesser et al., 2016) and key information about how to promote PrEP uptake and adherence. One US study found that PrEP adherence decreased among adolescent men who have sex with men (MSM) as the frequency of follow-up visits decreased (Hosek et al., 2017). A study in South Africa also found decreased adherence over time (Gill et al., 2017) and no evidence of increased risky sexual behaviour (which was a possibility if individuals felt PrEP completely prevented HIV infection) over a three-month period on PrEP among male and female adolescents (Maljaars et al., 2017).

There are multiple barriers to PrEP uptake for adolescents (Koechlin et al., 2017). On the one hand, service providers have difficulties in identifying PrEP-eligible adolescents and can be reluctant to prescribe without parental consent. On the other hand, adolescents' own discomfort and lack of confidence can constrain them from seeking use of PrEP. Long-term adherence may be a major challenge because of developmental issues, but this is not yet known.

Voluntary medical male circumcision (VMMC)

VMMC was associated with an approximate 60% reduction in HIV acquisition in RCTs in SSA (Auvert et al., 2005; Bailey et al., 2007; Gray et al., 2007). Expansion of VMMC is an essential component of the joint UNAIDS strategy for ending AIDS by 2030 (UNAIDS, 2014; Hines et al., 2017; UNAIDS and WHO, 2018). Nearly 15 million VMMCs in 14 ESA countries were performed between 2007 and 2017 and are expected to avert over 500,000 new infections by 2030.

Overall, younger men seem to have more favourable attitudes towards VMMC. This has been evident in the numbers of younger men undergoing circumcision in Tanzania, Eswatini, Kenya and Uganda (Westercamp et al., 2012; Ashengo et al., 2014; Hines et al., 2017). Studies have shown that acceptability among young people is highest when the targeted age groups conform to those ages among whom traditional circumcision is usually performed (Ngalande et al., 2006). Following evidence that uptake was considerably higher in 10–14-year-old boys than in older males, in 2016 the WHO and UNAIDS developed a new strategy that incorporates VMMC as an integral component of public health services for young men. Similar to HIV testing and accessing PrEP, this shift in prioritization of age groups has required changes to consent laws in some ESA countries, reducing the requirements for parental permission (Herman-Roloff et al., 2011). For some ABYM, VMMC is an entry point for accessing other health services.

Peers and trusted adults may be able to encourage ABYM to take up VMMC by emphasizing the ancillary benefits that some endorse, most commonly penile hygiene (Weiss et al., 2008; Mbonye et al., 2016) and sexual potency (Peltzer and Kanta, 2009). These benefits are often part of promotional campaigns, such as the Make-the-Cut-Plus trial in Zimbabwe, a sports campaign designed to increase VMMC uptake among secondary school boys aged 14–20 (DeCelles et al., 2016). Both this study and a Uganda study (Miiro et al., 2017) found that strong bonding between interested boys and a circumcised coach, who discussed circumcision and its health benefits, was important to the motivation of ABYM to undergo VMMC. In other studies, the social network of the ABYM was demonstrated to be an influential source regarding the decision to undergo VMMC, particularly for adolescents, and peers have been shown to alleviate concerns about pain and to promote the benefits in terms of sexual pleasure (Montaño et al., 2014; Osaki et al., 2015; Lilleston et al., 2017). Some studies have shown that parents and other family members also wield influence on young ABYM decisions on VMMC (Mugwanya et al., 2011; Jayeoba et al., 2012). In Botswana, after an informational session, most parents encouraged VMMC for their sons (Jayeoba et al., 2012), although the majority felt that the son should be the principal decision-maker. Conversely, in other studies, parents found it challenging to support VMMC and were reluctant to counsel due in part to their discomfort in talking about sex with their sons as well as concern that their sons would be stigmatised if VMMC was conditional upon HIV testing (Dam et al., 2018). For example, in a study in Uganda, most parents preferred infant circumcision, with only 5% wanting 11–15-year-olds to be circumcised (Mugwanya et al., 2011). The contexts for parental influence remain unclear but deserve further evaluation.

Barriers to accessing VMMC services can depend on age, as concerns about VMMC among older ABYM differ from those of younger ABYM, where the latter seem to worry primarily about pain (George et al., 2014), time away from school, and poor quality or unsafe services. Among older, married ABYM, wives are an important source of influence, and some of these men report that their wives may refuse to have sex with uncircumcised partners (Price et al., 2014; Osaki et al., 2015; Lilleston et al., 2017).

Older ABYM also worried about costs and time not working (Evens et al., 2014), as well as that the recovery time would give their spouses licence to engage in sexual activity outside the partnership. All ABYM indicated concern about long-term erectile problems (Jayeoba et al., 2012). Financial incentives have had some success in supporting older ABYM to miss work to undergo the procedure; it is unclear if these are as effective in younger males. Finally, some data suggest that beliefs about upholding traditional circumcision affect acceptability and uptake of VMMC; for example if VMMC is performed in a hospital, it is difficult to perform traditional circumcision rituals (Mshana et al., 2011).

Despite concerns about sexual risk compensation (increase in risky behaviours after circumcision), evidence-based research in real-world settings does not appear to support this. For example, a study in KwaZulu-Natal found no evidence of increased sexual risk behaviours (number of sex partners, condom use, transactional sex) or decreased HIV risk perception in a 12-month period following VMMC among secondary school male students (Govender et al., 2018).

Interventions to increase testing rates among ABYM

A number of studies have evaluated the impact of door-to-door, home-based HIV testing on HIV testing rates. Results show that making HIV testing available at home increases testing rates substantially among adolescents as well as adults and also seems to decrease gender disparities in testing. Studies of door-to-door HIV testing campaigns with ABYM from South Africa, Malawi, Zambia and Uganda have shown high acceptance rates, ranging from 85.6% to 99% (Were et al., 2006; Angotti et al., 2009; Isingo et al., 2012; Naik et al., 2012; Govindasamy et al., 2015; Shanaube et al., 2017).

A study conducted among 15–24-year-old AGYW and ABYM in Tanzania showed significant differences in the effectiveness of two different methods of HIV testing but no substantive gender differences in testing uptake. The study offered HIV testing after conducting interviews with participants in a central location within the community, either using an opt-out approach that involved the interviewer offering HIV counselling and testing immediately following the interview, which individuals could decline, or an opt-in approach, in which after completing the interview, participants were told that they could access HIV testing in a room down the hall. Among both ABYM and AGYW and across age bands, the opt-out approach was associated with much higher testing rates than the opt-in approach (Baisley et al., 2012).

HIV self-testing (HIVST) may be an approach to increase testing coverage among adolescents. A study that recruited adolescents from two schools in Mozambique and offered them directly assisted oral HIVST through two youth-friendly clinics found that although not statistically significant, females were more likely to test than males (OR = 1.30, 95% CI = 0.79–2.13) (Hector et al., 2018).

Interventions to alter behaviours or exposures that increase risk

Interventions to reduce IPV

Although a number of systematic reviews of interventions to address IPV have been conducted, of the interventions included in these reviews, only the Stepping Stones intervention in South Africa reported data for young men (Jewkes et al., 2008). An evaluation of this program, which used participatory learning to improve HIV prevention practices and enhance relationship skills, found that the intervention lowered the incidence of herpes infection (HSV-2) among men and women and decreased reported IPV perpetration, transactional sex, and problem drinking after a 12-month period among men but had no effect on lowering HIV incidence among men and women. An intervention that combined Stepping Stones with an economic empowerment component in Uganda (SHARE) and that included participants aged 15–49 showed a reduction in IPV and overall HIV incidence over a 16-month period (Wagman et al., 2015). Of the 4746 male participants, approximately 27% (n = 1305) were aged 15–24. Even though SHARE did not stratify results by age, the large proportion of young men and the promising reductions in IPV and HIV incidence suggest that this intervention may be effective among ABYM. Interventions in Ethiopia and Kenya have reported changes in HIV risk behaviours for young men, for example, increased HIV knowledge, improved condom negotiations, reductions in partner violence, and endorsement of more equitable gender norms (Pulerwitz, Michaelis, Verma et al., 2010; Pulerwitz, Michaelis, Weiss et al., 2010).

School-based interventions

Sexuality education, either as part of the standard school curriculum or through focused HIV risk-reduction interventions in school settings, has long been viewed as an excellent approach for transmitting the knowledge, attitudes and skills necessary to reduce HIV-related risk behaviours to adolescents in low- and middle-income countries (Kirby et al., 2006, 2007; Adelekan, 2017). School-based interventions have the potential to reach large numbers of young people, to influence social norms of an entire youth cohort, and to alter key determinants of risk before youth become sexually active.

Systematic reviews of school-based interventions in SSA, both in earlier (Gallant and Maticka-Tyndale, 2004; Paul-Ebhohimhen et al., 2008; Harrison et al., 2010; Michielsen et al., 2010; Napierala Mavedzenge et al., 2011) and more recent years (Sani et al., 2016), have concluded that school-based interventions can be effective at increasing knowledge, positive attitudes towards protective sexual behaviours and self-efficacy to enact these behaviours, and there is some evidence that they have a positive effect on self-reported protective sexual behaviours (Sani et al., 2016). In a recent meta-analysis, effective school-based interventions were more often adapted from other programmes, were theory-based, included provision of health services and activities outside school, and were monitored to ensure they were implemented according to protocol (Sani et al., 2016). Despite the encouraging results of this meta-analysis, one-half of the school-based interventions included in the review did not show statistically significant positive effects on protective sexual behaviours. Identified reasons for the limited effectiveness of programs included teacher resistance and/or poor skills to teach sexuality-focused curricula and limited ability of schools alone to alter deeply ingrained cultural norms and values around sexual behaviour (Maticka-Tyndale et al., 2007; Adelekan, 2017).

Few school-based interventions have evaluated effects on STI or other biological outcomes. A recent Cochrane review and meta-analysis (not restricted to SSA) concluded that six studies with these outcomes (three of which were in SSA) provided no demonstrable evidence of an effect on prevalence of HIV or other STIs (Mason-Jones et al., 2016).

Whether school-based interventions have differential effects for young men versus young women is unknown. Curricula for school-based interventions typically are the same for both girls and boys, and the intervention is delivered to girls and boys together, although results may be reported separately by gender. We reviewed 20 school-based interventions that were conducted in ESA in 2005 or later, which were identified from among those included in the two most recent systematic reviews of such interventions (Mason-Jones et al., 2016; Sani et al., 2016) and two identified elsewhere (Harrison et al., 2012; Maticka-Tyndale et al., 2014). Of these, nine reported results disaggregated by gender or tested if an intervention effect was present for both boys and girls. Even though an earlier review and meta-analysis reported that condom use at last sex only increased among males (Michielsen et al., 2010), we found no consistent pattern of differential intervention effects by gender.

Cash transfers

Interventions using cash transfers – either an unconditional benefit or a benefit conditional on achieving a specific behaviour or outcome – have often been adopted to mitigate the effects of poverty and gender inequalities on elevated risk for HIV infection among AGYW (United Nations Development Programme, 2014). Only a few studies have been conducted to assess the effects of these programs on boys. Considering unconditional cash transfers, three studies have evaluated whether state-sponsored social benefits programs, which provide cash to low-income households with eligible children, affect youth sexual risk behaviours. Two studies found significant effects among girls but not among boys. These included a study of Kenya's cash transfer program for orphans and vulnerable children, which observed that girls in cash-transfer households delayed sexual debut, and a South African study, which found lower prevalence and incidence of transactional and age-disparate sex among girls in households receiving cash transfers (Cluver et al., 2013). However, the third study found that whereas cash transfers along with provision of free school meals and/or food gardens reduced HIV risk behaviours among girls but not boys, an intervention that also included positive parenting and teacher support components led to substantial reductions in HIV risk behaviours among both girls and boys (Cluver et al., 2014).

Considering conditional cash transfer (CCT) interventions, the Rewarding Sexually Transmitted Infection Prevention and Control in Tanzania (RESPECT) project randomized 2399 rural Tanzanians aged 18–30 (and spouses aged 16 or over) to one of two conditions that provided cash incentives dependent on negative test results from periodic screenings for curable STIs (de Walque et al., 2014). The intervention demonstrated that compared with those in the control arm (no incentives), those in the arm that received a thrice-yearly $20 incentive for remaining STI-negative had lower incidence of STIs, but those that received a $10 incentive did not. There was no difference in effect between males and females, but significantly, a follow-up survey one year after completion of the intervention showed sustained effectiveness among young men but not among young women (de Walque et al., 2014). In contrast, a study in Malawi that provided cash on the condition that individuals stayed HIV-negative over the course of one year had no significant effect on remaining HIV-negative (Kohler and Thornton, 2012). However, the cash incentives in this study were smaller than those in RESPECT, which might account for the lack of effect. Yet shortly after the final payment, men who had received the incentive increased risky sex, whereas women decreased risky sexual behaviour. An RCT in Lesotho also produced mixed results. It involved 3426 young adults, men and women, who were randomly assigned to a control arm or to one of two intervention arms. Both intervention arms provided participants with a lottery ticket every four months with a chance to win either $50 (low-incentive arm) or $100 (high-incentive arm) conditional on testing negative for curable STIs (Björkman Nyqvist et al., 2015). An evaluation after two years of implementing the intervention revealed an overall 21.4% reduction in HIV incidence as well as reductions in curable STIs. However, there was no significant reduction in HIV incidence in men alone, although the study was not well-powered to detect differences by gender.

Moving forward to address gaps

Achieving an AIDS-free generation requires actively engaging ABYM in HIV prevention interventions that have optimal impact, documenting unmet prevention needs, and outlining an onward blueprint for research. Regrettably, there are many research and programmatic gaps.

The following list highlights key gaps and suggests some strategies to address them.

1 Analytic shortcomings contribute to lack of understanding of the determinants of risk behaviours among ABYM (Amoateng et al., 2013; Tenkorang and Maticka-Tyndale, 2014b). Few studies provide gender- and age-disaggregated data and other contextual factors, making it difficult to identify salient beliefs, attitudes, and behaviours to target among ABYM overall and among specific age groups, and to design gender-, age- and developmentally-appropriate HIV prevention strategies. Specifically, analyses of disaggregated age data across five-year age bands (10–14, 15–19, and 20–24) and by gender are needed to allow for more nuanced understanding of risk and prevention practices of ABYM for the design of HIV programmes and tackling the adolescent AIDS epidemic – a need underscored by UNICEF and UNAIDS (UNAIDS, 2016a; UNICEF, 2016c).
2 There is a dearth of studies of sub-populations of ABYM, especially adolescents 10–14 years of age. Young adolescents may be neglected because of age of consent requirements for research participation without parental permission (often 18 years and older), making it more cumbersome for researchers to obtain ethics approval, and by adolescents' unwillingness to participate due to confidentiality concerns. Additionally, studies are few among sexual minority adolescents, especially among young men who have sex with men, which is perhaps not surprising given the stigmatisation of homosexuality in most ESA countries (Carroll and Mendos, 2017).
3 Across SSA, adolescents have less access to HIV testing and counselling than adults because the legal age of consent for HIV testing is a barrier (Fox et al., 2013; WHO et al., 2013). However, ABYM are even less likely to access HIV testing compared to their female counterparts (UNICEF, 2013; Idele et al., 2014; UNICEF, 2016a). Pregnancy at an early age may explain some of this discrepancy as it circumvents the age of consent for girls in some countries (MacPhail et al., 2009; Fox et al., 2013; Idele et al., 2014), but health-seeking behaviour is another likely explanation. Interventions that make HIV testing immediately available at home have generally been associated with high uptake and little or no gender disparity (Were et al., 2006; Angotti et al., 2009; Naik et al., 2012; Govindasamy et al., 2015), whereas interventions that require young people to go to a clinic for directly assisted oral HIV self-testing yielded non-statistically significant but lower uptake among boys than girls (Hector et al., 2018).

   More research is needed to identify barriers and facilitators to HIV testing among ABYM in order to develop interventions to increase their testing rates, decrease gender disparities and initiate positive HIV testing habits that may continue throughout life (Govindasamy et al., 2015). Tailored interventions to make testing more accessible and friendly to ABYM, such as home-based testing, and in social contexts where ABYM congregate, such as sports fields, workplace, and secondary schools and tertiary institutions, may be effective in increasing uptake of testing and counselling services by ABYM. At the same time, ongoing training of healthcare providers is essential to creating a conducive environment for ABYM-friendly services.

4 Most studies of adolescent sexual behaviour in ESA focus on individual-level risk factors and behaviour. While some studies recognize the importance of contextual factors, few examine how factors such as parental monitoring, interactions with peers and teachers, family structure and family socio-economic status influence sexual risk.
5 Targeting adolescent boys at ages when they are developing behavioural patterns that will endure throughout adulthood is essential for transforming masculinity from harmful masculine practices and enacting positive gender-equitable social norms. With transition to adulthood, adolescents begin to develop an understanding of their current and future roles and responsibilities in society (Erikson, 1959). It is at this critical transitional juncture that they develop the behaviours – including risky and sometimes violent as well as protective practices – which they may continue to engage in throughout their adult lives. For younger adolescent boys, we need to understand their experiences with masculine norms and focus interventions around the time of sexual debut. Interventions that address sexual health communications between parents/guardians and adolescents might be a pragmatic approach.
6 To support the global movement to expand and upgrade comprehensive sexuality education for youth, additional research is needed to identify curricula that, beyond improving knowledge, can alter skills and behaviours (UNFPA, 2015). Special attention needs to be given to identifying and addressing the unmet sexual health needs of young men and to promoting gender-equitable norms among both young men and women.
7 More research is needed on the differential effects among girls and boys on cash incentives to promote staying in school and performing specific health-related behaviours.
8 Addressing the gap in IPV and HIV research among ABYM is critical given gender differences in adolescent development and HIV risk. Research on IPV has shown that it is easier to prevent than treat. A series of interventions has targeted women and men, but less research has focused on ABYM. Therefore, it is vital to offer interventions that target and are tailored to ABYM at a young age (O'Leary et al., 2012). Future research should report age-stratified findings to determine what IPV interventions may be most effective for ABYM.

In addition, IPV among MSM and transgender youth has been understudied, especially in ESA. Research in South Africa has included predominantly adult MSM, primarily of White/European racial identity and gay sexual identity (Stephenson et al., 2011). Strategies are needed to ascertain the prevalence of IPV (both experience and perpetration) among non-white MSM in ESA, especially those under 18 years of age.

9 Interventions for ABYM must be youth-centric and grounded in the realities of youth's lives, fully engaging and mobilizing them in intervention development. A youth-centred design strategy, which entails understanding user needs and insights, ideation (brainstorming creative solutions, building representation of ideas [prototypes]) and implementation (sharing prototypes with users and obtaining feedback and refining intervention) to co-design innovative interventions with youth, is increasingly being applied in global health programs and should become the norm (IDEO.org, 2014; Vechakul et al., 2015).
10 Use of male peer-driven and social network intervention models may be effective in reaching ABYM given the importance of peer norms. AGYW could also serve as champions for their male partners' health, encouraging them to seek prevention services.
11 Establishment of dedicated male sexual health clinics may be an effective way to reach ABYM who have sex with men and who would otherwise forgo seeking public health services.
12 As part of combination HIV prevention, PrEP should be integrated into ABYM-friendly sexual health services, with outreach to older at-risk youth in sports clubs and youth centres.
13 The association of anxiety and depression with lower condom use and greater likelihood of sexual partner concurrency highlights the need for addressing mental health issues and for exploring the feasibility of integrating mental health components into HIV prevention interventions for ABYM.
14 Anal sex needs to be explicitly discussed in age-appropriate adolescent HIV prevention and sexual health programming (Ybarra et al., 2018).

In sum, ABYM must be part of the solution to interrupt the cycle of HIV transmission. Even though ABYM are at lower risk than AGYW for HIV acquisition, they are not at zero risk due to their risk-taking behaviours. Culturally reinforced masculinities that encourage male dominance, along with men's inability to uphold these gendered expectations within the context of structural inequalities, ultimately contribute to HIV risk among both ABYM and AGYW. As adolescent boys grow older, their risk of HIV exposure and transmission increases. Given that gender socialization occurs during early adolescence, it is important to target boys to engender sexual health and equitable gender norms.

The new MenStar Coalition launched by Sir Elton John and the Duke of Sussex in 2018 at the 22nd International AIDS Conference in Amsterdam specifically seeks to engage men in HIV epidemic control, and it is supported by committed funding of over USD 1.2 billion (MenStar Coalition, 2018). No single intervention will likely suffice to stem the HIV epidemic. Rather, a combination of biomedical, behavioural and structural interventions that target not only HIV risk behaviours but also upstream factors associated with risk behaviour, such as poverty and harmful masculine norms, will be needed. A recent editorial in the *Lancet* reminds us that "being gender blind benefits neither men nor women" and calls attention to how machismo can increase risk-taking behaviour and deter boys and men from accessing health services ("Gender and health," 2018).

References

Adelekan, M. (2017) 'A critical review of the effectiveness of educational interventions applied in HIV/AIDS prevention no title', *Patient Education and Counseling*, 100(Suppl. 1), pp. S11–S16. doi.org/10.1016/j.pec.2015.12.004.

Amoateng, A., Kalule-Sabiti, I. and Arkaah, Y. (2013) 'Social structure and sexual behaviour of Black African adolescents in the North West Province, South Africa', *South African Review of Sociology*, 44(1), pp. 131–157. doi:10.1080/21528586.2013.784453.

Anderson, K. G., Beutel, A. M. and Maughan-Brown, B. (2007) 'HIV risk perceptions and first sexual intercourse among youth in Cape Town South Africa', *International Family Planning Perspectives*, 33(3), pp. 98–105. doi:10.1363/3309807.

Angotti, N. et al. (2009) 'Increasing the acceptability of HIV counseling and testing with three C's: Convenience, confidentiality and credibility', *Social Science and Medicine*, 68(12), pp. 2263–2270. doi:10.1016/j.socscimed.2009.02.041.

Armstrong, A. et al. (2018) 'A global research agenda for adolescents living with HIV', *JAIDS: Journal of Acquired Immune Deficiency Syndromes*, 78(Suppl. 1), pp. S16–S21. doi:10.1097/QAI.0000000000001744.

Ashengo, T. A. et al. (2014) 'Voluntary medical male circumcision (VMMC) in Tanzania and Zimbabwe: Service delivery intensity and modality and their influence on the age of clients', *PLoS One*, 9(5), p. e83642. doi:10.1371/journal.pone.0083642.

Auvert, B. et al. (2005) 'Randomized, controlled intervention trial of male circumcision for reduction of HIV infection risk: The ANRS 1265 trial', *PLoS Medicine*, 3(5), p. e298. doi:10.1371/journal.pmed.0020298.

Baggaley, R. F., White, R. G. and Boily, M. C. (2010) 'HIV transmission risk through anal intercourse: Systematic review, meta-analysis and implications for HIV prevention', *International Journal of Epidemiology*, 39(4), pp. 1048–1063. doi:10.1093/ije/dyq057.

Bailey, R. C. et al. (2007) 'Male circumcision for HIV prevention in young men in Kisumu, Kenya: A randomised controlled trial', *Lancet*, 369(9562), pp. 643–656. doi:10.1016/S0140-6736(07)60312-2.

Baisley, K. et al. (2012) 'Uptake of voluntary counselling and testing among young people participating in an HIV prevention trial: Comparison of opt-out and opt-in strategies', *PLoS One*, 7(7), p. e42108. doi:10.1371/journal.pone.0042108.

Barker, G. and Ricardo, C. (2005) 'Young men and the construction of masculinity in sub-Saharan Africa: Implications for HIV/AIDS, conflict and violence', *Social Development Papers: Conflict Prevention and Reconstruction*. Available at: http://www-wds.worldbank.org/servlet/WDSContentServer/WDSP/IB/2005/06/23/000012009_20050623134235/Rendered/PDF/327120rev0PAPER0AFR0young0men0WP26.pdf.

Björkman Nyqvist, M. et al. (2015) *Using lotteries to incentivize safer sexual behavior: Evidence from a randomized controlled trial on HIV prevention.* World Bank Policy Research Working Paper. Washington, DC: World Bank.

Boerma, J.T. et al. (2002) 'Sociodemographic context of the AIDS epidemic in a rural area in "Tanzania" with a focus on people's mobility and marriage', *Sexually Transmitted Infections,* 78(Suppl. 1), pp. i97–i105. doi:10.1136/sti.78.suppl_1.i97.

Brewer, N.T. et al. (2004) 'Risk perceptions and their relation to risk behavior', *Annals of Behavioral Medicine,* 27(2), pp. 125–130. doi:10.1207/s15324796abm2702_7.

Bronfenbrenner, U. and Ceci, S.J. (1994) 'Nature-nurture reconceptualized in developmental perspective: A bioecological model', *Psychological Review,* 101(4), pp. 568–586. doi:10.1037/0033-295X.101.4.568.

Camlin, C.S. et al. (2014) ' "She mixes her business": HIV transmission and acquisition risks among female migrants in Western Kenya', *Social Science and Medicine,* 102, pp. 146–156. doi:10.1016/j.socscimed.2013.11.004.

Capaldi, D.M. et al. (2012) 'A systematic review of risk factors for intimate partner violence', *Partner Abuse,* 3(2), pp. 231–280. doi:10.1891/1946-6560.3.2.e4.

Carroll, A. and Mendos, L. (2017) *State-sponsored homophobia 2017: A world survey of sexual orientation laws: Criminalisation, protection and recognition.* International Lesbian, Gay, Bisexual, Trans and Intersex Association. Available at: https://ilga.org/downloads/2017/ILGA_State_Sponsored_Homophobia_2017_WEB.pdf.

Choudhry, V. et al. (2014) 'Giving or receiving something for sex: A cross-sectional study of transactional sex among Ugandan university students', *PLoS One,* 9(11), p. 112431. doi:10.1371/journal.pone.0112431.

Choudhry, V. et al. (2015) 'Transactional sex and HIV risks – evidence from a cross-sectional national survey among young people in Uganda', *Global Health Action,* 8, p. 27249. doi:10.3402/gha.v8.27249.

Closson, K. et al. (2018) 'Sexual self-efficacy and gender: A review of condom use and sexual negotiation among young men and women in sub-Saharan Africa', *Journal of Sex Research,* 55(4–5), pp. 522–539. doi:10.1080/00224499.2017.1421607.

Cluver, L., Orkin, M., Boyes, M., Gardner, F., Meinck, F. Transactional sex amongst AIDS-orphaned and AIDS-affected adolescents predicted by abuse and extreme poverty. *JAIDS: Journal of Acquired Immune Deficiency Syndromes,* 2011, 58 (3), pp. 336–343.

Cluver, L.D. et al. (2013) 'Child-focused state cash transfers and adolescent risk of HIV infection in South Africa: A propensity-score-matched case-control study', *Lancet Global Health,* 1(6), pp. e362–e370. doi:10.1016/S2214-109X(13)70115-3.

Cluver, L.D. et al. (2014) 'Cash plus care: Social protection cumulatively mitigates HIV-risk behaviour among adolescents in South Africa', *AIDS,* 28(Suppl. 3), pp. S389–S397. doi:10.1097/QAD.0000000000000340.

Cornell, M. and Dovel, K. (2018) 'Reaching key adolescent populations', *Current Opinion in HIV and AIDS,* 13(3), pp. 274–280. doi:10.1097/COH.0000000000000457.

Dam, K.H. et al. (2018) 'Parental communication, engagement, and support during the adolescent voluntary medical male circumcision experience', *Clinical Infectious Diseases,* 66(S3), pp. S189–S197. doi:10.1093/cid/cix970.

DeCelles, J. et al. (2016) 'Process evaluation of a sport-based voluntary medical male circumcision demand-creation intervention in Bulawayo, Zimbabwe', *Journal of Acquired Immune Deficiency Syndromes,* 72(Suppl 4), pp. S304–S308. doi:10.1097/QAI.0000000000001172.

Devries, K.M. et al. (2013) 'Intimate partner violence and incident depressive symptoms and suicide attempts: A systematic review of longitudinal studies', *PLoS Medicine,* 10(5), p. e1001439. doi:10.1371/journal.pmed.1001439.

de Walque, D., Dow, W.H. and Nathan, R. (2014) *Rewarding safer sex: Conditional cash transfers for HIV/STI prevention.* Washington, DC: World Bank.

DiCarlo, A.L. et al. (2014) ' "Men usually say that HIV testing is for women": Gender dynamics and perceptions of HIV testing in Lesotho', *Culture, Health and Sexuality,* 16(8), pp. 867–882. doi:10.1080/13691058.2014.913812.

Dietrich, J. et al. (2011) ' "Group sex" parties and other risk patterns: A qualitative study about the perceptions of sexual behaviours and attitudes of adolescents in Soweto, South Africa', *Vulnerable Children and Youth Studies,* 6(3), pp. 244–254. doi:10.1080/17450128.2011.597796.

Dovel, K. et al. (2015) 'Men's heightened risk of AIDS-related death: The legacy of gendered HIV testing and treatment strategies', *AIDS (London, England),* 29(10), pp. 1123–1125. doi:10.1097/QAD.0000000000000655.

Dovel, K. et al. (2016) 'Prioritizing strategies to reduce AIDS-related mortality for men in sub-Saharan Africa: Authors' reply', *AIDS (London, England) DS,* 30(1), pp. 158–159. doi:10.1097/QAD.0000000000000898.

Doyle, A.M. et al. (2012) 'The sexual behaviour of adolescents in sub-Saharan Africa: Patterns and trends from national surveys', *Tropical Medicine and International Health,* 17(7), pp. 796–807. doi:10.1111/j.1365-3156.2012.03005.x.

Duby, Z. and Colvin, C. (2014) 'Conceptualizations of heterosexual anal sex and HIV risk in five East African communities', *Journal of Sex Research,* 51(8), pp. 863–873. doi:10.1080/00224499.2013.871624.

Dude, A.M. (2011) 'Spousal intimate partner violence is associated with HIV and other STIs among married Rwandan women', *AIDS and Behavior,* 5(1), pp. 142–152. doi:10.1007/s10461-009-9526-1.

Dunkle, K.L. and Decker, M.R. (2013) 'Gender-based violence and HIV: Reviewing the evidence for links and causal pathways in the general population and high-risk groups', *American Journal of Reproductive Immunology,* 69(Suppl. 1), pp. 20–26. doi:10.1111/aji.12039.

Dunkle, K.L. et al. (2006) 'Perpetration of partner violence and HIV risk behaviour among young men in the rural Eastern Cape, South Africa', *AIDS,* 20(16), pp. 2107–2114. doi:10.1097/01.aids.0000247582.00826.52.

Dunkle, K.L. et al. (2007) 'Transactional sex with casual and main partners among young South African men in the rural Eastern Cape: Prevalence, predictors, and associations with gender-based violence', *Social Science and Medicine,* 65(6), pp. 1235–1248. doi:10.1016/j.socscimed.2007.04.029.

Durowade, K.A. et al. (2017) 'Early sexual debut: Prevalence and risk factors among secondary school students in Ido-Ekiti, Ekiti state, South-West Nigeria', *African Health Sciences,* 17(3), pp. 614–622. doi:10.4314/ahs.v17i3.3.

Elsesser, S.A. et al. (2016) 'Seasons of risk: Anticipated behavior on vacation and interest in episodic antiretroviral pre-exposure prophylaxis (PrEP) among a large national sample of U.S. men who have sex with men (MSM)', *AIDS and Behavior,* 20(7), pp. 1400–1407. doi:10.1007/s10461-015-1238-0.

Erikson, E.H. (1959) *Identity and the life cycle: Selected papers.* New York: International University Press.

Evens, E. et al. (2014) 'Identifying and addressing barriers to uptake of voluntary medical male circumcision in Nyanza, Kenya among men 18–35: A qualitative study', *PLoS One,* 9(6), p. e98221. doi:10.1371/journal.pone.0098221.

Folayan, M.O. et al. (2014) 'Differences in sexual behaviour and sexual practices of adolescents in Nigeria based on sex and self-reported HIV status', *Reproductive Health*, 11, 83. doi:10.1186/1742-4755-11-83.

Fonck, K. et al. (2005) 'Increased risk of HIV in women experiencing physical partner violence in Nairobi, Kenya', *AIDS and Behavior*, 9(3), pp. 335–339. doi:10.1007/s10461-005-9007-0.

Fortenberry, J.D. (2017) 'The visible man: Gendering health care services to improve young men's sexual health', *Journal of Adolescent Health*, 61(1), pp. 3–5. doi:10.1016/j.jadohealth.2017.05.002.

Fox, K. et al. (2013) 'Adolescent consent to testing: A review of current policies and issues in sub-Saharan Africa', in *HIV and adolescents: Guidance for HIV testing and counselling and care for adolescents living with HIV*. Available at: http://www.ncbi.nlm.nih.gov/books/NBK217954/pdf/Bookshelf_NBK217954.pdf.

Francis, D. (2010) '"They should know where they stand": Attitudes to HIV voluntary counselling and testing amongst a group of out-of-school youth', *South African Journal of Education*, 30(3), pp. 327–342. Available at: http://ez.lshtm.ac.uk/login?url=http://search.proquest.com/docview/761041825?accountid=130503%5Cnhttp://lshtmsfx.hosted.exlibrisgroup.com/lshtm?url_ver=Z39.88-2004&rft_val_fmt=info:ofi/fmt:kev:mtx:journal&genre=article&sid=ProQ:ProQ%3Aibssshell&atitle=%60.

Gallant, M. and Maticka-Tyndale, E. (2004) 'School-based HIV prevention programmes for African youth', *Social Science and Medicine*, 58(7), pp. 2764–2789. doi:10.1016/S0277-9536(03)00331-9.

Gari, S. et al. (2014) 'Sex differentials in the uptake of antiretroviral treatment in Zambia', *AIDS Care – Psychological and Socio-Medical Aspects of AIDS/HIV*, 26(10), pp. 1258–1262. doi:10.1080/09540121.2014.897911.

Gass, J.D. et al. (2011) 'Gender differences in risk for intimate partner violence among South African adults', *Journal of Interpersonal Violence*, 26(14), pp. 2764–2789. doi:10.1177/0886260510390960.

'Gender and health are also about boys and men.' (2018). *Lancet*, 392, p. 188. Available at: www.thelancet.com/pdfs/journals/lancet/PIIS0140-6736(18)31610-6.pdf.

George, G. et al. (2014) 'Barriers and facilitators to the uptake of voluntary medical male circumcision (VMMC) among adolescent boys in KwaZulu-Natal, South Africa', *African Journal of AIDS Research*, 13(2), pp. 179–187. doi:10.2989/16085906.2014.943253.

Gibbs, A., Govender, K. and Jewkes, R. (2016) 'An exploratory analysis of factors associated with depression in a vulnerable group of young people living in informal settlements in South Africa', *Global Public Health*,13(7), pp. 788–803. doi:10.1080/17441692.2016.1214281.

Gibbs, A., Sikweyiya, Y. and Jewkes, R. (2014) '"Men value their dignity": Securing respect and identity construction in urban informal settlements in South Africa', *Global Health Action*, 7, p. 23676. doi:10.3402/gha.v7.23676.

Gilead Sciences (2018) 'U.S. food and drug administration approves expanded indication for Truvada® (emtricitabine and tenofovir disoproxil fumarate) for reducing the risk of acquiring HIV-1 in adolescents', *Business Wire*. Available at: www.businesswire.com/news/home/20180515006187/en/U.S.-Food-Drug-Administration-Approves-Expanded-Indication (Accessed: 15 June 2018).

Gill, K. et al. (2017) *Pluspills: An open label, safety and feasibility study of oral pre-exposure prophylaxis (PrEP) in 15–19 year old adolescents in two sites in South Africa.*

International AIDS Society. Available at: http://programme.ias2017.org/PAG Material/PDF/Tuesday.pdf.

Godia, P.M. et al. (2013) 'Sexual reproductive health service provision to young people in Kenya; health service providers' experiences', *BMC Health Services Research*, 13, p. 476. doi:10.1186/1472-6963-13-476.

Govender, K. et al. (2018) 'Risk compensation following medical male circumcision: Results from a 1-year prospective cohort study of young school-going men in KwaZulu-Natal, South Africa', *International Journal of Behavioral Medicine*, 25(1), pp. 123–130. doi:10.1007/s12529-0179673-0.

Govindasamy, D. et al. (2015) 'Uptake and yield of HIV testing and counselling among children and adolescents in sub-Saharan Africa: A systematic review', *Journal of the International AIDS Society*,18, p. 20812. doi:10.7448/IAS.18.1.20182.

Gray, R.H. et al. (2007) 'Male circumcision for HIV prevention in men in Rakai, Uganda: A randomised trial', *Lancet*, 369(9562), pp. 657–666. doi:10.1016/S0140-6736(07)60313-4.

Hargreaves, J.R. and Glynn, J.R. (2002) 'Educational attainment and HIV-1 infection in developing countries: A systematic review', *Tropical Medicine and International Health*, 7(6), pp. 489–498. doi:10.1046/j.1365-3156.2002.00889.x.

Hargreaves, J.R. et al. (2008) 'Systematic review exploring time trends in the association between educational attainment and risk of HIV infection in sub-Saharan Africa', *AIDS (London, England)*, 22(3), pp. 403–414. doi:10.1097/QAD.0b013e3282f2aac3.

Hargreaves, J.R. et al. (2015) 'Trends in socioeconomic inequalities in HIV prevalence among young people in seven countries in Eastern and Southern Africa', *PLoS One*, 10(3), p. e0121775. doi:10.1371/journal.pone.0121775.

Harling, G. et al. (2014) 'Do age-disparate relationships drive HIV incidence in young women? Evidence from a population cohort in rural KwaZulu-Natal, South Africa', *JAIDS: Journal of Acquired Immune Deficiency Syndromes*, 66(4), pp. 443–451. doi:10.1097/QAI.0000000000000198.

Harrison, A. et al. (2006) 'Young men's HIV risks in South Africa: The importance of multiple risk behaviors', *AIDS*, 20(1), pp. 1467–1468. doi:10.1097/01.aids.0000233588.33080.00.

Harrison, A. et al. (2010) 'HIV prevention for South African youth: Which interventions work? A systematic review of current evidence', *BMC Public Health*, 10, p. 102. doi:10.1186/1471-2458-10-102.

Harrison, A. et al. (2012) 'Gender, peer and partner influences on adolescent HIV risk in rural South Africa', *Sexual Health*, 9(2), pp. 178–186. doi:10.1071/SH10150.

Hector, J. et al. (2018) 'Acceptability and performance of a directly assisted oral HIV self-testing intervention in adolescents in rural Mozambique', *PLoS One*, 13(4), p. e0195391. doi:10.1371/journal.pone.0195391.

Herman-Roloff, A. et al. (2011) 'Implementing voluntary medical male circumcision for HIV prevention in Nyanza Province, Kenya: Lessons learned during the first year', *PLoS One*, 6(4), p. e18299. doi:10.1371/journal.pone.0018299.

Hill, L.M. et al. (2017) 'Anxiety and depression strongly associated with sexual risk behaviors among networks of young men in Dar es Salaam, Tanzania', *AIDS Care*, 29(2), pp. 1–7. doi:10.1080/09540121.2016.1210075.

Hines, J.Z. et al. (2017) 'Scale-up of voluntary medical male circumcision services for HIV prevention – 12 countries in Southern and Eastern Africa, 2013–2016', *MMWR: Morbidity and Mortality Weekly Report*. doi:10.15585/mmwr.mm6647a2.

Hladik, W. et al. (2017) 'Men who have sex with men in Kampala, Uganda: Results from a bio-behavioral respondent driven sampling survey', *AIDS and Behavior*, 21(5), pp. 1478–1490. doi:10.1007/s10461-016-1535-2.

Hoffman, S. et al. (2017) 'Sexual and reproductive health risk behaviours among South African university students: Results from a representative campus-wide survey', *African Journal of AIDS Research*, 16(1), pp. 1–10. doi:10.2989/16085906.2016.1259171.

Hosek, S.G. et al. (2017) 'An HIV preexposure prophylaxis demonstration project and safety study for young MSM', *Journal of Acquired Immune Deficiency Syndromes*, 74(1), pp. 21–29. doi:10.1097/QAI.0000000000001179.

Idele, P. et al. (2014) 'Epidemiology of HIV and AIDS among adolescents: Current status, inequities, and data gaps', *Journal of Acquired Immune Deficiency Syndromes*, 66(Suppl. 2), pp. S144–S153. doi:10.1097/QAI.0000000000000176.

IDEO.org (2014) *The field guide to human-centered design*. doi:10.1007/s13398-014-0173-7.2. Available at: https://bestgraz.org/wp-content/uploads/2015/09/Field-Guide-to-Human-Centered-Design_IDEOorg.pdf.

Isingo, R. et al. (2012) 'Trends in the uptake of voluntary counselling and testing for HIV in rural Tanzania in the context of the scale up of antiretroviral therapy', *Tropical Medicine and International Health*, 17(8), pp. e15–e25. doi:10.1111/j.1365-3156.2011.02877.x.

Jayeoba, O. et al. (2012) 'Acceptability of male circumcision among adolescent boys and their parents, Botswana', *AIDS and Behavior*, 16(2), pp. 340–349. doi:10.1007/s10461-011-9929-7.

Jewkes, R. et al. (2008) 'Impact of stepping stones on incidence of HIV and HSV-2 and sexual behaviour in rural South Africa: Cluster randomised controlled trial', *British Medical Journal*, 337, p. a506. doi:10.1136/bmj.a506.

Jewkes, R. et al. (2011) 'Gender inequitable masculinity and sexual entitlement in rape perpetration South Africa: Findings of a cross-sectional study', *PLoS One*, 6(12), p. e29590. doi:10.1371/journal.pone.0029590.

Joint United Nations Programme on HIV/AIDS and UNAIDS (Joint United Nations Programme on HIV/AIDS) (2014) *Fast track-ending the AIDS epidemic by 2030*. UNAIDS. ISBN:978-92-9253-063-1. Available at: https://www.unaids.org/sites/default/files/media_asset/JC2686_WAD2014report_en.pdf.

Kagaayi, J. et al. (2014) 'Indices to measure risk of HIV acquisition in Rakai, Uganda', *PLoS One*, 9(4), p. e92015. doi:10.1371/journal.pone.0092015.

Kågesten, A. et al. (2016) 'Understanding factors that shape gender attitudes in early adolescence globally: A mixed-methods systematic review', *PLoS One*, 11(6), p. e0157805. doi:10.1371/journal.pone.0157805.

Kalichman, S.C. et al. (2007) 'Alcohol use and sexual risks for HIV/AIDS in sub-Saharan Africa: Systematic review of empirical findings', *Prevention Science*, 8(2), pp. 141–151. doi:10.1007/s11121-006-0061-2.

Kalichman, S.C. et al. (2009) 'Heterosexual anal intercourse among community and clinical settings in Cape Town, South Africa', *Sexually Transmitted Infections*, 85(6), pp. 411–415. doi:10.1136/sti.2008.035287.

Kalichman, S.C. et al. (2011) 'Heterosexual anal intercourse and HIV infection risks in the context of alcohol serving venues, Cape Town, South Africa', *BMC Public Health*, 11, p. 807. doi:10.1186/1471-2458-11-807.

Kayibanda, J.F., Bitera, R. and Alary, M. (2012) 'Violence toward women, men's sexual risk factors, and HIV infection among women: Findings from a national household survey in Rwanda', *Journal of Acquired Immune Deficiency Syndromes*, 59(3), pp. 300–307. doi:10.1097/QAI.0b013e31823dc634.

Kirby, D.B., Laris, B.A. and Rolleri, L.A. (2007) 'Sex and HIV education programs: Their impact on sexual behaviors of young people throughout the world', *Journal of Adolescent Health*, 40(3), pp. 206–217. doi:10.1016/j.jadohealth.2006.11.143.

Kirby, D.B., Obasi, A. and Laris, B. (2006) *The effectiveness of sex education and HIV education interventions in schools in developing countries*. Technical Report Series. Geneva: World Health Organization.

Koechlin, F.M. et al. (2017) 'Values and preferences on the use of oral pre-exposure prophylaxis (PrEP) for HIV prevention among multiple populations: A systematic review of the literature', *AIDS and Behavior*, 21(5), pp. 1325–1335. doi:10.1007/s10461-016-1627-z.

Kohler, H.P. and Thornton, R.L. (2012) 'Conditional cash transfers and HIV/AIDS prevention: Unconditionally promising?', *World Bank Economic Review*, 26(2), pp. 165–190. doi:10.1093/wber/lhr041.

Koole, O. et al. (2014) 'Retention and risk factors for attrition among adults in antiretroviral treatment programmes in Tanzania, Uganda and Zambia', *Tropical Medicine and International Health*, 19(12), pp. 1397–1410. doi:10.1111/tmi.12386.

Kouyoumdjian, F.G. et al. (2013) 'Intimate partner violence is associated with incident HIV infection in women in Uganda', *AIDS*, 3(1), pp. e23–e33. doi:10.1097/QAD.0b013e32835fd851.

Kreniske, P., Grilo, S., Nalugoda, F., Wolfe, J. and Santelli, J. (2019) 'Narrating the transition to adulthood for youth in Uganda: Leaving school, mobility, risky occupations, and HIV', *Health Education & Behavior*, 46(4), pp. 550–558. doi:10.1177/1090198119829197.

Lane, T. et al. (2006) 'Heterosexual anal intercourse increases risk of HIV infection among young South African men', *AIDS*, 20(1), pp. 123–125. doi:10.1097/01.aids.0000198083.55078.02.

Langhaug, L.F. et al. (2010) 'High prevalence of affective disorders among adolescents living in rural Zimbabwe', *Journal of Community Health*, 35(4), pp. 355–364. doi:10.1007/s10900-010-9261-6.

Lightfoot, M., Dunbar, M. and Weiser, S.D. (2017) 'Reducing undiagnosed HIV infection among adolescents in sub-Saharan Africa: Provider-initiated and opt-out testing are not enough', *PLoS Medicine*, 14(7), p. e1002361. doi:10.1371/journal.pmed.1002361.

Lilleston, P.S. et al. (2017) 'Multilevel influences on acceptance of medical male circumcision in Rakai district, Uganda', *AIDS Care – Psychological and Socio-Medical Aspects of AIDS/HIV*, 29(8), pp. 1049–1055. doi:10.1080/09540121.2016.1274014.

Lloyd, C.B. (2005) 'Growing up global', *National Research Council and Institute of Medicine, Panel on Transitions to Adulthood in Developing Countries*. doi:10.17226/11174.

MacPhail, C. et al. (2009) 'Factors associated with HIV testing among sexually active South African youth aged 15–24 years', *AIDS Care – Psychological and Socio-Medical Aspects of AIDS/HIV*, 21(4), pp. 456–467. doi:10.1080/09540120802282586.

Magadi, M.A. (2013) 'Migration as a risk factor for HIV infection among youths in sub-Saharan Africa: Evidence from the DHS', *Annals of the American Academy of Political and Social Science*, 648(1), pp. 136–158. doi:10.1177/0002716213482440.

Magidson, J.F. et al. (2017) 'Psychosocial correlates of alcohol and other substance use among low-income adolescents in peri-urban Johannesburg, South Africa:

A focus on gender differences', *Journal of Health Psychology*, 22(11), pp. 1415–1425. doi:10.1177/1359105316628739.

Maljaars, L.P. et al. (2017) 'Condom migration after introduction of pre-exposure prophylaxis among HIV-uninfected adolescents in South Africa: A cohort analysis', *Southern African Journal of HIV Medicine*, 18(1), p. 712. doi:10.4102/sajhivmed.v18i1.712.

Maman, S. et al. (2002) 'HIV-positive women report more lifetime partner-violence: Findings from a voluntary counseling and testing clinic in Dar es Salaam, Tanzania', *American Journal of Public Health*, 92(8), pp. 1331–1337. doi:10.2105/AJPH.92.8.1331.

Mason-Jones, A.J. et al. (2016) 'School-based interventions for preventing HIV, sexually transmitted infections, and pregnancy in adolescents', *Cochrane Database of Systematic Reviews*. doi:10.1002/14651858.CD006417.pub3.

Maswanya, E.S. et al. (2012) 'Sexual behavior and condom use among male students in Dar-Es-Salaam, Tanzania with emphasis on contact with barmaids', *East African Journal of Public Health*, 9(1), pp. 39–43.

Maticka-Tyndale, E., Mungwete, R. and Jayeoba, O. (2014) 'Replicating impact of a primary school HIV prevention programme: Primary school action for better health, Kenya', *Health Education Research*, 29(4), pp. 611–623. doi:10.1093/her/cyt088.

Maticka-Tyndale, E. and Tenkorang, E.Y. (2010) 'A multi-level model of condom use among male and female upper primary school students in Nyanza, Kenya', *Social Science & Medicine*, 71(3), pp. 616–625. doi 10.1016/j.socscimed.2010.03.049.

Maticka-Tyndale, E., Wildish, J. and Gichuru, M. (2007) 'Quasi-experimental evaluation of a national primary school HIV intervention in Kenya', *Evaluation & Program Planning*, 30(2), pp. 172–186. doi:10.1016/j.evalprogplan.2007.01.006.

Mbonye, M. et al. (2016) 'Voluntary medical male circumcision for HIV prevention in fishing communities in Uganda: The influence of local beliefs and practice', *African Journal of AIDS Research*, 15(3), pp. 1–8. doi:10.2989/16085906.2016.1179652.

MenStar Coalition (2018) *Global partners pledge over $1.2 billion to launch the MenStar coalition*. Available at: www.menstarcoalition.org/menstar.pdf.

Michielsen, K. et al. (2010) 'Effectiveness of HIV prevention for youth in sub-Saharan Africa: Systematic review and meta-analysis of randomized and nonrandomized trials', *AIDS*, 24(8), pp. 1193–1202. doi:10.1097/QAD.0b013e3283384791.

Miiro, G. et al. (2017) 'Soccer-based promotion of voluntary medical male circumcision: A mixed-methods feasibility study with secondary students in Uganda', *PLoS One*,12(10), p. e0185929. doi:10.1371/journal.pone.0185929.

Miller, C.L. et al. (2017) 'The Botsha Bophelo adolescent health study: A profile of adolescents in Soweto, South Africa', *Southern African Journal of HIV Medicine*, 18(1), p. a731. doi:10.4102/sajhivmed.v18i1.731.

Montaño, D.E. et al. (2014) 'Evidence-based identification of key beliefs explaining adult male circumcision motivation in Zimbabwe: Targets for behavior change messaging', *AIDS and Behavior*, 18(5), pp. 885–904. doi:10.1007/s10461-013-0686-7.

Mshana, G. et al. (2011) 'Traditional male circumcision practices among the Kurya of North-Eastern Tanzania and implications for national programmes', *AIDS Care – Psychological and Socio-Medical Aspects of AIDS/HIV*, 23(9), pp.1111–1116. doi:10.1080/09540121.2011.554518.

Mugwanya, K.K. et al. (2011) 'Circumcision of male children for reduction of future risk for HIV: Acceptability among HIV serodiscordant couples in Kampala, Uganda', *PLoS One*, 6(7), p. e22254. doi:10.1371/journal.pone.0022254.

Mulawa, M. et al. (2018) 'Perpetration and victimization of intimate partner violence among young men and women in Dar es Salaam, Tanzania', *Journal of Interpersonal Violence*, 33(16), pp. 2486–2511. doi:10.1177/0886260515625910.

Müller, A. et al. (2018) 'The no-go zone: A qualitative study of access to sexual and reproductive health services for sexual and gender minority adolescents in Southern Africa', *Reproductive Health*, 15(12). doi:10.1186/s12978-018-0462-2.

Mullinax, M. et al. (2017) 'HIV-risk behaviors of men who perpetrate intimate partner violence in Rakai, Uganda', *AIDS Education and Prevention*, 29(6), pp. 525–539. doi:10.1521/aeap.2017.29.6.527.

Naik, R. et al. (2012) 'Client characteristics and acceptability of a home-based HIV counselling and testing intervention in rural South Africa', *BMC Public Health*, 12, p. 824. doi:10.1186/1471-2458-12-824.

Napierala Mavedzenge, S.M., Doyle, A.M. and Ross, D.A. (2011) 'HIV prevention in young people in sub-Saharan Africa: A systematic review', *Journal of Adolescent Health*, 49(6), pp. 568–586. doi:10.1016/j.jadohealth.2011.02.007.

Ngalande, R.C., Levy, J., Kapondo, C. and Bailey, R. (2006) 'Acceptability of male circumcision for prevention of HIV infection in Malawi', *AIDS and Behavior*, 10(4), pp. 377–385. doi:10.1007/s10461-006-9076-8.

Nyblade, L. et al. (2017) 'Perceived, anticipated and experienced stigma: Exploring manifestations and implications for young people's sexual and reproductive health and access to care in North-Western Tanzania', *Culture, Health and Sexuality*, 19(10), pp. 1092–1107. doi:10.1080/13691058.2017.1293844.

Ochieng-Ooko, V. et al. (2010) 'Influence of gender on loss to follow-up in a large HIV treatment programme in Western Kenya', *Bulletin of the World Health Organization*, 88(9), pp. 681–688. doi:10.2471/BLT.09.064329.

Olawore, O. et al. (2018) 'Migration and risk of HIV acquisition in Rakai, Uganda: A population-based cohort study', *Lancet HIV*, 5(4), pp. e181–e189. doi:10.1016/S2352-3018(18)30009-2.

O'Leary, K., Slep, D. and Smith, A. (2012) 'Prevention of partner violence by focusing on behaviors of both young males and females', *Prevention Science*, 13(4), pp. 329–339. doi:10.1007/s11121-011-0237-2.

Onoya, D. et al. (2015) 'Determinants of multiple sexual partnerships in South Africa', *Journal of Public Health*, 37(1), pp. 97–106. doi:10.1093/pubmed/fdu010.

Osaki, H. et al. (2015) ' "If you are not circumcised, I cannot say yes": The role of women in promoting the uptake of voluntary medical male circumcision in Tanzania', *PLoS One*,10(9), p. e0139009. doi:10.1371/journal.pone.0139009.

Owen, B.N. et al. (2017) 'How common and frequent is heterosexual anal intercourse among South Africans? A systematic review and meta-analysis', *Journal of the International AIDS Society*, 20(1), p. 21162. doi:10.7448/IAS.20.1.21162.

Pace, J. (2018) *A systematic review of associations between education and HIV infection for young people living in low- and middle-income countries.* Unpublished manuscript.

Paul-Ebhohimhen, V.A., Poobalan, A. and van Teijlingen, E. (2008) 'A systematic review of school-based sexual health interventions to prevent STI/HIV in sub-Saharan Africa', *BMC Public Health*, 7(8), p. 4. doi:10.1186/1471-2458-8-4.

Peltzer, K. and Kanta, X. (2009) 'Medical circumcision and manhood initiation rituals in the Eastern Cape, South Africa: A post intervention evaluation', *Culture, Health and Sexuality*, 11(1), pp. 83–97. doi:10.1080/13691050802389777.

Peltzer, K. and Matseke, G. (2013) 'Determinants of HIV testing among young people aged 18–24 years in South Africa', *African Health Sciences*, 13(4), pp. 1012–1020. doi:10.4314/ahs.v13i4.22.

Pettifor, A. et al. (2005) 'Young people's sexual health in South Africa: HIV prevalence and sexual behaviors from a nationally representative household survey', *AIDS*, 19(4), pp. 1525–1534.

Price, J.E. et al. (2014) 'Behavior change pathways to voluntary medical male circumcision: Narrative interviews with circumcision clients in Zambia', *PLoS One*, 9(12), p. e116361. doi:10.1371/journal.pone.0111602.

Pulerwitz, J., Michaelis, A., Verma, R.K. et al. (2010) 'Addressing gender dynamics and engaging men in HIV programs: Lessons learned from horizons research', *Public Health Reports*,125, pp. 282–292. doi:10.1177/003335491012500219.

Pulerwitz, J., Michaelis, A., Weiss, E. et al. (2010) 'Reducing HIV-related stigma: Lessons learned from horizons research and programs', *Public Health Reports*, 125, pp. 272–281. doi:10.1177/003335491012500218.

Ramirez-Avila, L. et al. (2012) 'Routine HIV testing in adolescents and young adults presenting to an outpatient clinic in Durban, South Africa', *PLoS One*, 7(9), p. e45507. doi:10.1371/journal.pone.0045507.

Ramsoomar, L. and Morojele, N.K. (2012) 'Trends in alcohol prevalence, age of initiation and association with alcohol-related harm among South African youth: Implications for policy', *South African Medical Journal*, 102(7), pp. 609–612. doi:10.7196/samj.5766.

Richter, L. et al. (2015) 'Early sexual debut: Voluntary or coerced? Evidence from longitudinal data in South Africa – the birth to twenty plus study', *South African Medical Journal*, 105(4), pp. 304–307. doi:10.7196/SAMJ.8925.

Rotheram-Borus, M.J. et al. (2016) 'Feasibility of using soccer and job training to prevent drug abuse and HIV', *AIDS and Behavior*, 20(9), pp. 1841–1850. doi:10.1007/s10461-015-1262-0.

Roye, C.F., Tolman, D.L. and Snowden, F. (2013) 'Heterosexual anal intercourse among black and Latino adolescents and young adults: A poorly understood high-risk behavior', *Journal of Sex Research*, 50(7), pp. 715–722. doi:10.1080/00224499.2012.719170.

Sani, A.S. et al. (2016) 'School-based sexual health education interventions to prevent STI/HIV in sub-Saharan Africa: A systematic review and meta-analysis', *BMC Public Health*,16(1), p. 1069. doi:10.1186/s12889-016-3715-4.

Santelli, J.S. et al. (2013) 'Behavioral, biological, and demographic risk and protective factors for new HIV infections among youth in Rakai, Uganda', *Journal of Acquired Immune Deficiency Syndromes*, 63(3), pp. 393–400. doi:10.1097/QAI.0b013e3182926795.

Schaefer, R. et al. (2017) 'Age-disparate relationships and HIV incidence in adolescent girls and young women: Evidence from Zimbabwe', *AIDS*, 31(10), pp. 796–807. doi:10.1097/QAD.0000000000001506.

Schuyler, A.C. et al. (2017) 'Mobility among youth in Rakai, Uganda: Trends, characteristics, and associations with behavioural risk factors for HIV', *Global Public Health*, 12(8), pp. 1033–1050. doi:10.1080/17441692.2015.1074715.

Serwadda, D. M. et al. (1992) 'HIV risk factors in three geographic strata of rural Rakai district, Uganda', *AIDS*, 6(9), pp. 983–990. doi:10.1097/00002030-199209000-00012.

Shai, N.J. et al. (2012) 'Masculinities and condom use patterns among young rural South Africa men: A cross-sectional baseline survey', *BMC Public Health*, 12, p. 462. doi:10.1186/1471-2458-12-462.

Shanaube, K. et al. (2017) 'Community intervention improves knowledge of HIV status of adolescents in Zambia: Findings from HPTN 071-PopART for youth study', *AIDS*, 31 (Suppl 3), pp. S221–S232. doi:10.1097/QAD.0000000000001530.

Singh, S. et al. (2000) 'Gender differences in the timing of first intercourse: Data from 14 countries', *International Family Planning Perspectives*, 26(1), pp. 21–28+43. doi:10.2307/2648286.

Skovdal, M. et al. (2011) 'Masculinity as a barrier to men's use of HIV services in Zimbabwe', *Global Health*, 7, p. 13. doi:10.1186/1744-8603-7-13.

Staveteig, S. et al. (2017) 'Reaching the "first 90": Gaps in coverage of HIV testing among people living with HIV in 16 African countries', *PLoS One*, 12(10), p. e0186316. doi:10.1371/journal.pone.0186316.

Stephenson, R., de Voux, A. and Sullivan, P.S. (2011) 'Intimate partner violence and sexual risk-taking among men who have sex with men in South Africa', *Western Journal of Emergency Medicine*, 12(3), pp. 343–347. doi:10.5811/westjem.2011.5.6700.

Stoebenau, K. et al. (2016) 'Revisiting the understanding of "transactional sex" in sub-Saharan Africa: A review and synthesis of the literature', *Social Science and Medicine*, 168, pp. 186–197. doi:10.1016/j.socscimed.2016.09.023.

Sun, C.J. et al. (2018) 'Gender differences in sexual and reproductive health protective and risk factors of Batswana adolescents: Implications for parent and adolescent interventions', *AIDS Education and Prevention*, 30(1), pp. 35–46. doi:10.1521/aeap.2018.30.1.35.

Tenkorang, E.Y. and Maticka-Tyndale, E. (2014a) 'Assessing young people's perceptions of HIV risks in Nyanza, Kenya: Are school and community level factors relevant?', *Social Science and Medicine*, 116, pp. 93–101. doi:10.1016/j.socscimed.2014.06.041.

Tenkorang, E.Y. and Maticka-Tyndale, E. (2014b) 'Individual- and community-level influences on the timing of sexual debut among youth in Nyanza, Kenya', *International Perspectives on Sexual and Reproductive Health*, 40(2), pp. 68–78. doi:10.1363/4006814.

UNAIDS (2017a) *Addressing a blind spot in the response to HIV – reaching out to men and boys*. Available at: www.unaids.org/sites/default/files/media_asset/blind_spot_en.pdf.

UNAIDS (2017b) *Start free stay free AIDS free 2017 progress report no title*. Available at: https://www.unaids.org/en/resources/documents/2018/start-free-stay-free-aids-free-2017-progress-report.

UNAIDS (2016a) *Ending the AIDS epidemic for adolescents, with adolescents: A practical guide to meaningfully engage adolescents in the AIDS response*. Available at: www.unaids.org/sites/default/files/media_asset/ending-AIDS-epidemic-adolescents_en.pdf%0A%0A.

UNAIDS (2016b) *Global AIDS response progress reporting 2016*. Available at: https://aidsreportingtool.unaids.org/static/docs/GARPR_Guidelines_2016_EN.pdf.

UNAIDS (2017) *UNAIDS data 2017.* UNAIDS. doi:10.1007/BF01110555. Available at: https://www.unaids.org/sites/default/files/media_asset/20170720_Data_book_2017_en.pdf.

UNAIDS (no date) *2017 estimates.* Online 2017. Available at: http://aidsinfo.unaids.org (Accessed: 31 August 2018).

UNAIDS and WHO (2018) 'Miles to go: Closing gaps breaking barriers righting injustices', *UNAIDS.* doi:10.1111/j.1600-6143.2011.03542.x.

UNFPA (2015) *Emerging evidence, lessons and practice in comprehensive sexuality education, a global review.* Paris. Available at: www.unfpa.org/publications/emerging-evidence-lessons-and-practice-comprehensive-sexuality-education-global-review.

UNICEF (2013) *Towards an AIDS-free generation – children and AIDS: Sixth stocktaking report.* New York: UNICEF.

UNICEF (2016a) *For every child end AIDS-seventh stocktaking report, 2016.* Available at: www.childrenandaids.org/sites/default/files/2017-08/For Every Child%2C EndAIDS-SeventhStocktakingReport-2016.pdf.

UNICEF (2016b) *Towards an AIDS-free generation – children and AIDS.* Seventh Stocktaking Report. Available at: https://www.unicef.org/reports/every-child-end-aids-seventh-stocktaking-report-2016.

UNICEF (2016c) *Collecting and reporting of sex- and age-disaggregated data on adolescents at the sub-national level.* Available at: https://childrenandaids.org/sites/default/files/2017-03/DataAbstractionGuidedraftNovember2016.pdf.

UNICEF (2018) *Turning the tide against AIDS will require more concentrated focus on adolescents and young people.* New York: UNICEF.

United Nations Development Programme (2014) *Discussion paper: Cash transfers and HIV prevention.* Available at: https://ipcig.org/pub/eng/WP184_HIV_inclusive_and_sensitive_cash_transfer_initiatives.pdf.

Varga, C.A. (2001) 'The forgotten fifty per cent: A review of sexual and reproductive health research and programs focused on boys and young men in sub-Saharan Africa', *African Journal of Reproductive Health*, 5(3), pp. 175–195. doi:10.2307/3583334.

Vechakul, J., Shrimali, B. and Sandhu, J. (2015) 'Human-centered design as an approach for place-based innovation in public health: A case study from Oakland, California', *Maternal and Child Health Journal*, 19(2), pp. 2552–2559. doi:10.1007/s10995-015-1787-x.

Wagman, J.A. et al. (2015) 'Effectiveness of an integrated intimate partner violence and HIV prevention intervention in Rakai, Uganda: Analysis of an intervention in an existing cluster randomised cohort', *Lancet Global Health*, 3(1), pp. e23–e33. doi:10.1016/S2214-109X(14)70344-4.

Wagner, A.D. et al. (2018) 'Disclosure, consent, opportunity costs, and inaccurate risk assessment deter pediatric HIV testing: A mixed-methods study', *Journal of Acquired Immune Deficiency Syndromes*, 77(7), pp. 393–399. doi:10.1097/QAI.0000000000001614.

Wamoyi, J. et al. (2016) 'Transactional sex and risk for HIV infection in sub-Saharan Africa: A systematic review and meta-analysis', *Journal of the International AIDS Society*, 19, p. 20992. doi:10.1016/0167-4838(89)90134-9.

Weine, S.M. and Kashuba, A.B. (2012) 'Labor migration and HIV risk: A systematic review of the literature', *AIDS and Behavior*, 16(6), pp. 1605–1621. doi:10.1007/s10461-012-0183-4.

Weiss, H. A. et al. (2008) 'Circumcision among adolescent boys in rural Northwestern Tanzania', *Tropical Medicine and International Health*, 13(8), pp. 1054–1061. doi:10.1111/j.1365-3156.2008.02107.x.

Were, W. A. et al. (2006) 'Undiagnosed HIV infection and couple HIV discordance among household members of HIV-infected people receiving antiretroviral therapy in Uganda', *Journal of Acquired Immune Deficiency Syndromes*, 43(1), 91–95. doi:10.1097/01.qai.0000225021.81384.28.

Westercamp, M. et al. (2012) 'Circumcision preference among women and uncircumcised men prior to scale-up of male circumcision for HIV prevention in Kisumu, Kenya', *AIDS Care – Psychological and Socio-Medical Aspects of AIDS/HIV*, 24(2), pp. 157–166. doi:10.1080/09540121.2011.597944.

WHO, UNICEF and UNAIDS (2013) *Global update on HIV treatment 2013: Results, impact and opportunities.* Geneva: World Health Organization. ISBN:978-92-4-150573-4.

Wilson, K. S. et al. (2017) ' "At our age, we would like to do things the way we want": A qualitative study of adolescent HIV testing services in Kenya', *AIDS*, 31(Suppl 3), pp. S213–S220. doi:10.1097/QAD.0000000000001513.

Wood, K. and Jewkes, R. (2006) 'Blood blockages and scolding nurses: Barriers to adolescent contraceptive use in South Africa', *Reproductive Health Matters*, 14(27), pp. 109–118. doi:10.1016/S0968-8080(06)27231-8.

Woog, V. and Kagesten, A. (2017) *The sexual and reproductive health needs of very young adolescents in developing countries.* Guttmacher Institute. Available at: www.guttmacher.org/fact-sheet/srh-needs-very-young-adolescents-in-developing-countries.

World Health Organization (2016) *Appropriate medicines: Options for pre-exposure prophylaxis.* Available at: http://apps.who.int/iris/bitstream/handle/10665/273934/WHO-CDS-HIV-18.22-eng.pdf.

Wyrod, R. (2011) 'Masculinity and the persistence of AIDS stigma', *Culture, Health and Sexuality*, 13(4), pp. 443–456. doi:10.1080/13691058.2010.542565.

Ybarra, M., Price-Feeney, M. and Mwaba, K. (2018) 'Prevalence and correlates of anal sex among secondary school students in Cape Town, South Africa', *AIDS Care*, 30(7), pp. 821–829. doi:10.1080/09540121.2018.1426824.

10 *Things less spoken* – HIV research with adolescent boys and young men

Implications for theory, policy and practice

Lesley Gittings, Rebecca Hodes, Christopher J. Colvin and Nompumelelo Zungu

Introduction

There is an increasing acknowledgement that men and boys must be better engaged in HIV prevention and treatment initiatives. Improving men's access to prevention and treatment services would result in a 'triple dividend', benefitting boys and men themselves, their sexual partners and their families (UNAIDS, 2017).

Although girls and women are biologically and socially more vulnerable to acquiring HIV, men access HIV prevention and treatment services less and at a later stage of disease progression and are more likely to die whilst on ART than women (Cornell, McIntyre and Myer, 2011; Johnson et al., 2013).

The adolescent HIV epidemic presents further challenges. AIDS-related illness is the leading cause of death among adolescents in Eastern and Southern Africa (ESA), and these deaths have tripled among adolescents since 2000 while declining in all other age groups (WHO, 2015). Adolescent boys have significantly lower HIV prevalence in late adolescence and early adulthood than adolescent girls and young women (AGYW). However, adolescent boys experience sharp increases in HIV prevalence in the years that follow, suggesting that adolescence may be a critical time where boys form risk behaviours and are exposed to new vulnerabilities.

Despite a growing number of interventions that work with men and boys, there is limited research that explores the processes, politics, limitations and challenges of such work (Gibbs, Vaughan and Aggleton, 2015). This chapter responds to this gap by presenting some methodological and ethical considerations in working with adolescent boys and young men (ABYM).

The first sections of this chapter provide a theoretical and conceptual overview and outline some current debates within masculinities research and HIV social science. The findings comprises three main components, each detailing a particular occurrence from Gittings' doctoral research (supervised by Hodes and Colvin), which focused on the health beliefs and experiences of ABYM (aged 13–24) living with HIV in South Africa's Eastern

Cape province. It is a sub-study of Mzantsi Wakho, a mixed-methods, longitudinal community-traced study of adolescents living with HIV ($n = 1057$).

The findings section begins by asking, 'Who is best placed to work with adolescent boys and young men?', highlighting the significance of positionality and intersubjectivity. The section then explores the strategies of engagement used by young male researchers working with adolescent boys. It employs the dual interpretive frameworks of 'hegemonic masculinities' and the conceptualisation of both dominant and alternative masculinities bound up in Xhosa masculine identities. It focuses on how considered, contextually grounded performances of masculinity may encourage boys to move beyond dominant masculine scripts and allow for greater honesty, vulnerability and the enactment of alternative masculine norms. The section then considers potential opportunities, as well as pitfalls and challenges, of interventions and research focusing specifically on ABYM.

This chapter highlights some methodological and ethical considerations for working with this diverse group and challenges dominant assumptions about masculinity.

Theory, concepts and definitions

This chapter acknowledges the social construction of gender as a binary, which separates certain behaviours and attitudes into those deemed 'feminine' or 'masculine'.

Hegemonic masculinity has been described as the dominant form of an idealised masculinity within a society, which imposes meanings about the position and identity of other forms of masculinity and femininity (Connell, 2005). In many settings, the hegemonic forms of masculinity promote values and practices of independence, physical strength, sexual prowess and restraint in displays of emotion or vulnerability. These values and practices are, in turn, seen to act as powerful barriers to avoiding health risks and managing health problems effectively when they do emerge (Courtenay, 2000). This understanding of the potential links between hegemonic forms of masculinity and poor health has been applied to the field of HIV and health research as a way to understand men's poorer engagement in health services, risky sexual practices and poorer HIV-related outcomes (Gibbs, Vaughan and Aggleton, 2015).

The concept of hegemonic masculinity encompasses diverse behaviours and identities, produced contextually and relationally (Wetherell and Edley, 2014). This chapter recognises the malleability and the multiplicity of masculinities while acknowledging the limitations of the concept. We use hegemonic masculinities as an interpretive framework through which to view the beliefs and behaviours of boys and young men, specifically in relation to their participation in the research at the centre of this chapter. We explore how hegemonic masculine norms were practiced within the study context among Xhosa men and adapted through the processes of engaging with this research project.

Social scientists in Southern Africa have a rich history of emphasising the importance of context in limiting or enabling the effectiveness of HIV interventions (Hodes and Morrell, 2018). In his theoretical work on Xhosa masculinity, Mfecane (2016) argues that 'Western'[1] gender theories are limited in their understanding of Xhosa masculinity, in which the concept of *indoda*[2] is central. Similarly, in her work on social representations of AIDS and narratives of risk, Zungu (2013) found that the meanings of some HIV prevention messages as constructed within a 'Western' paradigm may be in conflict with meanings within other contexts. Oyěwùmí (1997) posits that dominant gender narratives and interpretations of the social world 'cannot be assumed uncritically for other cultures' in her writing about her work in Nigeria. The message here is that the ways that gender and masculinity are understood locally must be central to the design and evaluation of research and interventions.

This chapter employs notions of both hegemonic masculinities and Xhosa masculine identities encapsulated within the terms *indoda* and *inkwenkwe* to examine how boys and young men perform, reconstruct and resist masculine norms in the study context. Despite some suggested theoretical tensions between Mfecane's work on Xhosa masculinities and Connell's hegemonic masculinit(ies), this chapter employs the work of both scholars, with the understanding that the concept of hegemonic masculinities is expansive enough to include these contextual masculine norms. Hegemonic masculinities may be a useful concept to characterise the construction of gender norms and practices, and in particular the stark distinction between manhood and boyhood within the study context.

This chapter also draws on central tenets of feminism and gender studies, emphasising the multiplicity of gendered power dynamics and their interrelationship with health. The concepts of positionality and reflexivity are also used to reflect on the workings of embedded agency in interactions between researchers and participants. Reflexivity has been described as 'the project of examining how the researcher and intersubjective elements impinge on, and even, transform research' (Finlay, 2002). It is a systematic, conscious reflection on research design, methods and findings to provide insight into the subjective aspects of a study and to enable validation of the experiential data provided by study participants. We use the term 'positionality' to describe aspects of identities including race, gender and class, not as essential qualities but as indicators of relational positions (Maher and Tetreault, 1993).

Background: adolescence, health and masculinity

Given that adolescence is a period marked by multiple physical and psychosocial changes, this time represents an often risky period in young people's lives. It may also be a crucial time in which to intervene to influence the development of health, gendered and sexual behaviours. A growing evidence base suggests that gender transformative work with men and boys has the potential to shift harmful gendered norms and practices that might put men and their partners at risk of contracting HIV and having poor AIDS-related outcomes (Dworkin, Fleming and Colvin, 2015). Gender transformative approaches aim to alter discriminatory gender practices, policies, beliefs and ideas, recognising the benefits that gender-equitable environments have for health (Betron et al., 2012).

It has been theorised that men's poorer health outcomes are a result of hegemonic masculine norms, which have a negative effect on health-seeking and protective behaviours. While acknowledging how hegemonic masculine norms vary by context and shift throughout time, commonalities in global hegemonic masculine constructs include courage, independence and self-sufficiency, toughness, emotional and physical strength, sex with multiple partners, fearlessness and control over other men and women (Courtenay, 2000; Mfecane, 2008; Lindegger and Quayle, 2009). In an attempt to perform to these ideals embedded in hegemonic masculinity, it may be difficult for men to seek or accept healthcare, including HIV prevention, testing and treatment services and other forms of support (Colvin, Robins and Leavens, 2010; Mfecane, 2010). Institutional supply-side barriers relating to the availability and delivery of healthcare services are also a significant factor in men's poorer HIV-related health outcomes (Dovel et al., 2015).

There is a growing literature in the ESA region on childhood and adolescent masculinities that considers the pressures exerted on young males to perform to hegemonic masculine norms in contexts underlain by HIV, disempowerment and poverty (Langa, 2010; Govender, 2011; Hensels et al., 2016). This work highlights the vulnerability and uncertainty of ABYM and the importance of better understanding this group, rather than simply framing them in contrast to vulnerable AGYW. Childhood exposure of ABYM to familial, community and structural violence may be internalised and find expression in harmful performances of masculinity, violence perpetration and behaviours that increase HIV acquisition risk (Jewkes et al., 2011; Mathews, Jewkes and Abrahams, 2011).

These texts, alongside critiques of traditional approaches to behaviour change in the context of HIV, suggest that group participatory identity construction work, and initiatives to address social and community-level factors, are better placed than individual-level initiatives that focus on individual behaviour change as a result. Similarly, a focus on attitudes in behaviour change may result in failure to consider important institutional and structural factors that shape behaviours (Pease and Flood, 2008).

Findings and discussion

Who is best placed to work with adolescent boys and young men? Positionality and intersubjectivity

This section focuses on positionality and explores the ways in which intersubjective factors and identities shape HIV work with ABYM. Such factors include demographic similarity and difference, personality and context. We suggest that it is important to take stock of the many intersecting factors that will shape interactions with participants, and that reflexivity is crucial in HIV prevention research and programming. We also interrogate the assumption that certain aspects of demographic 'sameness', such as geographic proximity, ethnicity or gender concurrence, mean that such interactions will be simpler. The following story explores how aspects of identity, alongside contextual issues, can shape engagements with ABYM.

The Ezobudoda (translated from isiXhosa as 'manhood things') sub-study focused on HIV-positive adolescent boys and young men's engagement with traditional and biomedical health services. While establishing Ezobudoda, Gittings asked the research team for help determining the selection criteria for hiring researchers who would work on this project. After three years of data collection, the research team had extensive experience speaking with adolescents and young people about HIV and sexual and reproductive health. Among key requirements for these positions were the need to be 'good with young people', fluency in local languages and the commitment to the research team as a collective. In addition, the research staff suggested – without prompting – certain demographic requirements.

The researchers should be male, they explained, because there are things that participants would not say to female researchers. Part of their argument was based on their perception that certain things are spoken about only by men. They described how certain traditional practices, including *ulwaluko*,[3] a month-long initiation into manhood, are highly secretive and that it is a taboo to discuss them with women. Given that there were things about which Gittings, as a woman, should not have knowledge, they suggested that the male research assistants could also act as ethical advisors and mediators, controlling the flow of secretive information from research participants. Beyond collecting data, the researchers would also be crucial in supporting its interpretation due to their proximity to the topic.

They also suggested that it would be easier for male researchers to build relationships with participants and that that these interviews would generate richer and more honest narratives (for an example image of an interview, see the life history interview in Figure 10.1). This belief was based on the assumption that participants are generally more comfortable sharing intimate information with someone of the same gender, due to the perception that they have shared similar experiences.

That speaking about health may be more difficult for men is not surprising given expressions of physical or emotional vulnerability are delimited by hegemonic masculine norms (Connell, 2005). In order to collect richer and more accurate evidence, it would be important for participants to 'open up' and speak freely. Southern African interventions, such as Stepping Stones, Brothers for Life and One Man Can, are premised on the idea that gender-equitable beliefs and practices are better for the health and well-being of men as well as their families and communities. These interventions are centred on in-depth work with men, usually facilitated by other

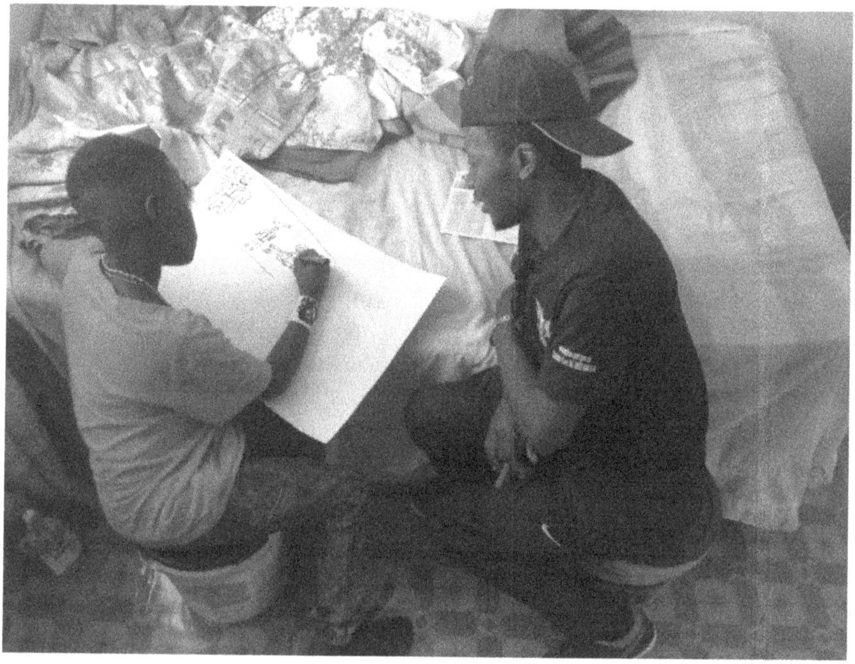

Figure 10.1 Ulwazi (13) conducting a pilot life history interview with researcher Zukolwethu Jantjies, 26 November 2016

men who encourage more gender-equitable practices and enact these practices themselves. They have drawn on certain 'health-promoting' aspects of hegemonic masculinities, such as taking responsibility for the welfare of others (Colvin, Robins and Leavens, 2010). Such campaigns have not been without critique. It has been suggested that certain aspects of these campaigns may reify harmful hegemonic masculine norms (Fleming, Lee and Dworkin, 2014). Despite these potential shortfalls, the lesson we draw here is the way in which positionality may be an important consideration in who does the work with adolescent boys and young men.

A male identity was not the only demographic characteristic advised by researchers as a necessity in their work. They also believed that age was important, and recommended that researchers should be no younger than 25. They reasoned that if the older participants saw the researchers as their peers, they would not be taken seriously. At the same time, they advised that the successful candidates should be no older than 45, because if participants saw them as elders, they would not feel open to speak frankly to them. They explained that age-based hierarchy is an important factor, especially in a place where issues of sexuality are not usually discussed directly with elders. They also recommended that the candidate(s) should be isiXhosa speaking, to circumvent the additional challenges of translation, and that they should themselves be *indoda*, having followed local traditions and customs of *ulwaluko*.

What was clear from these discussions was that the research team saw the positionality of the research assistant to be of vital importance and that intersubjective identities were a crucial component of the research and analysis process.

As a result of this planning, the Mzantsi Wakho study hired two 29-year-old isiXhosa-speaking men. Mhlabeni was from Ginsberg, a township directly outside of King William's Town, and Mene was from Dimbaza, a larger urban location a bit further outside of King William's Town.[4] When the new researchers were deciding which participants they would work with, they requested that they not work with participants in the communities in which they live. They suggested that Mhlabeni interview participants in Dimbaza, where Mene is from, and vice versa. The reason, they explained, was that the social proximity between residents in their communities meant that participants might not feel as safe speaking about intimate issues for fear that others would find out.

In this context, the concern was that participants might be uncomfortable during or after the interview or less likely to open up for fear of unwanted disclosure of their HIV status or personal issues. Unspoken here was also that the researchers may also have been uncomfortable having in-depth and sensitive discussions with fellow community members, as these could complicate personal and professional boundaries. These findings align with evidence suggesting that geographic and social proximity may affect uptake and retention in HIV testing and care services, and that people may choose to visit healthcare providers or institutions in other localities in an attempt to maintain confidentiality (Mhode and Nyamhanga, 2016). This literature contrasts claims that long travel distances to clinics are a key factor in non-adherence. It suggests that in proximate health services, patients fear their HIV status will be disclosed and their confidentiality breached, which may negatively impact on accessing health services.

Researchers calibrated certain types of similarity and difference within the research encounter. Despite believing that linguistic and gendered similarities could support the research aims, they also recommended some distance in terms of age and geographic proximity. In doing so, they challenged a popular assumption that differences between researchers and participants are complicating factors in the research encounter. The next section of this chapter further explores how 'insider' and 'outsider' roles shaped this research.

The ways in which different forms of identity shape interactions was also evident in an unanticipated aspect of the study. As hoped, participants were opening up to the researchers. They were also asking them to act beyond their research role. While drafting the protocol for the study, the ethical and methodological challenges and responsibilities that could be encountered were carefully considered, including when participants ask for help. Challenges of working with a group of vulnerable young people in an environment where social services are limited and inconsistent have been documented by Cluver and colleagues (2014). In one week alone, one of the researchers (Mene) encountered a few self-referral cases where ABYM disclosed that they were struggling with drug addiction and requested help. This type of referral was relatively uncommon in the Mzantsi Wakho quantitative survey. Mzantsi Wakho quantitative researchers more frequently encountered participants sharing accounts of violence and hunger, and the established response protocol upheld the ethical commitments and legal requirements of the study. However, accounts of substance abuse were shared more openly and frequently by the participants in the Ezobudoda sub-study. These referrals raised several questions: Was it because the participants were getting older? Was this a gender issue (i.e. more common with boys than with girls)?

Our hypothesis was that while age and gender played a role, it was possible that participants also felt comfortable sharing this type of challenge with Mene because they (rightly) assumed that he would be unlikely to judge or scold them. As someone with a laid-back demeanour and relaxed style, Mene may have given them this impression.

Mhlabeni's referrals were often different in nature. Participants sought assistance for multiple challenges, ranging from intimate subjects such as navigating romantic relationships and material concerns about securing food and work to technology challenges such as how to fix a broken television. Boys frequently asked him for guidance on how to access social services (apply for social grants), and for advice related to circumcision and becoming a man. As someone who appeared to perform to Xhosa notions of being *indoda* in terms of his presentation, lifestyle and communication style, boys regarded Mhlabeni as an authority on masculine rites of passage.

Cluver and colleagues (2014) suggest that the presence of a caring, attentive adult is a reason why adolescent participants may open up and ask for help. Among study participants, many of whom did not have present fathers, being interviewed by a young man might have also been a rare occasion to have the positive attention of an engaged male figure. The requests for help made by the young men in this study may be attributed to a number of other interrelated factors. The research design saw researchers build relationships with participants over multiple interviews. These encounters also encouraged participants to speak freely and provided opportunities for them to ask questions and direct the conversation based on their interests. An additional factor may have been that participants demonstrated creativity and resilience by leveraging the research encounter as an opportunity to mobilise resources, a phenomenon that has been documented by Vale and Thabeng (2015). In the mix of all of these factors, given the different nature of referral cases that Mhlabeni and Mene met, a number of elements may have played a role in what participants felt comfortable to disclose. These may have included participants' perceptions of the researchers' interest in them and how they perceived the researchers' authority, expertise, abilities and personalities.

One finding here, which can be directly applied to HIV prevention research and programming, is that demographic factors coalesce with individual subjectivities and contextual circumstances in shaping interactions between adolescents and adults and between participants and researchers/programmers. The preceding case study suggests that a close, reflexive consideration of how intersubjective identities operate alongside the research or programmatic aims is warranted in working with adolescent boys and young men. Contextual factors, such as access to social support and engagement with caring adult male figures, may powerfully influence interactions with participants.

Careful consideration should also be given to the contexts and needs of participants and how to respond to requests for support. Researchers and programmers must undertake adequate planning and training prior to beginning a project, so that they are well-equipped to respond to the ethical and methodological imperatives of the work. Managing participant expectations and upholding the ethical commitments made are crucial steps to mitigating any mistrust or disappointment among participants and to guard against producing false expectations and empty promises. This process is especially important when working with adolescent boys and men in contexts of constraint and vulnerability.

Performing masculinit(ies) – strategies for engaging adolescent boys

These cases in some ways challenge the conventional belief that men do not seek care and support. One can infer that the participants had neither adequate access to social services and resources nor people who could effectively refer them. But was there something beyond the researchers' positionality that allowed participants to express themselves? How did these relationships form? In this section, we explore strategies to create more comfortable spaces for participants and argue that performances of both hegemonic and alternative masculine norms can foster the formation of such key relationships. We document how Mene and Mhlabeni performed to hegemonic masculine norms to gain trust and respect, and how they created spaces for alternative forms of expression by making boys feel comfortable.

While observing the researchers' engagements with participants, it became clear that they curated their performances of masculinity in order to make them feel comfortable and free to share. In the research setting, boys are often subject to instruction by older men and women, and a person is considered to be *indoda* only after completing *ulwaluko*. His age as a man begins from this point and is an organising factor that manifests in everyday interactions and traditional ceremonies alike. The process of initiation, and the time following, is often marked by instruction and testing by 'older' young men.

At the beginning of our research, 17 participants had undergone *ulwaluko*, mostly within the last year or two. This meant that even the 'oldest' participants were much younger, and in a different stage of life, than the researchers. The remainder were considered *amakhwenkwe* (translated from isiXhosa as 'boys') because they had not undergone *ulwaluko*.

Despite this evident hierarchy, in conversations with participants, the researchers often used descriptors such as 'my man', 'boss', *bhuti* ('brother' in isiXhosa) and 'my brother', treating participants in a manner that acknowledged their identities as emerging adult men. This approach affirmed participants' masculine identities and conveyed a sense of respect, familiarity, legitimacy and confidence. Although the researchers did not develop friendships per se with participants, they leveraged a different type of social capital that drew on their identities as employed, 'cool' young men to achieve the research aims. Making participants feel comfortable in this way supported the collection of rich data. However, this strategy also posed possible ethical challenges, including blurring boundaries between research and personal relationships and demonstrating simultaneous authority and familiarity that may have made it difficult for participants to set the terms of engagement.

Also relevant here are the ways that researchers perform to 'insider' and 'outsider' roles, in order to encourage participants to speak openly. In her work on Xhosa men's narratives of HIV risk, Zungu (2013) leveraged her outsider role (as woman of Zulu ethnicity) to probe sensitive matters that could not be spoken about in the presence of a Xhosa female. Despite speaking isiXhosa, and having worked for years in her research area, this outsider role allowed her to engage participants as authorities and informers of the subject.

By contrast, Mene and Mhlabeni leveraged their role as insiders by nature of having been legitimised as men by undergoing the process of *ulwaluko*. However, they also used the authority that having gone through this process bestowed upon them. These masculine performances were employed as a way to legitimise participants' masculine identities and establish familiarity with them. Although seemingly counterintuitive, such performances were the starting point for participants to become comfortable expressing more personal experiences and vulnerabilities. Despite the benefits of this approach, careful consideration should be given to avoiding further entrenching hegemonic masculine gender norms and to minimising social desirability bias.

Many participants in this sample have demonstrated creativity, agency and resilience in moving through precarious and challenging situations. This experience was evident in the ways that boys navigated health facility attendance and medicine-taking, responded to difficult social and familial situations and excelled in multiple areas of their lives. At the same time, they faced multiple intersecting challenges and vulnerabilities as (mostly) poor, HIV-positive and 'Black'[5] young people, growing up in contexts of precarity and constraint.

That people have lived experiences that are informed by multiple intersecting privileges and marginalisations (Crenshaw, 1991) is relevant here. By engaging with boys' masculine social capital[6] as an entry point, Mhlabeni and Mene discussed participants' structural, relational and personal vulnerabilities with them.

A methodological lesson from observing the researchers was that through performing to participants' masculinities (an area where participants held power), an entry point was created to express vulnerability. By engaging participants in a way that made them feel comfortable and validated, the researchers created a starting place to encourage them to speak about more challenging aspects of their identities and lives. This approach fits within a multi-level approach to children and resilience – one which considers social, material and relational factors that may affect their well-being while also recognising their agency and life skills (Skovdal and Daniel, 2012).

The ways in which male community health workers engage men living with HIV bear some similarity. In a previous study, we observed that male community health workers acted in a warm and informal way towards their clients and indirectly broached sensitive subjects (Gittings, 2016). In addition to employing these strategies with participants, Mene and Mhlabeni drew on their social capital as 'older' young men who were employed and 'cool'. They performed to hegemonic masculine norms as a way to gain respect and trust from male participants. This careful strategy, when performed properly, often made boys feel comfortable.

This groundwork, in turn, allowed for expressions of vulnerability and emotion – typically performances associated with alternative masculine norms. Participants spoke extensively about personal issues related to health services engagement and intimate relationships and expressed opinions that might be seen as controversial. Heartache, anger and fear were present in many participants' narratives. As discussed earlier, some also asked for advice and help.

While recognising the value of HIV research and programming work with ABYM, we must remain mindful of the pull of patriarchy, which privileges the perspectives and the needs of men above women and gender nonconforming people, and of heterosexual men above gay and transgendered men. Meeting men and boys 'where they are at', while at the same time not reifying gender binaries and harmful gender norms, is a challenge. If the goal is healthier individuals and societies and gender transformation, engaging strategies that draw on masculine norms and identities is not an end in itself but rather a means towards furthering research and programming practice for better health and gender equity outcomes. We explore this in the final section, which focuses on opportunities, pitfalls and challenges of such work. The strategies outlined above engaged aspects of hegemonic masculine identity and drew on their authority and resonance in fostering engagements with greater depth, trust and honesty.

Not all participants felt open to, or comfortable with, Mene and Mhlabeni's strategic performances of masculinity. For example, one participant who Mhlabeni believed to be 'gay' (his word) chose not to do a second interview. Another participant whose father was from Ghana openly questioned Xhosa notions of masculinity; Mene responded to this interaction neutrally, but he later disclosed that the experience had bothered him. These situations demonstrate the limitations of gender norms and scripts. In other words, formulaic performances to engage with participants are not always effective, and adolescent boys and young men require engagements that resonate with them.

However, the strategies that Mhlabeni and Mene employed worked relatively well most of the time. Almost all participants were willing to participate in a second and third interview, and some asked – unprompted – for the researchers to come back. In expressing their vulnerabilities, they demonstrated an ability and openness to alternative masculine performances. Their feeling comfortable was in part due to Mene's and Mhlabeni's strategies that drew on the authority offered by hegemonic masculine norms in order to acknowledge them as 'men'. This required delicately deploying hegemonic masculine norms without at the same time further entrenching them. In this context, being *indoda* by nature of having completed the process of *ulwaluko* allowed them to occupy the most honoured type of masculinity (Mfecane, 2016).

Outlined above are considerations of positionality, context and strategies for engaging boys and young men in HIV research and programming. The final section traces the contours of some of the debates around work with men and boys by drawing on case studies alongside the substantial and growing academic and programmatic literature that interrogates the meanings, benefits and challenges of such work.

Working with adolescent boys and young men – opportunities, pitfalls and challenges

While recruiting research assistants, we asked value-based and situational questions with the aim of determining if the interviewees held gender-equitable beliefs. Both researchers responded in a way that was in line with the values and skills we were looking for.

Over the period of a year, Gittings, Mene and Mhlabeni took many long drives together to visit participants, during which they would explore different ideas, happenings and theories together and co-analyse emergent findings. In conversations about gender, sex and intimacy they would usually speak indirectly, zig-zagging around the boundaries of the professional and the personal. As they learned more about each other's communication styles, they also began to fill in the spaces of what was not said. After working together closely over a period of many months, Mene and Mhlabeni started to demonstrate certain gender-inequitable beliefs.

One day, ten months into working together, Mhlabeni expressed his belief that women aren't good drivers, which surprised Gittings, because he would often ask her to drive. Mene responded by quipping that he didn't see a difference between men's and women's driving abilities. An animated discussion ensued. Gittings asked Mhlabeni why he asked her to drive if, as a woman, he believed she could not be a good driver. 'It's different with you because I'm used to it', he answered.

In a team meeting with a group of approximately 15 researchers, Gittings led an activity as an icebreaker where the team was read a list of yes/no/maybe questions about beliefs. 'Yes' was signaled by standing up with their arms above their heads, 'no' by sitting down on their chair, and a 'maybe' was displayed by standing with their arms at their sides.

They started with simple statements such as 'I had a nice weekend' and 'It is rude not to greet when you see someone'. After warming up, they engaged with more complex, and potentially more controversial statements. One such statement was 'Women are responsible for cooking and cleaning'. Mhlabeni and Mene stood up and stretched their hands over their heads, while the rest of the team sat down. Everyone else looked up at them, chuckling from their seats – partly in discomfort, and partly because of the irony of the only two staff members directly conducting gender research displaying this belief. The idea that women can be responsible for certain activities is not, in itself, gender inequitable. However, the (unequal) burden of labour and value placed on men's and women's work, combined with the team's different answers when asked about typical 'masculine' responsibilities, meant that these responses likely drew on a gender-inequitable belief about women's labour.

Why had they demonstrated this belief, given their awareness about gender equality and their interview responses a year earlier, in which they recounted different perspectives about men's and women's roles? Had their work, though aiming to understand boys' and young men's beliefs and actions, somehow cemented hegemonic masculine norms for them? Did being part of a sub-study that allowed the researchers more flexibility and privileges due to its design reinforce patriarchal norms that men and boys are superior, both as researchers and research participants? Or had the comfort, familiarity and trust the team had built created a space in which they felt open to share their gender-inequitable beliefs? And if the latter was the case, was it a 'good' thing, a step towards, or away from, the gender-transformative objectives of the research?

While not wanting to over-estimate the role of these interactions and their work as researchers on their belief systems, they had actively and continuously engaged about issues of gender over an extended period of time. Their speaking openly about beliefs that were professionally undesirable, and their sharing opinions that were different to Gittings's, suggests that relationships had been built where a certain degree of sharing, comfort and ability to express and manage conflicting beliefs was present.

A few days later Gittings asked Mhlabeni and Mene about the opinions they had shared. They said that they felt comfortable displaying their perspectives because, as a function of having frequent and frank conversations about gender, they were more comfortable talking about their beliefs than before. By contrast, they suggested that for the others in the room, their lived practice was also one where women were responsible for domestic work in their homes. They thought that their colleagues may have felt uncomfortable to express their belief that women should be responsible for domestic work in a group setting because they felt it socially unacceptable to do so.

The other potential explanation that Mene and Mhlabeni offered was that their colleagues might hold a different belief in theory, but not in practice, or hold different gendered beliefs for different spheres of their lives – in this case, work and home. This echoes Ratele's (2014) assertion that people might support gender equality in the abstract, but that this might not translate behaviourally. He posits that gender equality discourse may influence men's support of gender equality 'in the abstract' but that 'men's positive, but ambivalent and resistant gender attitudes' prevail (Ratele, 2014, p. 510). In a review of the evidence on work with men and boys, Gibbs and colleagues (2015) point out that such work does not always lead to behaviour changes that support gender equality. The processes and contexts in which work is implemented play a role in intervention effectiveness (Dworkin, Treves-Kagan and Lippman, 2013).

Were Mene and Mhlabeni's choices to display gender-inequitable beliefs in conflict with, ambivalent to or part of a gender-transformative process? Shifting socialised gender norms can be a lengthy and elusive endeavour (Gibbs, Vaughan and Aggleton, 2015). Is performing to socially acceptable gendered beliefs (while not believing them) better than burying gender-inequitable beliefs? In terms of Ratele's (2014) assertion that gender-equitable beliefs can exist in the abstract but not in practice, was it possible that Mhlabeni and Mene had 'broken the bubble' of the abstract but not shifted into practice? And was this the same as going back to explicit gender-inequitable beliefs or towards conscientization?

These questions and examples are raised as part of broader debates around working with ABYM for HIV prevention. As described earlier, gender inequality is a driver of HIV transmission, and ART initiation and retention in care are mediated by hegemonic masculine norms. For these reasons, questions of gender-equitable belief and practice are important to research and interventions focusing specifically on HIV and ABYM. It has been suggested that it is through practice that new ways of relating are produced (Sideris, 2004), and that it is necessary to create lived experiences of gender equality through structural and policy approaches as well as programmatic initiatives that change attitudes (Levtov et al., 2014).

As the preceding case studies and reflections demonstrate, the work of gender transformation is neither straightforward nor formulaic. We suggest that approaches that create space for dialogue and reflection, and that focus on processes (rather than solely on endpoints), are important components in the often complicated work of exploring and challenging gender norms.

Finally, as highlighted by scholars such as Mfecane (2016), Zungu (2013), Oyěwùmí (1997) and Hodes and Morrell (2018), the broader gendered context in which HIV work with men and boys takes place is important to consider. How do we engage with context-specific gendered constructs to support men's improved health outcomes? And what does it mean to be working with men and boys for HIV prevention in a context where women and girls are more biologically and socially at risk to HIV acquisition? Scholars such as Gupta et al. (2008) have mapped out the importance of multilayered and systematic approaches in addressing the multiple, overlapping structural and power dynamics that fuel the HIV epidemic. However, work with men and boys may still raise ethical and political considerations, given that it may be seen to compete for resources and attention with work with women and girls. It is therefore critical that gender-transformative research and practice with men and boys be able to articulate how its methods and objectives line up with broader feminist principles and goals.

Conclusion

Using case studies of HIV research with ABYM, this chapter raises questions about addressing gendered power imbalances and reducing HIV risks and poor health behaviours within this group.

Given the relational nature of gendered power and HIV risk, it is crucial to work with ABYM in order to improve population health outcomes (UNAIDS, 2017). Interventions to reduce the material vulnerabilities of adolescents have demonstrated efficacy in reducing HIV risk behaviours among adolescent girls, but not boys, suggesting the differently gendered relationships between material vulnerability and risky sexual behaviour (Cluver et al., 2013). This is relevant given that HIV risk increases for ABYM as they enter their twenties and thirties. Efforts and strategies for working with ABYM to prevent them from acquiring HIV, and from transmitting it onwards, require further elucidation.

In feminist and participatory research, the processes through which evidence is gathered are important. The lessons derived from this research point to the need for consideration of positionality and intersubjectivity, and the importance of considering the unique and intersecting identities, especially for those living in contexts of racialisation and discrimination, precarity and poverty. We suggest that careful consideration of demographic and personal qualities of facilitators, researchers and programme workers are important. Engagements can be radically shaped by elements of 'sameness', 'difference' and geographic proximity. Findings suggest that demographic factors should be carefully considered in deciding who conducts HIV work with ABYM, that sameness is not always more effective and that considerations of positionality are strongly mediated by context. Drawing on the expertise of participants and local researchers and programmers can help navigate these complexities.

Research and programming that aims to conduct in-depth work with ABYM must also consider the intersecting vulnerabilities and privileges of participants. The same structural factors that inform HIV risk will be present in aspects of participants' lives. During project development, consideration of how to respond to participant needs and requests for help that are beyond the context of the programme/research are essential, especially in contexts of precarity and constraint.

This chapter has described strategies for working with ABYM – including partially leveraging hegemonic masculine interactions – to creating the trusting and open relationships that support in-depth research and interventions to promote health and gender-equitable practice. We found that affirming aspects of participant masculine identities can be a starting point for alternative forms of engagement. This process requires delicate consideration of how to make participants feel safe while not reifying harmful hegemonic masculine norms and rigid gender binaries. In the complicated work of exploring and challenging gender norms, creating space for dialogue and reflection and the use of multiple methods to introduce different perspectives may guard against such risks.

Ideally, research and programming should be framed within conducive policy frameworks and a commitment to changing harmful gendered beliefs in practice. The process of meaningfully engaging men for HIV prevention efforts is informed by a variety of factors, including the very gendered power dynamics that are being challenged.

In a context in which little is known about gender transformation, the work of engaging with hegemonic masculine norms is complicated, with 'progress' being difficult to measure. The complexities and dynamics of gender work with ABYM are reflective of broader workplace and societal dynamics. Building and documenting relationships over time that allow for ongoing, continuous and non-judgemental engagement may provide some clues as to the pathways towards gender equity.

This chapter has drawn on case studies with qualitative researchers to consider some ethical and methodological aspects of HIV work with ABYM. In doing so, it aims to contribute to the movement for engaging men and to raise some theoretical, ethical and practical questions to add to our notions of young masculinities and HIV risk. The case studies have aimed to provide a window into how ABYM experience, manage and perform masculinity and to ultimately add depth to what we understand about this group.

Acknowledgements

This evidence was gathered within the auspices of a large longitudinal study on medicine-taking in the Eastern Cape, the Mzantsi Wakho study. We are grateful to co-principal investigators Professor Lucie Cluver and Dr Elona Toska, study collaborators at the Universities of Cape Town and Oxford, and the researchers who supported data collection and analysis as well as the research participants for sharing their perspectives and experiences that formed the basis of this research. Thank you also to Mlamli Mayosi for reviewing and providing input into the early drafts of this chapter and to Kaymarlin Govender, Andrew Gibbs and Timothy Quinlan for their detailed review and comments.

Thank you for the financial support provided by Evidence for HIV Prevention in Southern Africa (EHPSA), a DFID programme managed by Mott MacDonald (MM/EHPSA/UCT/05150014). In addition to EHPSA, Lesley Gittings was a supported by the South African National Research Foundation (NRF) Innovation scheme for doctoral student funding, the University of Cape Town AIDS and Society Research Unit (ASRU), the South African Social Science and HIV (SASH) Programme, an initiative funded by the Eunice Kennedy Shriver National Institute of Child Health and Human Development of the National Institutes of Health (Award #R24HD077976), the South African National Research Foundation travel funding for postgraduate students, and the University of Cape Town's Max and Lille Sonnenberg Scholarship for international travel.

Christopher J. Colvin was supported by the US National Institute of Mental Health and the South African Medical Research Council (SAMRC) [#1R01 MH106600]. This content is solely the responsibility of the authors and does not necessarily represent the official views of the aforementioned funders.

Data collection support was provided by the Mzantsi Wakho Study, funded by the Nuffield Foundation [CPF/41513], but the views expressed are those of the authors and not necessarily those of the Foundation; Evidence for HIV Prevention in Southern Africa (EHPSA), a UK aid programme managed by Mott MacDonald; Janssen Pharmaceutica N.V., part of the Janssen Pharmaceutical Companies of Johnson & Johnson; the Regional Inter-Agency Task Team for Children Affected by AIDS – Eastern and Southern Africa (RIATT-ESA); UNICEF Eastern and Southern Africa Office (UNICEF-ESARO); the International AIDS Society through the CIPHER grant [155-Hod; 2018/625-TOS], the views expressed in written materials or publications do not necessarily reflect the official policies of the International AIDS Society; Oxford University Clarendon-Green Templeton College Scholarship; Claude Leon Foundation [F08 559/C]; the Leverhulme Trust [PLP-2014–095]; the Oak Foundation [R46194/AA001], [OFIL-20-057]/GCRF "Accelerating Violence Prevention in Africa"; the University of Oxford's ESRC Impact Acceleration Account [K1311-KEA-004]; and the John Fell Fund [103/757; 161/033].

Notes

1 The limitations of literal and/or simplistic interpretations of geographical terms have been noted by scholars such as the Comaroff and Comaroff (2012), who suggest that power and marginality are important considerations in interpretation.
2 Constructs of masculinity in the research site hold a strong distinction between a 'boy' (in isiXhosa *inkwenkwe*, 'uncircumcised boy') and a 'man' (in isiXhosa *indoda*, a traditionally circumcised person), which are defined by whether a person has completed the process of *ulwaluko*.
3 Referred to throughout this chapter as *ulwaluko* (isiXhosa), or traditional initiation/circumcision. A rite of passage, *ulwaluko* is a powerful organising factor in constructions of masculinity among the amaXhosa (Mfecane, 2016; Mager, 1998).
4 Pseudonyms have been used for researcher and participant names throughout this chapter.
5 Racial identifiers, when used within this chapter, are put within quotation marks to denote that these categories are socially constructed. As much as possible, this work aims to avoid reproducing these categories while acknowledging these historical and ongoing constructs when relevant to this study. We aim to consider race-related power alongside other intersecting factors of power and marginalisation such as class identity, foreign status, language, HIV status and age.
6 Putnam (1993, p. 35) defines social capital as 'features of social organizations such as networks, norms and trust that facilitate action and cooperation for mutual benefit'.

References

Betron, M., Barker, G., Contreras, J. & Peacock, D., 2012. *Men, Masculinities and HIV/AIDS: Strategies for Action.* Available at: https://s28691.pcdn.co/wp-content/uploads/2014/12/Men-Masculinities-and-HIV-AIDS-Strategies-for-Action.pdf.

Cluver, L. et al., 2013. Child-Focused State Cash Transfers and Adolescent Risk of HIV Infection in South Africa: A Propensity-Score-Matched Case-Control Study. *The Lancet Global Health,* 1, pp. e362–e370.

Cluver, L. et al., 2014. The Cost of Action: Large Scale, Longitudinal Quantitative Research with AIDS-Affected Children in South Africa. In D. Posel & F. Ross, eds. *Ethical Quandaries in Social Research.* Cape Town: HSRC Press, pp. 41–56.

Colvin, C.J., Robins, S. & Leavens, J., 2010. Grounding "Responsibilisation Talk": Masculinities, Citizenship and HIV in Cape Town, South Africa. *Journal of Development Studies,* 46(7), pp. 1179–1195.

Comaroff, J. & Comaroff, J., 2012. *Theory from the South: Or, How Euro-America Is Evolving Toward Africa.* London: Paradigm Publishers.

Connell, R.W., 2005. *Masculinities.* Cambridge: Polity.

Cornell, M., McIntyre, J. & Myer, L., 2011. Men and Antiretroviral Therapy in Africa: Our Blind Spot. *Tropical Medicine and International Health,* 16(7), pp. 828–829.

Courtenay, W.H., 2000. Constructions of Masculinity and Their Influence on Men's Well-Being: A Theory of Gender and Health. *Social Science & Medicine,* 50(10), pp. 1385–1401.

Crenshaw, K., 1991. Mapping the Margins: Intersectionality, Identity Politics, and Violence Against Women of Color. *Stanford Law Review,* 43(6), pp. 1241–1299.

Dovel, K. et al., 2015. Men's Heightened Risk of AIDS-Related Death: The Legacy of Gendered HIV Testing and Treatment Strategies. *AIDS,* 29(10), pp. 1123–1125.

Dworkin, S. L., Fleming, P.J. & Colvin, C.J., 2015. The Promises and Limitations of Gender-Transformative Health Programming with Men: Critical Reflections from the Field. *Culture, Health & Sexuality*, 17(Suppl 2), pp. 128–143.

Dworkin, S. L., Treves-Kagan, S. & Lippman, S., 2013. Gender-Transformative Interventions to Reduce HIV Risks and Violence with Heterosexually-Active Men: A Review of the Global Evidence. *AIDS Behaviour*, 17(9), pp. 2845–2863.

Finlay, L., 2002. Negotiating the Swamp: The Opportunity and Challenge of Reflexivity in Research Practice. *Qualitative Research*, 2(2), pp. 209–230.

Fleming, P.J., Lee, J. G. L. & Dworkin, S. L., 2014. "Real Men Don't": Constructions of Masculinity and Inadvertent Harm in Public Health Interventions. *American Journal of Public Health*, 104(6), pp. 1029–1035.

Gibbs, A., Vaughan, C. & Aggleton, P., 2015. Beyond "Working with Men and Boys": (Re)defining, Challenging and Transforming Masculinities in Sexuality and Health Programmes and Policy. *Culture, Health & Sexuality*, 17(Suppl 2), pp. 85–95.

Gittings, L., 2016. "When You Visit a Man You Should Prepare Yourself": Male Community Care Worker Approaches to Working with Men Living with HIV in Cape Town South Africa. *Culture, Health & Sexuality*, 18(8), pp. 936–950.

Govender, K., 2011. The Cool, the Bad, the Ugly, and the Powerful: Identity Struggles in Schoolboy Peer Culture. *Culture, Health & Sexuality*, 13(8), pp. 887–901.

Gupta, G.R. et al., 2008. Structural Approaches to HIV Prevention. *Lancet*, 372(9640), pp. 764–775.

Hensels, I.S. et al., 2016. Do Not Forget the Boys – Gender Differences in Children Living in High HIV-Affected Communities in South Africa and Malawi in a Longitudinal, Community-Based Study. *AIDS Care*, 28, pp. 100–109.

Hodes, R. & Morrell, R., 2018. Incursions from the Epicentre: Southern Theory, Social Science, and the Global HIV Research Domain. *African Journal of AIDS Research*, 17(1).

Jewkes, R. et al., 2011. Gender Inequitable Masculinity and Sexual Entitlement in Rape Perpetration South Africa: Findings of a Cross-Sectional Study B.J. Shea, ed. *PLoS One*, 6(12), p.e29590.

Johnson, L. F. et al., 2013. Life Expectancies of South African Adults Starting Antiretroviral Treatment: Collaborative Analysis of Cohort Studies. *PLoS Medicine*, 10(4).

Langa, M., 2010. Adolescent Boys' Talk About Absent Fathers. *Journal of Psychology in Africa*, 20(4), pp. 519–526.

Levtov, R.G. et al., 2014. Pathways to Gender- Equitable Men: Findings from the International Men and Gender Equality Survey in Eight Countries. *Men and Masculinities*, 17(5), pp. 467–501.

Lindegger, G. & Quayle, M., 2009. Masculinity and HIV/AIDS. In P. Rohleder et al., eds. *HIV/AIDS in South Africa 25 Years on: Psychosocial Perspectives*. New York: Springer-Verlag.

Mager, A., 1998. Youth Identities and Construction of Masculine Identities in Ciskei and Transkei, 1945–1960. *Journal of Southern African Studies*, 24(4), pp. 653–667.

Maher, F. A. & Tetreault, M.K., 1993. Frames of Positionality: Constructing Meaningful Dialogues About Gender and Race. *Anthropological Quarterly, Feminism and Postmodernism in Anthropology and the Academy*, 66(3 Part 2), pp. 118–126.

Mathews, S., Jewkes, R. & Abrahams, N., 2011. "I Had a Hard Life": Exploring Childhood Adversity in the Shaping of Masculinities Among Men Who Killed an Intimate Partner in South Africa. *British Journal of Criminology*, 51(6), pp. 960–977.

Mfecane, S., 2008. Living with HIV as a Man: Implications for Masculinity. *Psychology in Society*, 36(Special Issue on Masculinities 2), pp. 45–59.
Mfecane, S., 2010. *Exploring Masculinities in the Context of ARV Use: A Study of Men Living with HIV in a South African Village.* Johannesburg: University of Witwatersrand.
Mfecane, S., 2016. "Ndiyindoda" [I am a Man]: Theorising Xhosa Masculinity. *Anthropology Southern Africa*, 39(3), pp. 204–214.
Mhode, M. & Nyamhanga, T., 2016. Experiences and Impact of Stigma and Discrimination among People on Antiretroviral Therapy in Dar es Salaam: A Qualitative Perspective. *AIDS Research and Treatment.* https://doi.org/10.1155/2016/7925052
Oyěwùmí, O., 1997. *The Invention of Women: Making an African Sense of Western Gender Discourses.* Minneapolis: University of Minnesota Press.
Pease, B. & Flood, M., 2008. Rethinking the Significance of "Attitudes" in Challenging Men's Violence Against Women. *Australian Journal of Social Issues*, 43, pp. 547–561.
Putnam, R., 1993. The Prosperous Community. *The American Prospect*, 4(13), pp. 35–42.
Ramose, M. B., 1999. *African Philosophy Through Ubuntu.* Harare: Mond Books.
Ratele, K., 2014. Gender Equality in the Abstract and Practice. *Men and Masculinities*, 17(5), pp. 510–514.
Sideris, T., 2004. Men, Identity and Power. A Case Study of the Re-Invention of "Tradition": Implications for Involving Men in Training and Education About Gender. *Agenda*, 60, pp. 37–41.
Skovdal, M. & Daniel, M., 2012. Resilience Through Participation and Coping-Enabling Social Environments: The Case of HIV-Affected Children in Sub-Saharan Africa. *African Journal of Agricultural Research*, 11(3), pp. 153–164.
UNAIDS, 2017. *Blind Spot: Reaching Out to Men and Boys, Addressing a Blind Spot in the Response to HIV.* Geneva: UNAIDS.
Vale, B. & Thabeng, M., 2015. Mobilising AID(S)? Contesting HIV as a Social and Economic Resource Among Youth in South Africa's Eastern Cape. *Journal of Southern African Studies*, 41(4), pp. 797–813.
Wetherell, M. & Edley, N., 2014. A Discursive Psychological Framework for Analyzing Men and Masculinities. *Psychology of Men & Masculinity*, 15(4), pp. 355–364.
WHO, 2015. *Estimates for 2000–2012: Disease Burden.* Geneva: WHO.
Zungu, N., 2013. *Social Representations of AIDS and Narratives of Risk Among Xhosa Men.* Cape Town: University of Cape Town.

11 Closing the gap in programming for adolescents living with HIV in Eastern and Southern Africa

The role of social protection in positive prevention

Nompumelelo Zungu, Elona Toska, Lesley Gittings and Rebecca Hodes

Introduction

The Eastern and Southern Africa (ESA) region has a high burden of HIV and AIDS, with an estimated 19.6 million people living with the virus (UNAIDS, 2018). All countries in the region have 'generalised' epidemics, with an adult prevalence of 6.8% among those aged 15–49 (greater variations are observed between countries). HIV incidence and prevalence tends to be concentrated in particular sub-populations such as adolescent girls and young women (AGYW), men who have sex with men (MSM), transgender people, people who sell sex, prisoners and people who inject drugs (UNAIDS, 2018). According to UNICEF, 2.1 million adolescents aged 10–19 were living with HIV globally in 2016. Furthermore, 590,000 young people between the ages of 15 and 24 were newly infected with HIV, of whom 250,000 were adolescents between the ages of 15 and 19 in 2017 (UNAIDS, 2018). AGYW aged 15–24 are the most affected by HIV: HIV prevalence among this population in the ESA region was double that among adolescent boys and young men (ABYM) in 2016 (3.4% vs 1.6%) (UNAIDS, 2017; Govender et al., 2018). Furthermore, while HIV incidence rates are generally decreasing, they are still high in many ESA countries (UNAIDS, 2017). It is estimated that new HIV infections declined by 56% among children (aged 14 or younger) to 77,000 between 2010 and 2016 (UNAIDS, 2017). Among adults, declines were estimated at 29% over the same period, although significant variations are observed between countries.

In light of the foregoing, UNICEF (2017) has estimated that, without concerted action, the actual number of new adolescent infections will increase steadily in the next decade. In addition, in the last decade, reductions in AIDS-related sickness and death among children and adolescents in the region have demonstrated the vital impact of national ART programmes. While remarkable progress has been made in preventing paediatric HIV through the provision of prevention of mother-to-child transmission treatment, HIV testing and ART initiation and adherence, support for children and adolescents is lacking. Figures from UNICEF (2017) suggest that only 43% of infants exposed to HIV are tested within two months, and that only 43% of the 2.1 million children living with HIV globally are receiving ART. Thus, while HIV testing and treatment for infants has improved in recent years, the benefits of these programmes tapers off for older children and adolescents.

Limited available data for adolescents suggest worrisome trends regarding treatment access and AIDS-related deaths (UNAIDS, 2017). According to UNAIDS (2018), only 67 countries worldwide reported disaggregated adolescent treatment data. Among these, median ART coverage was low, at 20% in 2016. These data suggest that adolescents in ESA are the only population group in the region among which AIDS-related morbidity and mortality continues to grow (UNAIDS, 2018). The total numbers of adolescents living with HIV are growing, with a greater proportion of those infected through mother-to-child transmission surviving into adulthood due to improved access to ART, while new infections among 15–24-year-olds persist (UNAIDS, 2017).

The findings of the HPTN052 study (showing that ART can prevent onward transmission among HIV-discordant individuals) have challenged the assumption that HIV treatment and prevention are distinct, with a growing body of research demonstrating how effective HIV treatment and prevention are intrinsically connected (Cohen et al., 2013). This evidence, coupled with the UNAIDS 90–90–90 targets and the recent move to adopt a 'test and treat' approach in many countries with high HIV prevalence and incidence, has led to the promotion of ART as means of enabling 'positive prevention' among key populations and vulnerable groups such as AGYW aged 15–24. The current, burgeoning evidence base on associations between social protection and improvements in health outcomes among HIV-positive children and adolescents opens up a new field of prospective enquiry and promising prospective interventions.

There is growing evidence that social protection programmes have the potential to reduce HIV transmission through promoting safer sexual behaviours among adolescents and promoting adherence to ART. UNICEF defines social protection as 'a set of public and private policies and programmes aimed at preventing, reducing and eliminating economic and social vulnerabilities to poverty and deprivation' (UNICEF, 2015). It includes both formal and informal initiatives that provide social assistance to extremely poor individuals and households, with an aim of mitigating risks and related consequences (Devereux and Sabates-Wheeler, 2004). Social protection can be provided through public (governmental and non-governmental) and private institutions and may fulfil protective, promotive, preventative or transformative capacities. In this chapter, social protection is conceptualised broadly to include many possible interventions and components that fall under this umbrella term. Specifically, this chapter focuses on the burgeoning evidence base on associations between access to social grants and other forms of social protection and the improved positive health outcomes among ALHIV. A transdisciplinary research base that captures the impact of social protection initiatives on health behaviours demonstrates the intertwining of health and social domains in global development, and the responsiveness of each to boundary-spanning interventions that may target either health or social development, but whose benefits ripple widely from their central location to other dimensions of life, well-being and livelihood.

We employ a twofold conceptualisation of HIV prevention, treatment and care package for adolescents living with HIV (Gittings et al., 2016), as both the prevention of new HIV-infections among those previously HIV-negative and as the prevention of onward transmission of HIV – 'positive prevention'. This chapter makes the case for elaborating the positive protection approach, drawing on existing HIV-oriented social protection programmes. The chapter draws on previous work about the potential of social protection to support positive prevention and adherence to ART for children and adolescents living with HIV (Gittings et al., 2016; Toska et al., 2017a). In doing so, it highlights the urgent need for flexible, inclusive and responsive social protection mechanisms as a promising and productive means of promoting improved health outcomes and reducing risk behaviours among ALHIV.

ART adherence, sexual practices and reproductive health among ALHIV in ESA

A growing evidence base shows that biomedical interventions combined with social programmes are the best means of reducing new HIV infections and, ultimately, turning the tide of the AIDS epidemic (Padian et al., 2010), especially among young people (Cluver et al., 2016a). However, while reducing incidence through keeping adolescents HIV-free is critical, it is also important to support those already living with HIV to lead safe and healthy lives, including through viral suppression, engaging in safer sex and having planned, safe pregnancies and parenthoods. This section briefly reviews factors related to non-adherence and sexual risk-taking among adolescents living with HIV. It describes how different forms of social protection may help to support ART-adherence and reduce sexual risk-taking among adolescents in hyper-endemic contexts.

ART offers an opportunity for the survival and long-term well-being of people living with HIV. Yet many of the estimated 1.2 million children and adolescents living with HIV in ESA struggle to initiate and remain on ART. Once initiated on ART, 80%–95% adherence is required to avoid medication resistance, meaning that even occasional lapses in adherence to the ART regimen could reduce its efficacy (Paterson et al., 2000). Promisingly, increased linkages to ensure that adolescents access both sexual and reproductive health (SRH) and HIV services have been shown to increase

HIV-positive adolescents' access to and use of treatment services (UNICEF, 2015) and healthcare (Hodes et al., 2018a, 2018b).

Understanding the sexual practices and reproductive health needs of adolescents living with HIV remains critical for positive prevention. A recent systematic review focusing on sexual risk-taking among adolescents found mostly cross-sectional evidence on eight sexual risk-taking outcomes in 13 ESA countries (Toska et al., 2017b). Studies reported widely varying rates of sexual risk-taking, with nearly half of adolescents being sexually active, 33%–50% reporting unprotected sex, and 10%–66% reporting other sexual risk practices such as transactional sex, multiple sexual partners in the last year or sex with older men (Toska et al., 2017b). Adolescent girls living with HIV reported higher prevalence of transactional sex, unprotected sex and sex with older partners, though adolescent boys were more likely to report early sexual debut and multiple sexual partners.

Social, economic and structural drivers of sexual risk behaviours and non-adherence to ART

The limited research on adolescent ART adherence shows that many adolescents struggle to comply with ART regimens (Auld et al., 2014) and reveals exceptionally low rates of children and adolescents maintaining ART adherence (Cluver et al., 2016b; Hudelson & Cluver, 2015; Nachega et al., 2009). Evidence suggests that a combination of factors, including lack of social support, disclosure challenges, food insecurity and the costs of clinic attendance make it difficult for adolescents to initiate and remain on treatment (Cluver et al., 2016b; Hudelson & Cluver, 2015; Nachega et al., 2009). A burgeoning literature documents the additional, various experiential, clinical and operational challenges that adolescents living with HIV face in engaging with health programmes (Bernays et al., 2016; Delany-Moretlwe et al., 2015; Toska et al., 2015; Vale, Hodes & Cluver, 2017; Visser, Zungu & Ndala-Magoro, 2015).

Drivers of ART non-adherence and sexual risk-taking among adolescents living with HIV include (1) social, economic and structural issues; (2) non-disclosure, stigma and discrimination; (3) caregiver well-being, disrupted family structures and caregiver-child relationships; and (4) healthcare services and health systems factors (Campbell et al., 2012; Gittings et al., 2016; Hudelson & Cluver, 2015). A growing literature also demonstrates the interconnections between structural deprivations, non-adherence to ART and sexual risk-taking (Kidman et al., 2018; Toska & Cluver, 2018). This evidence is presented below, providing an overview on how structural drivers, stigma and discrimination, caregiver relationships and family structure, and health services are linked to both poor ART adherence and sexual risk outcomes.

Social, economic, and structural drivers – Poverty and related food insecurity are known barriers to ART adherence. Many adolescents living with HIV in ESA face food insecurity, and believe that these medicines must be taken with food (Gittings et al., 2016; WHO, 2015). Food insecurity and poverty are also known drivers of HIV risk behaviours for adolescent girls because they promote high-risk relationships with older partners, in which transactional sex provides the means of subsistence or survival for girls and young women. These vulnerabilities are mutually reinforcing, fostering a concatenation of risky behaviours, including unprotected sex and ART non-adherence. Understanding the gendered dimension of ART non-adherence for adolescents is also important because certain social protection interventions may affect boys and girls differently (Cluver et al., 2016b; Handa et al., 2014), and a higher proportion of new adolescent infections occur in girls (UNAIDS, 2017). Given that age-disparate sex is a driver of these infections, work with their older male partners on safer sexual practices and improved ART adherence is also warranted.

A recent study found that exposure to violence – at home and school and in clinics – was strongly linked with increased ART non-adherence, as shown in Figure 11.1 (Cluver et al., 2018), with exposure to multiple types of violence associated with higher levels of ART non-adherence. The study focuses on the detrimental effects of clinic victimisation in particular, identifying the negative impact that punitive, debasing and violent healthcare services have on both healthcare attendance and compliance with medical regimens among adolescents. Regarding other forms of violent victimisation beyond healthcare facilities, several studies in Uganda and Kenya reported that gender-based violence was linked with unintended pregnancies (Nhamo, 2013; Obare, Birungi & Kavuma, 2011) and transactional sex (Nhamo, 2013). The association between violence and ART non-adherence requires further investigation.

Disclosure, stigma and discrimination – Social barriers to treatment must be challenged, particularly HIV-related stigma and discrimination and legislation addressing the criminalisation of HIV non-disclosure, onward transmission, and age of consent to access testing services and criminalising same-sex practices through legislation. Evidence from community-based HIV testing programmes suggests that removing such barriers would encourage more people to get tested and seek out treatment (Iwuji et al., 2018; Orne-Gliemann et al., 2015). For fear of unwanted disclosure, some adolescents and young adults may not adhere to medicines when they are in situations where they might be seen taking medicines (leading to unintended HIV-positive serostatus disclosure) – such as in public, or even in social situations and with friends, family members or intimate partners (Hodes et al., 2018a). This issue may be compounded by fear of loss of material support in situations in which adolescents are also receiving material support from their partners (Toska et al., 2015) and family or community members.

Negative effects on adherence have also been seen in children and adolescents who have not been disclosed to at an appropriate age, defined by WHO as starting at the age of 10 and completed by the age of 12 (Cluver et al., 2015; Hudelson & Cluver, 2015). This may be due to poor understanding of

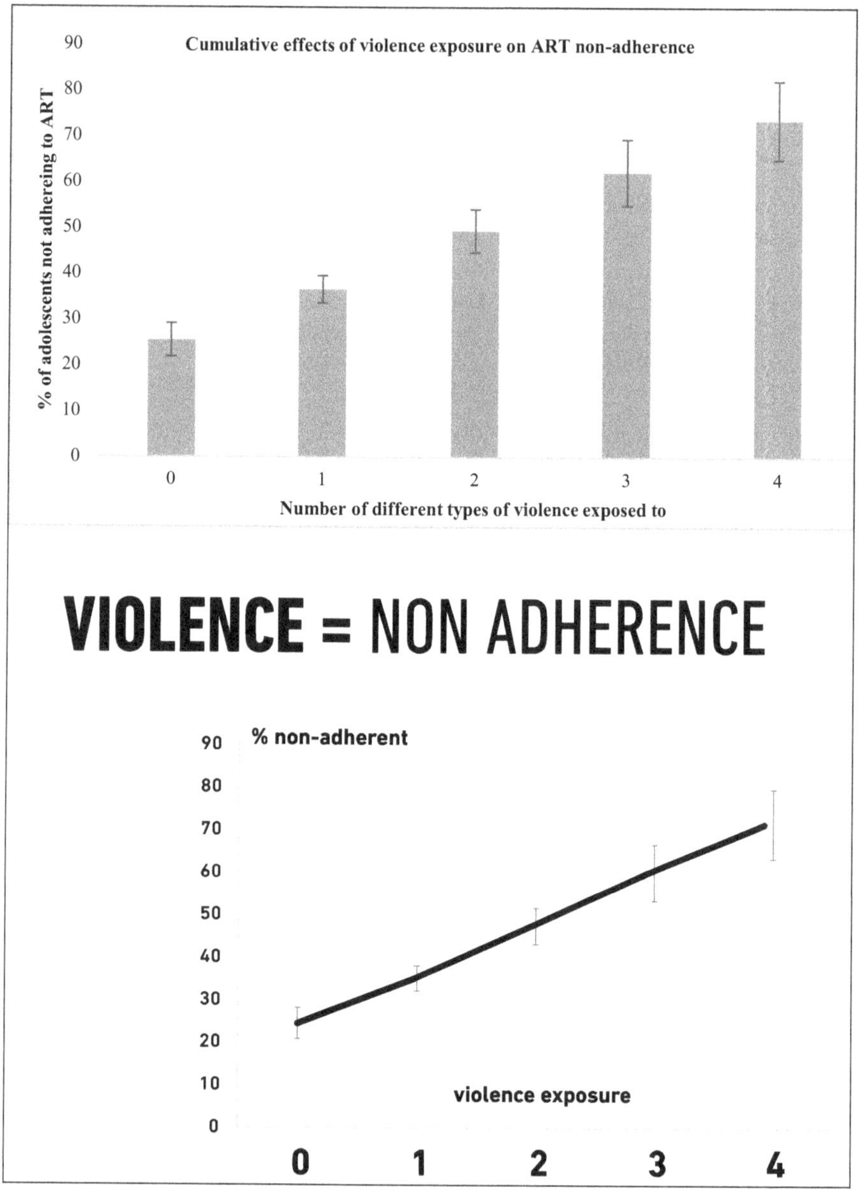

Figure 11.1 Marginal effects model testing for additive effect of violence on adolescent ART adherence (Cluver et al., *2018* – figure INCLUDED with AUTHOR permission).

Source: Cluver et al. (2018).

the reasons for which they are taking medication or issues with acceptance of their HIV-positive status. By contrast, adolescents who were disclosed to early, and in a sensitive and supportive way, achieve better adherence and sexual health outcomes (Cluver et al., 2015; Toska et al., 2015).

Caregiver relationships and family structures – Living alone or with a partner (compared to living with a caregiver) were strongly associated with sexual risk-taking among adolescents living with HIV in two studies in Uganda (Baryamutuma et al., 2010; Mbalinda et al., 2015). Moreover, caregiver monitoring is closely linked to safe sexual practices among adolescents living with HIV (Toska et al., 2017a). For this reason, it has been suggested that caregiver psychosocial and physical well-being is fundamental to supporting ART adherence and safe sexual practices (Cluver et al., 2018; Hudelson & Cluver, 2015; Toska et al., 2017a; WHO, 2015).

Healthcare services and system factors – There are also many documented healthcare-related barriers to ART adherence, including treatment costs, travel costs and distances to clinics and transition between paediatric and adult care (Cluver et al., 2018; Hudelson & Cluver, 2015; PATA & WHO, 2015). Additionally, accessing HIV and reproductive health services separately can be stigmatising, which is a core reason for integration of HIV and sexual healthcare to support all SRH services to be HIV-inclusive rather than HIV-specific[1] (Hodes, 2013; Gittings et al., 2016). HIV-related stigma and discrimination can exacerbate social exclusion and create barriers to the uptake of health services, particularly among adolescents. Transformative social protection aims to create enabling legal and normative environments for the delivery of provisions that address stigma and reduce barriers to uptake of health services (Gittings et al., 2016).

Syndemic risk factors for ART adherence and sexual risk-taking – The research among ALHIV in ESA outlined in the section below suggests a strong overlap between factors shaping ART adherence, sexual risk-taking and retention in HIV/SRH care in this vulnerable group of young people. Many of these factors are shared for both of these health outcomes and are closely linked to structural vulnerabilities. Given that non-adherence combined with risky sexual practices fosters high-risk situations for HIV onward transmission, efforts to improve adherence must go hand in hand with those aimed at promoting safer sex.

Social protection to interrupt pathways for non-adherence and sexual risk-taking – a review of the evidence

A growing body of literature demonstrates that social protection is a critical enabler for HIV prevention outcomes through interrupting pathways for non-adherence and sexual risk-taking (Baird et al., 2012; Gittings et al., 2016). There is also a strong evidence base that shows the impacts of social protection on HIV and risky-sex pathways such as food insecurity, early marriage, economic migration, transactional sex, early pregnancy, early sexual debut and school dropout (Gittings et al., 2016; Shisana et al., 2014; UNICEF, 2015). This section provides an overview of this evidence.

In 2016, a review was conducted on the role of social protection for improved adherence and HIV-related health outcomes among children and adolescents in ESA that extended and detailed these findings. The review found 11 programmes, including one RCT (Ssewamala et al., 2018), one pre-post pilot (Bhana et al., 2014), one pre-post small-scale pilot RCT (Snyder et al., 2014), two quantitative (Grimwood et al., 2012; Van Winghem et al., 2008) and six qualitative studies (Busza et al., 2014; Denison et al., 2015; Mupambireyi et al., 2014; O'Hare et al., 2005; Strasser & Gibbons, 2014) for which there was evidence of ART adherence outcomes among children aged 15 or younger) and/or adolescents (aged 10–19). The majority of these included adherence alongside other outcomes, such as HIV treatment knowledge, psychosocial well-being and retention in care (Gittings et al., 2016).

A more recent systematic review of ART adherence interventions among adolescents living with HIV found only one additional new programme to support ART adherence among adolescents living with HIV, although a study conducted in Thailand provided useful insights into the potential of group-based adherence counselling (Ridgeway et al., 2018).

A 2017 systematic review of programmes to prevent or respond to sexual risk-taking among adolescents living with HIV located four interventions. Three of the included intervention studies were individual-level randomised controlled trials (Lightfoot, Rotheram-Borus & Tevendale, 2007; Nhamo, 2013; Senyonyi et al., 2012), with one pre- and post-test experimental design study (Snyder et al., 2014). All four studies reported increases in condom use following the intervention; however, these were only significant in one intervention (Nhamo, 2013). The social protection interventions included in these studies were group-based support, livelihoods training, and integrated HIV/SRH services.

What types of social protection work?

Among different types of social protection, cash transfers have received significant attention, and there is a rich multidisciplinary literature on their efficacy. 'Cash transfers', in the form of social support grants, travel vouchers to get to facilities and school lunch programmes, can support adherence by addressing poverty-related factors, such as food insecurity and household unemployment (Cluver et al., 2018). In addition, evidence demonstrates that social transfers in the form of transport costs and food can have an effect on adult ART adherence (UNAIDS, 2014). However, the current literature is unclear on whether 'cash-only' social protection interventions directly impact adolescent adherence to ART. The only intervention that focused on ART adherence is a cash plus care plus capability intervention trial in Uganda, which focuses directly on adherence and viral suppression

(Bermudez et al., 2018; Ssewamala et al., 2018). Two additional pre- and post-test small-scale trials including adherence outcomes had promising results (Bhana et al., 2013; Snyder et al., 2014). Cross-sectional analyses from a large cohort in South Africa found that improving food security was associated with reduced ART non-adherence (Cluver et al., 2016b). Within this study, having sufficient funding to get to the clinic was also associated with improved retention on treatment (Cluver et al., 2018).

Among trials and evaluations of social cash transfers, seven studies found improvements in HIV-related treatment knowledge and adherence (Gittings et al., 2016). Twelve studies included children and adolescents living with HIV, and two of these were quantitative studies of care only that focused on improving ART-related outcomes (Grimwood et al., 2012; Van Winghem et al., 2008). The other two were pre-post pilot studies of care-only interventions (Bhana et al., 2013; Snyder et al., 2014). One trial among adolescent girls living with HIV in Zimbabwe combined cash with care interventions (Nhamo, 2013), resulting in improved condom use and reduced transactional sex. Additional analyses from a large cohort in South Africa suggests that attending fee-free schools combined with care interventions at home and clinics was strongly associated with reduced unprotected sex, especially among adolescent girls living with HIV (Toska et al., 2017a). These last two studies demonstrate associations between social protection interventions and the enhanced capacity for 'positive prevention' among ALHIV.

Beyond cash social protection, care mechanisms offer value in several ways: through directly benefitting recipients, acting as flexible mechanisms that can respond to their shifting, complex needs, in supporting the uptake and retention of other types of social protection (Gittings et al., 2016). Care provisions improved adherence in two pre- and post-test small-scale pilot trials (Bhana et al., 2013; Snyder et al., 2014), three quantitative studies (Cluver et al., 2016a; Grimwood et al., 2012; Van Winghem et al., 2008) and six qualitative studies (Busza et al., 2014; Denison et al., 2015; Mupambireyi et al., 2014; Parker et al., 2013; Strasser and Gibbons, 2014).

The potential of home-based and community care interventions has been demonstrated. One study found an association between receiving a community care intervention and reduced probabilities of attrition and mortality (Grimwood et al., 2012). A study by Busza and colleagues found that home-based care support was positively received by families of children and younger adolescents living with HIV in Tanzania (Busza et al., 2014). HIV-specific support groups have shown increased linkages to healthcare for adolescents living with HIV (Snyder et al., 2014), and peer-education interventions have also demonstrated improved adherence support (Denison et al., 2015). Such home- and community-based care programmes may improve ART adherence by providing psychosocial support, replacing costs of traditional healthcare (facility-based care) and enabling beneficiaries access to livelihood opportunities and life-saving health services (Busza et al., 2014; Gittings et al., 2016; Grimwood et al., 2012). There is also a much larger literature on community and home-based care initiatives for HIV testing and treatment (Hodes and Naimak, 2011; Schneider, Hlophe and van Rensburg, 2008) preceded in South Africa by community-based healthcare interventions reaching back over half a century (Phillips, 2014).

Three group and individual counselling-based programmes to reduce sexual risk-taking among adolescents living with HIV in Kenya and Uganda showed promising reductions in unprotected sex and multiple sexual partners. Last, capability interventions (i.e. programmes that support skills development and advance livelihoods) demonstrate promise (Gittings et al., 2016). For some adolescents, accessing interventions that support their capabilities may support ART adherence through better financial outcomes and therefore improve food and clinic access and reduce riskier sex.

Evidence also demonstrates that social protection, particularly cash plus care provisions in combination, have greater potential for improved HIV-related health outcomes among adolescents than cash interventions alone (Bandiera et al., 2012; Cho et al., 2011; Cluver et al., 2016a; Duflo, Dupas & Kremer, 2011; Karim, 2015). It has been suggested that social protection interventions with multiple components have additive and possibly multiplicative effects (Cluver et al., 2016a) and are necessary to meet the complex psychosocial needs of adolescents living with HIV (Amzel et al., 2013). Combinations can respond to the manifold pathways to ART non-adherence, in acknowledgement of the myriad intersecting challenges that adolescents may face to adherence. Promisingly, there is evidence that improving food security alone, and combined with other forms of social protection, significantly affected adherence outcomes for adolescents living with HIV (Cluver et al., 2016b). Similarly, combining care interventions (good caregiver monitoring) with clinic care (adolescent-sensitive services) and cash interventions (access to fee-free schools) reduced unprotected sex reported by adolescent girls living with HIV (Gittings et al., 2016).

How affordable and feasible is social protection?

The relative affordability, acceptability and scalability of social protection provisions are common concerns for ESA governments and for bilateral agencies. Social protection initiatives for children and adolescents are an investment in their health and well-being. They are also a long-term cost-saving mechanism through off- setting the costs of poor health outcomes and capitalising further on earlier investments in public health (Remme etal., 2014). The World Bank Social Safety Nets report (2015) examined social assistance in 120 developing countries and suggested that well-designed social assistance programmes are cost-effective (between 1.5% and 1.9% of GDP). Social assistance in sub-Saharan Africa only covers one-tenth of the poorest 20% (Honorati, Gentilini & Yemtsov, 2015), and expanding social protection provisions is possible for most African countries (Garcia & Moore, 2012). Co-financing from multiple government departments (as demonstrated in the STRIVE consortium) can make budgetary commitments for social protection more manageable but requires integrating evaluations and budgeting mechanisms. It also requires a conceptual shift in the cost-benefit analysis of health and social programming, similar to what was required in the reconceptualisation of the global ART rollout as not just a social and medical good but an investment in public health which would benefit the fiscus over the long term. Recent cost-benefit modeling from South Africa suggests that an investment of ZAR 4154.22 (USD 299.73) per adolescent living with HIV per year would allow for 69.5% to be retained in care (Standish-White, 2018).

Conclusion and recommendations

In view of the potential linkages between poor adherence and sexual risk-taking among ALHIV (Kidman et al., 2018; Marhefka et al., 2010; Toska & Cluver, 2018), it is of crucial importance to identify policy and programmatic interventions that can address their vulnerabilities in order to improve their health and resilience and to prevent the onward transmission of HIV. Our analysis of key findings in the literature suggests that flexible and responsive social protection mechanisms can be an important component in the response to the complex causal pathways of HIV risk. Evidence on social protection programmes and policies highlights the potential for combinations of social protection interventions, particularly 'cash' combined with 'care' and 'capability', to interrupt pathways for sexual risk behaviours and non-adherence to ART and to foster resilience.

The focus of this chapter is not only on social protection programmes and policies that help HIV-negative children and adolescents stay healthy, but also that support children and adolescents living with HIV to take medication and prevent transmitting HIV onwards. There is a small body of literature on positive prevention, ART adherence and social protection among adolescents in ESA. However, a review of evidence suggests a number of overlapping mechanisms through which social protection may achieve these impacts: (1) poverty reduction and economic development (Gillespie et al., 2007; Nattrass & Gonsalves, 2009); (2) improved educational outcomes such as school retention for girls and young women (Pettifor et al., 2008; UNAIDS, 2014; UNICEF, 2015); (3) improved food security (Cluver et al., 2016b; Emenyonu et al., 2010); and (4) improved psychosocial outcomes (Govender et al., 2014). Investigating overlapping mechanisms and additive effects of health and social interventions signals a move away from single-source, siloed and isolated interventions towards a more comprehensive, collective and broadscale conceptualisation of the boundary-spanning, complementary and interlinked effects of development work across the domains of health and social development.

Available evidence indicates the potential of social protection for alleviating structural drivers of HIV risk, including poverty and unemployment, gender inequalities and social stigma and marginalisation. If social protection is to be effective for children and adolescents, it must be both HIV-inclusive and responsive to their developmental and contextual needs (Delany-Moretlwe et al., 2015; Pettifor et al., 2015). A key area for further inquiry is improving our understandings of how different combinations of social protection programmes can have the most impact for the prevention of new HIV infections as well as 'positive prevention' among adolescents living with HIV.

Global strategies such as the Fast Track targets and policy directives such as the Sustainable Development Goals offer a breadth of opportunity for scaling up more holistic forms of social protection. These development plans commit governments, donors and bilateral partners to ambitious, large-scale improvements in health and social service provision, and they are often echoed by the state's own policy provisions and commitments, reflected, for instance, in the objectives of South Africa's National Development Plan (National Planning Commission, 2012).

The literature surveyed in this chapter suggests that different forms of social protection can support improved ART adherence and reduce risky sexual practices among adolescents living with HIV. This is promising in achieving the dual objectives of keeping young people living with HIV healthy while reducing the risk of onward transmission. However, the potential pathways through which different types of social protection succeed for these adolescents requires further, careful elucidation. For policy and programming, questions about which forms of social protection offer the greatest benefit (and calculations of their cost-effectiveness) are pressing. Further research is urgently needed to address these questions. As a large cohort of HIV-affected children in sub-Saharan Africa reaches adolescence, social protection that improves the resilience of young people is also needed, particularly a combination of social protection which includes 'capabilities' (or skills building) components in addition to 'cash' and 'care' provisions.

While cash transfers have received much attention, this chapter argues for greater focus on care and capability interventions, either alone or in combination. Here, novel combinations of biomedical and social interventions that factor behavioural alongside structural, psychosocial and biomedical responses are a new direction in HIV research (Coates, Richter & Caceres, 2008), as seen in the DREAMS initiative (Gittings et al., 2016; PEPFAR, 2015). However, questions of scalability, flexibility and sustainability of such interventions remain (Delany-Moretlwe et al., 2015). Ensuring reach and uptake for the most vulnerable will be integral to ensuring that no child or adolescent is left behind in the future HIV response.

In conclusion, social protection's potential to address structural drivers of vulnerabilities places such provisions in a unique position to address multiple health outcomes for adolescents living with HIV in ESA. Additional empirical and programmatic evidence is needed to explore which combinations are most effective for different sub-groups of adolescents, including for highly vulnerable key populations which face additional structural and socio-legal barriers to accessing services. Such evidence should be complemented by rigorous cost-effectiveness analyses to support informed decision-making on which provisions are likely to have the highest return on investment, and an adaptive approach that matches social protection provisions to the profile and needs of each subgroup, shifting from care plus cash to care plus cash plus capability combinations, as children and adolescents living with HIV become older and aspire for a future in which they are not just surviving, but thriving.

Note

1 HIV-specific social protection is tailored specifically to HIV services, whereas HIV-inclusive social protection includes but is not limited specifically to HIV. For this reason, HIV-specific social protection can be stigmatizing.

References

Amzel, A., Toska, E., Lovich, R., Widyono, M., Patel, T., Foti, C., Dziuban, E.J., Phelps, B.R., Sugandhi, N., Mark, D. and Altschuler, J., 2013. Promoting a combination approach to paediatric HIV psychosocial support. *AIDS*, 27(Suppl 2), pp. S147–S157.

Auld, A.F., Agolory, S.G., Shiraishi, R.W., Wabwire-Mangen, F., Kwesigabo, G., Mulenga, M., Hachizovu, S., Asadu, E., Tuho, M.Z., Ettiegne-Traore, V. and Mbofana, F., 2014. Antiretroviral therapy enrollment characteristics and outcomes among HIV-infected adolescents and young adults compared with older adults – seven African countries, 2004–2013. *Morbidity and Mortality Weekly Report*, 63(47), pp. 1097–1103.

Baird, S.J., Garfein, R.S., McIntosh, C.T. and Özler, B., 2012. Effect of a cash transfer programme for schooling on prevalence of HIV and herpes simplex type 2 in Malawi: A cluster randomised trial. *Lancet*, 379(9823), pp. 1320–1329.

Bandiera, O., Buehren, N., Burgess, R., Goldstein, M., Gulesci, S., Rasul, I. and Sulaiman, M., 2012. *Empowering adolescent girls: Evidence from a randomized control trial in Uganda*. Washington, DC: World Bank.

Baryamutuma, R., Nabaggala, R., Muhairwe, L.B. and Baingana, F. 2010. *Factors influencing sexual behaviours among adolescents living with HIV and AIDS in Uganda*. 18th International AIDS Conference – AIDS2010, Vienna.

Bermudez, L. G., Ssewamala, F. M., Neilands, T. B., Lu, L., Jennings, L., Nakigozi, G., Mellins, C. A., Mckay, M. and Mukasa, M. (2018). Does economic strengthening improve viral suppression among adolescents living with HIV? Results from a cluster randomized trial in Uganda. *AIDS and Behavior*, 22(11), pp. 3763–3772.

Bernays, S., Paparini, S., Gibb, D. and Seeley, J., 2016. When information does not suffice: Young people living with HIV and communication about ART adherence in the clinic. *Vulnerable Children and Youth Studies*, pp. 1–9, February.

Bhana, A., Mellins, C.A., Petersen, I., Alicea, S., Myeza, N., Holst, H., Abrams, E., John, S., Chhagan, M., Nestadt, D.F. and Leu, C.S., 2014. The VUKA family program: Piloting a family-based psychosocial intervention to promote health and mental health among HIV infected early adolescents in South Africa. *AIDS Care*, 26(1), pp. 1–11.

Busza, J., Besana, G.V., Mapunda, P. and Oliveras, E., 2014. Meeting the needs of adolescents living with HIV through home based care: Lessons learned from Tanzania. *Children and Youth Services Review*, 45, pp. 137–142, February.

Campbell, C., Skovdal, M., Mupambireyi, Z., Madanhire, C., Nyamukapa, C. and Gregson, S., 2012. Building adherence-competent communities: Factors promoting children's adherence to anti-retroviral HIV/AIDS treatment in rural Zimbabwe. *Health and Place*, 18(2), pp. 123–131.

Cho, H., Hallfors, D.D., Mbai, I.I., Itindi, J., Milimo, B.W., Halpern, C.T. and Iritani, B.J., 2011. Keeping adolescent orphans in school to prevent human immunodeficiency virus infection: Evidence from a randomized controlled trial in Kenya. *Journal of Adolescent Health*, 48(5), pp. 523–526.

Cluver, L.D., Hodes, R.J., Toska, E., Kidia, K.K., Orkin, F.M., Sherr, L. and Meinck, F., 2015. "HIV is like a tsotsi. ARVs are your guns": Associations between HIV-disclosure and adherence to antiretroviral treatment among adolescents in South Africa. *AIDS*, 29, pp. S57–S65, April.

Cluver, L.D., Meinck, F., Toska, E., Orkin, F.M., Hodes, R. and Sherr, L., 2018. Multitype violence exposures and adolescent antiretroviral nonadherence in South Africa. *AIDS*, 32(8), pp. 975–983.

Cluver, L.D., Orkin, M.F., Yakubovich, A.R. and Sherr, L., 2016a. Combination social protection for reducing HIV-risk behavior amongst adolescents in South Africa. *Journal of Acquired Immune Deficiency Syndromes*, 72(1), p. 96.

Cluver, L.D., Toska, E., Orkin, F.M., Meinck, F., Hodes, R., Yakubovich, A.R. and Sherr, L., 2016b. Achieving equity in HIV-treatment outcomes: Can social protection improve adolescent ART-adherence in South Africa? *AIDS Care*, 28(Suppl 2), pp. 73–82.

Coates, T.J., Richter, L. and Caceres, C., 2008. Behavioural strategies to reduce HIV transmission: How to make them work better. *Lancet*, 372(9639), pp. 669–684.

Cohen, M.S., Smith, M.K., Muessig, K.E., Hallett, T.B., Powers, K.A. and Kashuba, A.D., 2013. Antiretroviral treatment of HIV-1 prevents transmission of HIV-1: Where do we go from here? *Lancet*, 382(9903). pp. 1515–1524.

Delany-Moretlwe, S., Cowan, F.M., Busza, J., Bolton-Moore, C., Kelley, K. and Fairlie, L., 2015. Providing comprehensive health services for young key populations: Needs, barriers and gaps. *JIAS: Journal of the International AIDS Society*, 18(2 Suppl 1), p. 19833.

Denison, J.A., Banda, H., Dennis, A.C., Packer, C., Nyambe, N., Stalter, R.M., Mwansa, J.K., Katayamoyo, P. and McCarraher, D.R., 2015. "The sky is the limit": Adhering to antiretroviral therapy and HIV self-management from the perspectives of adolescents living with HIV and their adult caregivers. *JIAS: Journal of the International AIDS Society*, 18(1), p. 19358.

Devereux, S. and Sabates-Wheeler, R., 2004. *Transformative social protection*. IDS working paper.

Duflo, E., Dupas, P. and Kremer, M., 2015. Education, HIV, and early fertility: Experimental evidence from Kenya. *American Economic Review*, 105(9), pp. 2757–2797.

Emenyonu, N., Muyindike, W., Habyarimana, J., Pops-Eleches, C., Thirumurthy, H., Ragland, K. and Bangsberg, D.R., 2010. *Cash transfers to cover clinic transportation costs improve adherence and retention in care in a HIV treatment program in rural Uganda*. 17th Conference on Retroviruses and Opportunistic Infections, San Francisco, CA.

Garcia, M. and Moore, C.M., 2012. *The cash dividend: The rise of cash transfer programs in sub-Saharan Africa*. Washington, DC: World Bank.

Gillespie, S., Kadiyala, S. and Greener, R., 2007. Is poverty or wealth driving HIV transmission? *AIDS*, 21(Suppl 7), pp. S5–S16.

Gittings, L., Toska, C., Hodes, R., Cluver, L., Zungu, N., Govender, K., Chademana, K.E. and Gutiérrez, V.E., 2016. *Resourcing resilience: The case for social protection for adherence and HIV-related outcomes in children and adolescents in Eastern and Southern Africa.* RIATT-ESA Report, June. Available at: https://ovcsupport.org/resource/resourcing-resilience-the-case-for-social-protection-for-adherence-and-hiv-related-outcomes-in-children-and-adolescents-in-eastern-and-southern/.

Govender, K., Masebo, W. G., Nyamaruze, P., Cowden, R. G., Schunter, B. T. and Bains, A., 2018. HIV prevention in adolescents and young people in the Eastern and Southern African region: A review of key challenges impeding actions for an effective response. *The Open AIDS Journal,* 12, p. 53.

Govender, K., Reardon, C., Quinlan, T. and George, G., 2014. Children's psychosocial wellbeing in the context of HIV/AIDS and poverty: A comparative investigation of orphaned and non-orphaned children living in South Africa. *BMC Public Health,* 14(1), p. 615.

Grimwood, A., Fatti, G., Mothibi, E., Malahlela, M., Shea, J. and Eley, B., 2012. Community adherence support improves programme retention in children on antiretroviral treatment: A multicentre cohort study in South Africa. *JIAS: Journal of the International AIDS Society,* 15(2), pp. 1–9.

Handa, T., Halpern, C. T., Pettifor, A. and Thirumurthy, H., 2014. The government of Kenya's cash transfer program reduces the risk of sexual debut among young people age 15–25. *PLoS One,* 9(1), p.e85473.

Hodes, R., 2013. "You know what a bad person you are?" HIV, abortion, and reproductive health care for women in South Africa. In R. A. Smith, ed. *Global HIV/AIDS politics, policy and activism: Persistent challenges and emerging issues.* Santa Barbara, CA: Praeger, pp. 233–252, 239–241.

Hodes, R., Doubt, J., Toska, E., Vale, B., Zungu, N. and Cluver, L., 2018b. The stuff that dreams are made of: HIV-positive adolescents' aspirations for development. *JIAS: Journal of the International AIDS Society,* 21(Suppl 1), p. e25057.

Hodes, R. and Naimak, T. 2011. Piloting antiretroviral therapy in South Africa: The role of partnerships in the Western Cape's provincial roll-out. *African Journal of AIDS Research,* 10(4), pp. 415–425.

Hodes, R., Vale, B., Toska, E., Cluver, L., Dowse, R. and Ashorn, M., 2018a. Yummy or crummy? The multisensory components of medicines-taking among HIV-positive youth. *Global Public Health,* 14(2), pp. 284–299.

Honorati, M., Gentilini, U. and Yemtsov, R. G., 2015. *The state of social safety nets 2015.* Washington, DC: International Bank for Reconstruction and Development / The World Bank. Available at http://documents.worldbank.org/curated/en/2015/07/24741765/state-social-safety-nets-2015

Hudelson, C. and Cluver, L. D., 2015. Factors associated with adherence to antiretroviral therapy among adolescents living with HIV/AIDS in low- and middle-income countries: A systematic review. *AIDS Care,* 27(7), pp. 805–816.

Iwuji, C. C., Orne-Gliemann, J., Larmarange, J., Balestre, E., Thiebaut, R., Tanser, F., Okesola, N., Makowa, T., Dreyer, J., Herbst, K. and McGrath, N., 2018. Universal test and treat and the HIV epidemic in rural South Africa: A phase 4, open-label, community cluster randomised trial. *Lancet HIV,* 5(3), pp. e116–e125.

Karim, Q. A., 2015. *Impact of conditional cash incentives on HSV-2 and HIV in rural high school students in South Africa: The CAPRISA 007 cluster randomized controlled trial.* 8th IAS Conference on HIV Pathogenesis, Treatment & Prevention, Vancouver, Canada.

Kidman, R., Nachman, S., Dietrich, J., Liberty, A. and Violari, A., 2018. Childhood adversity increases the risk of onward transmission from perinatal HIV-infected adolescents and youth in South Africa. *Child Abuse and Neglect,* 79, pp. 98–106.

Lightfoot, M.A., Rotheram-Borus, M.J. and Tevendale, H., 2007. An HIV-preventive intervention for youth living with HIV. *Behavior Modification*, 31, pp. 345–363.

Marhefka, S.L., Elkington, K., Dolezal, C. and Mellins, C., 2010. Transmission risk behaviour among youth living with perinatally acquired HIV: Are nonadherent youth more likely to engage in sexual behavior? *Society for Adolescent Medicine Annual Meeting Program Issue: Adolescent Clinical Care: Integrating Art & Science*, p. S29.

Mavhu, W., Berwick, J., Chirawu, P., Makamba, M., Copas, A., Dirawo, J., Willis, N., Araya, R., Abas, M.A., Corbett, E.L. and Mungofa, S., 2013. Enhancing psychosocial support for HIV positive adolescents in Harare, Zimbabwe. *PLoS One*, 8(7), p. e70254.

Mbalinda, S.N., Kiwanuka, N., Kaye, D.K. and Eriksson, L.E., 2015. Reproductive health and lifestyle factors associated with health-related quality of life among perinatally HIV-infected adolescents in Uganda. *Health and Quality of Life Outcomes*, 13(1), p. 170.

Mupambireyi, Z., Bernays, S., Bwakura-Dangarembizi, M. and Cowan, F.M., 2014. "I don't feel shy because I will be among others who are just like me . . .": The role of support groups for children perinatally infected with HIV in Zimbabwe. *Children and Youth Services Review*, 45, pp. 106–113.

Nachega, J.B., Hislop, M., Nguyen, H., Dowdy, D.W., Chaisson, R.E., Regensberg, L., Cotton, M. and Maartens, G., 2009. Antiretroviral therapy adherence, virologic and immunologic outcomes in adolescents compared with adults in Southern Africa. *Journal of Acquired Immune Deficiency Syndromes*, 51(1), pp. 65–71.

National Planning Commission, Department of the Presidency, Republic of South Africa, 2012. *National development plan 2030: Our future, make it work*. Available at www.gov.za/sites/default/files/gcis_document/201409/ndp-2030-our-future-make-it-workr.pdf, accessed 4 April 2019.

Nattrass, N. and Gonsalves, G., 2009. *Economics and the backlash against AIDS-specific funding*. Cape Town: University of Cape Town.

Nhamo, D., 2013. *Shaping the health of adolescents in Zimbabwe (SHAZ!) Key findings and recommendations from an economic and lifeskills intervention addressing SRH and HIV issues among female adolescents*. International AIDS Conference. Available at: https://www.avac.org/sites/default/files/event_files/SHAZ%21%20webinar%20slides.pdf.

Obare, F., Birungi, H. and Kavuma, L., 2011. Barriers to sexual and reproductive health programming for adolescents living with HIV in Uganda. *Population Research and Policy Review*, 30, pp. 151–163.

O'Hare, B.A., Venables, J., Nalubeg, J.F., Nakakeeto, M., Kibirige, M. and Southall, D.P., 2005. Home-based care for orphaned children infected with HIV/AIDS in Uganda. *AIDS Care*, 17(4), pp. 443–450.

Orne-Gliemann, J., Larmarange, J., Boyer, S., Iwuji, C., McGrath, N., Bärnighausen, T., Zuma, T., Dray-Spira, R., Spire, B., Rochat, T. and Lert, F., 2015. Addressing social issues in a universal HIV test and treat intervention trial (ANRS 12249 TasP) in South Africa: Methods for appraisal. *BMC Public Health*, 15(1), p. 209.

Padian, N.S., McLoy, S.I., Balkus, J.E. and Wasserheit, J.N., 2010. Weighing the gold in the gold standard: Challenges in HIV prevention research. *AIDS*, 24(5), pp. 621–635.

Paediatric AIDS Treatment for Africa & World Health Organization, 2015. *Adolescent Africa: A situational analysis of adolescent HIV-treatment and care in sub-Saharan Africa*. Cape Town: World Health Organization.

Parker, L., Maman, S., Pettifor, A., Chalachala, J.L., Edmonds, A., Golin, C.E., Moracco, K. and Behets, F., 2013. Adaptation of a U.S. evidence-based positive prevention intervention for youth living with HIV/AIDS in Kinshasa, democratic republic of the Congo. *Evaluation and Program Planning*, 36, pp. 124–135.

Paterson, D.L., Swindells, S., Mohr, J., Brester, M., Vergis, E.N., Squier, C., Wagener, M.M. and Singh, N., 2000. Adherence to protease inhibitor therapy and outcomes in patients with HIV infection. *Annals of Internal Medicine*, 133, pp. 21–30.

PEPFAR, 2015. *Preventing HIV in adolescent girls and young women: Guidance for PEPFAR country teams on the DREAMS partnership.* Washington, DC: PEPFAR.

Pettifor, A.E., Levandowski, B.A., MacPhail, C., Padian, N.S., Cohen, M.S. and Rees, H.V., 2008. Keep them in school: The importance of education as a protective factor against HIV infection among young South African women. *International Journal of Epidemiology*, 37(6), pp. 1266–1273.

Pettifor, A.E., Nguyen, N.L., Celum, C., Cowan, F.M., Go, V. and Hightow-Weidman, L., 2015. Tailored combination prevention packages and PrEP for young key populations. *Journal of the International AIDS Society*, 18(2), pp. 8–22.

Phillips, H. 2014. The return of the Pholela experiment: Medical history and primary health care in post-apartheid South Africa. *American Journal of Public Health*, 104(10), pp. 1872–1876.

Remme, M., Vassall, A., Lutz, B., Luna, J. and Watts, C., 2014. Financing structural interventions: Going beyond HIV-only value for money assessments. *AIDS*, 28(3), pp. 425–434.

Ridgeway, K., Dulli, L.S., Murray, K.R., Silverstein, H., Dal Santo, L., Olsen, P., de Mora, D.D. and McCarraher, D.R., 2018. Interventions to improve antiretroviral therapy adherence among adolescents in low- and middle-income countries: A systematic review of the literature. *PLoS One*, 13(1), p.e0189770.

Schneider, H., Hlophe, H. and van Rensburg, D. 2008. Community health workers and the response to HIV/AIDS in South Africa: Tensions and prospects. *Health Policy and Planning*, 23(3), pp. 179–187.

Senyonyi, R.M., Underwood, L.A., Suarez, E., Musisi, S. and Grande, T.L., 2012. Cognitive behavioral therapy group intervention for HIV transmission risk behavior in perinatally infected adolescents. *Health*, 4(12), pp. 1334–1345.

Shisana, O. et al., 2014. *South African national HIV prevalence, incidence and behaviour survey, 2012.* Cape Town: HSRC Press.

Snyder, K., Wallace, M., Duby, Z., Aquino, L.D., Stafford, S., Hosek, S., Futterman, D. and Bekker, L.G., 2014. Preliminary results from Hlanganani (coming together): A structured support group for HIV-infected adolescents piloted in Cape Town, South Africa. *Children and Youth Services Review*, 45, pp. 114–121.

Ssewamala, F. 2013. *Evaluating a youth-focused economic empowerment approach to HIV treatment adherence – study protocol.* Available at: https://clinicaltrials.gov/ct2/show/NCT01790373, accessed November 30, 2018.

Standish-White, J., 2018. *A cost-effectiveness analysis of stack: Maximising retention in care for adolescents living with HIV in South Africa.* Oxford: University of Oxford Press.

Strasser, S. and Gibbons, S., 2014. The development of HIV-related mental health and psychosocial services for children and adolescents in Zambia: The case for learning by doing. *Children and Youth Services Review*, 45, pp. 150–157.

Toska, E. and Cluver, L.D., 2018. *Barriers to U=U for adolescents living with HIV: Predictors of high HIV-transmission risk from a longitudinal cohort study.* 2nd International Workshop on HIV Adolescence – Challenges & Solutions, Reviews in Antiviral Therapy & Infectious Diseases, Cape Town, South Africa, p. 31.

Toska, E., Cluver, L.D., Boyes, M.E., Isaacsohn, M., Hodes, R. and Sherr, L., 2017a. School, supervision and adolescent-sensitive clinic care: Combination social protection and reduced unprotected sex among HIV-positive adolescents in South Africa. *AIDS and Behavior*, 21(9), 2746–2759.

Toska, E., Cluver, L.D., Hodes, R. and Kidia, K.K., 2015. Sex and secrecy: How HIV-status disclosure affects safe sex among HIV-positive adolescents. *AIDS Care*, 27(Supp 1), pp. 47–58.

Toska, E., Pantelic, M., Meinck, F., Keck, K., Haghighat, R. and Cluver, L., 2017b. Sex in the shadow of HIV: A systematic review of prevalence, risk factors, and interventions to reduce sexual risk-taking among HIV-positive adolescents and youth in sub-Saharan Africa. *PLoS One*, 12(6), p. e0178106. doi:10.1371/journal.pone.0178106.

UNAIDS, 2014. *HIV and social protection guidance note.* Geneva, Switzerland: UNAIDS.

UNAIDS, 2017. *UNAIDS data 2017.* Geneva, Switzerland: UNAIDS.

UNAIDS, 2018. *Miles to go: Closing gaps, breaking barriers, righting injustices.* Geneva, Switzerland: UNAIDS.

UNICEF, 2015. *Social protection evaluation synthesis UNICEF evaluation management response.* New York: UNICEF.

UNICEF, 2017. *Children and AIDS: Statistical update.* New York: UNICEF.

Vale, B., Hodes, R. and Cluver, L., 2017. Negotiations of blame and care among HIV-positive mothers and daughters in South Africa's Eastern Cape. *Medical Anthropology Quarterly*, 31(4), pp. 519–536.

Van Winghem, J., Telfer, B., Reid, T., Ouko, J., Mutunga, A., Jama, Z. and Vakil, S., 2008. Implementation of a comprehensive program including psycho-social and treatment literacy activities to improve adherence to HIV care and treatment for a pediatric population in Kenya. *BMC Pediatrics*, 8, p. 52.

Visser, M., Zungu, N. and Ndala-Magoro, N., 2015. ISIBINDI, creating circles of care for orphans and vulnerable children in South Africa: Post-programme outcomes. *AIDS Care: Psychological and Socio-Medical Aspects of AIDS/HIV*, 27(8), pp. 1014–1019.

WHO, 2015. *Guidelines on when to start antiretroviral therapy and on a pre-exposure prophylaxis for HIV.* Geneva, Switzerland: World Health Organization.

World Bank, 2015. *The state of social safety nets 2015.* Washington, DC: World Bank.

12 Progress and challenges with comprehensive sexuality education

What does this mean for HIV prevention in the ESA region?

Patricia Machawira, Chris Castle and Joanna Herat

Introduction

The Eastern and Southern Africa (ESA) region has 158 million young people aged 10–24, accounting for nearly 30% of the global population. This number is expected to rise to 281 million by 2050 (UNESCO, UNFPA and UNAIDS, 2016; AFIDEP and UNFPA, 2015). Unfortunately, a majority of these young people are facing significant sexual and reproductive health challenges. According to UNAIDS estimates (2016), less than 50% of young people demonstrate accurate knowledge about HIV prevention and transmission. Many studies emphasize that young adolescent girls in the region have very little knowledge about their sexual and reproductive health, in part due to social and cultural taboos against informing girls (and boys) about the changes to their bodies and relations as they mature. They are particularly at risk, not only for HIV but also early and unintended pregnancies (EUP), sexually transmitted infections (STIs), gender-based violence (GBV) and child marriage. Further research has shown that adolescent girls (15–19 years) in the sub-Saharan African region experience the highest rates of pregnancy in the world (UNFPA, 2013), often unintended, and largely because sex, marriage and pregnancy are often not consensual for them due to persisting gender-discriminatory norms and limited knowledge related to their sexuality.

Ensuring access to information and education on sexual health, power relations and gender norms is an essential component to address those issues. The shift from traditional forms of communication and learning within the extended family to a reliance on a mixture of family, school, peers and media has left an apparent gap in education that is relevant to young people in today's world in this region. The fear-based HIV prevention messages of the 1990s and 2000s have been shown to have little or no impact on the way that young people navigate their transition to adulthood, including their relationships. And in line with shifts in educational philosophy worldwide that prioritize the building of skills and critical thinking, education about health and HIV has undergone significant rethinking.

Comprehensive sexuality education (CSE) is the result of this process and empowers young people to make informed decisions about relationships and sexuality. Well-delivered CSE provides education about human rights, gender equality, relationships, reproduction, sexual behaviours, risks and prevention of ill health.

The newly revised UN International Technical Guidance on Sexuality Education defines CSE as a curriculum-based process of teaching and learning about the cognitive, emotional, physical and social aspects of sexuality (UNESCO, 2018a). It aims to equip children and young people with the knowledge, skills, attitudes and values that will empower them to realize their health, well-being and dignity; develop respectful social and sexual relationships; consider the well-being of others who are affected by their choices; and understand and ensure the protection of their rights throughout their lives. This definition of CSE stems from a human rights and empowerment-based approach essential to address sexual and reproductive health issues as well as gender inequality in ESA. It reflects development in the field, for example by integrating key structural issues of gender and power, which tend to be avoided in other definitions in the literature (Haberland, 2015).

Given the need for young people to realize their health in sexual relationships, this chapter will provide an overview on the evolution of sexuality education in the ESA region and assess the effectiveness of the CSE programmes on behavioural and biological indicators, notably with regards to HIV prevention, and their potential to bring broader social change. The chapter will end with the challenges raised by the scale-up of these programmes and a summary of the lessons learnt from implementing CSE programmes in ESA region.

History of CSE in the ESA region

From LSE to CSE

Since the early 1990s, ESA countries have been implementing life skills education (LSE) programmes supported by development partners, mostly as a response to HIV. The programmes did not have a common definition of life skills but rather included a range of generic personal, interpersonal, cognitive and psychosocial skills and knowledge. Similarly, the content, level of application and terminology used varied from country to country according to priorities and context.

The 2012 Global Evaluation of LSE Programmes found that in general LSE was relevant to national priorities and the lives of learners (UNICEF, 2012). However, while coverage was growing through integration into school curricula, implementation was a challenge. LSE was often squeezed out because of teacher shortages, overcrowded curricula, limited teaching material and the focus on traditional examinations. In addition, there were few opportunities for meaningful and systematic participation of learners' voices in designing interventions that take into account varying contexts, needs and interests. Most importantly, life skills prevention education was often sub-optimal because it failed to explore intersections between gender, sex and social relationships. Further, the content and delivery of LSE was restricted in its capacity to move beyond knowledge and into the development of psychosocial skills, attitudes and behaviours. The result is that many young people grow into adolescence and adulthood without the basic capabilities needed to access and utilize SRH services in an appropriate way.

Following the insights into the shortcomings of the LSE programmes, there was general realization that in their current form, the programmes had failed to equip young people with the adequate life skills (and at times basic knowledge) to enable appropriate decisions on sexual health and encourage more positive sexual behaviours. The weaknesses inherent in the current approach shifted the momentum towards a closer analysis of the role of sexuality education in promoting the well-being of adolescents with later agreements affirming the interrelations between sexual and reproductive health, gender equality and human rights (Haberland, 2015). Notably, the 1994 International Conference on Population and Development is seen as a key signpost for the introduction of this shift towards sexuality education and CSE.

This was strengthened by the 2009 introduction of the UN International Technical Guidance on Sexuality Education. For most countries, this document instigated a second generation of CSE programmes which often built on existing programmes and content. Some CSE topics are present in most school curriculums and there is a large overlap between CSE and LSE, dependent on each country context and the thematic areas of its LSE programme. Thus, the current programmes evolved from the strengthening of already existing LSE programmes through the enhancement of CSE content.

One of the major challenges has been to define sexuality education, particularly because the key elements stemmed from the different terminologies used across national policies and curricula. While CSE is the globally recognized term, in ESA and elsewhere the terminology varies. It is also known as prevention education, relationships and sexuality education, SRH education, population and family life education, life skills education, healthy lifestyles and the basics of life safety and so on. The differences of terminology have been accompanied with varying approaches, leading sometimes to a weakening of the CSE's contribution to the human rights–based agenda and the empowerment basis it is grounded on (UNESCO, 2017).

An internationally recognized guidance based on research and best practices to guide both essential content and methodology has been co-developed by UNESCO and other UN partners to serve as an educational resource, assisting decision-makers and programme designers in the conception of CSE curriculum. Many programmes in this region have used this guidance to inform the revision of their national curricula, and the publication of the revised edition in early 2018 offers an opportunity to review and strengthen these programmes. The revised International Technical Guidance on Sexuality Education recommends concepts and learning objectives that are logically staged, starting with developmentally appropriate concepts for younger children and building up to more complex concepts, information and activities for older children (UNESCO, 2018a). This ensures that when properly sequenced, CSE is in line with the age and cognitive abilities of learners with the following key eight concepts which are further delineated into three domains of learning *knowledge, attitudes* and *skills*:

1 Relationships
2 Values, rights, culture and sexuality
3 Understanding gender
4 Violence and staying safe
5 Skills for health and well-being
6 The human body and development
7 Sexuality and sexual behaviour
8 Sexual and reproductive health and HIV risk.

Each concept presents the opportunity to address different topics; for example, 'relationships' includes the topics of families, friendship, love and romantic relationships, tolerance and respect, long-term commitment to marriage, and parenting. Given that the SRH needs of young people vary among countries – and even communities – and that countries are governed by different laws and policies, topics and learning objectives should be adjusted to the context in which they are provided and based on available local, national and international evidence.

The ESA Ministerial Commitment: a tipping point for CSE

The endorsement of the ESA Ministerial Commitment by the region's leadership on 7 December 2013 has ushered in a strong movement in support of CSE. The ESA Commitment meant that the political will to ensure access to CSE has been affirmed at the highest decision-making level, explicitly prioritizing 'ensuring access to good quality, comprehensive, life skills-based HIV and sexuality education and youth-friendly sexual and reproductive health services for all adolescents and young people' (UNESCO, 2013). The ESA Commitment put the spotlight on young people and promoted inter-sectoral collaboration while rallying partners around four key results for adolescents and young people: reducing HIV infection, reducing early and unintended pregnancy, reducing gender-based violence and eliminating child marriage.

Seven years after its endorsement, the ESA Commitment is seen as a key driver with regards to scaling up CSE. The political momentum provided by the ESA commitment has led many governments to scale up delivery of CSE within the formal school curriculum, such that by the end of 2015, 14 out of 20 ESA countries reported providing CSE in 40% of schools, and all 20 countries declared having in-service teacher training programmes on CSE (UNESCO, UNFPA and UNAIDS, 2016).

Positive impacts of the ESA Commitment include providing a policy framework with set short- and long-term targets to facilitate the scale-up of CSE and helping to fast-track the process of strengthening CSE in existing policies, strategies and programs. It has also facilitated the strengthening of the collaboration between the Ministry of Education and Ministry of Health in the planning and delivery of CSE, improving collaboration between governmental and non-governmental stakeholders and mobilizing donors around a common agenda. The requirements for countries to periodically report on progress on the ESA Commitment targets, thus subjecting them to peer evaluation, has added impetus and consistency to the implementation of CSE. Similarly, the inclusion of CSE in other regional policy and technical guidance documents has provided a framework for country investments.

Most ESA countries are now embracing the concept of CSE and are engaged in strengthening its implementation at national level. In this regard, more attention has been given to review of national curricula to integrate CSE and scale-up of effective teacher training and investment in monitoring systems together with engagement of parents and communities. In concert with national governments and civil society, development partners (including the UNAIDS Joint Programme) are supporting countries in their efforts to develop curricula that reflects the country context and that will have a direct, beneficial impact on the HIV response and more widely on adolescent and young people's health.

While ESA has seen an increase in the provision of CSE in the curriculum, issues of quality become important. In 2015, UNESCO commissioned a five-country study to assess the quality of CSE curricula and delivery (Uganda, Zambia, Lesotho, Malawi, Namibia). The review used an in-depth assessment tool, the Sexuality Education Review and Assessment Tool (SERAT), completed with key stakeholders. SERAT results (see Figure 12.1) across all five countries revealed moderate to strong curriculum content for the 9–18 age range, and weak to no content for the 5–8 age range, with the exception of Malawi. In Lesotho, Uganda and Zambia, CSE is offered from age 10 onwards, and there is no CSE curriculum developed for the younger age group (5–8 years).

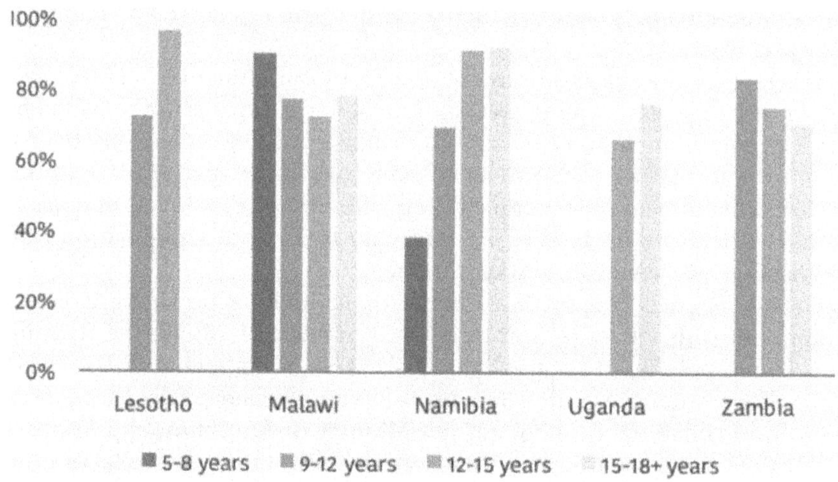

Figure 12.1 Average score of comprehensiveness of content in the CSE curriculum by age group

Analysis of effectiveness

CSE: an effective approach?

Whilst the rationale for delivering CSE to children and young people is partly situated within a rights-based framework, recognizing the right to a quality education and the right to information and education about SRH, the need for clear evidence on the effectiveness of CSE is nonetheless critical. Through two major reviews of evidence commissioned by UNESCO and conducted by independent experts, it is possible to understand the impact of sexuality education on some health-related outcomes (sexual behaviour, unintended pregnancy) as well as outcomes such as knowledge and attitudes, which are a pre-condition for healthy behaviours. These two reviews have considered the results of more than 150 studies from countries in the global north and the global south, including in sub-Saharan Africa (UNESCO, 2009, 2018c). The authors sought systematic reviews that included school-based CSE programmes ($N = 77$). Many of the reviews also included non-school-based programmes (in clinics or communities), and in some cases they performed direct comparisons between school-based and non-school-based programmes. The authors also sought systematic reviews that included at least some RCTs but often also included non-RCTs, case-control studies, before-after studies and cross-sectional surveys ($N = 65$).

Based on this evidence, curriculum-based sexuality education programmes are likely to contribute to the following outcomes:

- Delayed initiation of sexual intercourse (Guse et al., 2012)
- Decreased frequency of sexual intercourse
- Decreased unintended pregnancy
- Decreased number of sexual partners
- Reduced STIs
- Reduced risk-taking: increased use of condoms (Fonner et al., 2014) and increased use of contraception.

The evidence reviewed in 2018 also demonstrates that sexuality education leads to increased knowledge about different aspects of sexuality and behaviours, including risks of pregnancy and HIV and other STIs (Guse et al., 2012). Sexuality education is also strongly correlated with improved attitudes related to sexual and reproductive health, as shown for instance in a systematic review of the school programmes in Nigeria (Amaugo et al., 2014).

More generally, the evidence from sub-Saharan Africa has shown that the implementation of sexuality education has led to significant improvements in HIV-related knowledge and to delayed sexual debut (Ross et al., 2007). In Kenya, there was a significant positive difference in condom use between the intervention and control groups in the follow-up of a national primary school HIV intervention (Maticka-Tyndale, Wildish and Gichuru, 2010). Combining education with the provision of health services has shown positive effects on unintended pregnancy rates (Mavedzenge et al., 2011; Hindin et al., 2016) and/or delayed sexual debut. This approach highlights the importance of adopting an intersectoral efforts and recognizing that the mobilization of community and the provision of youth-friendly services alongside any school-based programme may be key drivers of its success.

In addition, CSE programmes have shown in some instances to be more effective than programmes only aiming at delaying sexual initiation after marriage on moral and/or public health grounds (Boonstra, 2011). Many studies assessing 'abstinence-only' programmes showed that this approach fails to increase the use of condoms, to avoid risk-taking attitudes or even to delay the date of sexual debut (Trenholm et al., 2007; Underhill, Operario and Montgomery, 2007). Besides, abstinence-only policies have the potential to be harmful for young people by depriving them of the basic information they need on HIV and sexuality – a critical issue in sub-Saharan Africa, where most young people have sex before the age of 18 (Amo-Adjei and Tuoyire, 2018).

The scope for improvement of CSE programmes

Despite the positive results of the implementation of CSE in the ESA region and worldwide, these conclusions must be nuanced. First, the outcomes observed on CSE are usually only slightly positive, and the quality and fidelity of the implementation play major roles here. Moreover, a third of the CSE programmes still have limited effect on the attitudes and behaviours of the targeted learners. Another challenge resides in the fact that it is still not possible to draw direct causal pathways between the delivery of sexuality education and biological outcomes such as reduced HIV/STIs or EUP. This is partly a result of the limited number of high-quality longitudinal trials and partly because of the range of confounding factors which are critical to HIV prevention efforts, such as the availability of services (including condoms), and the wider structural and behavioural factors which reduce agency or increase vulnerability. Hence, most of the studies only measure behavioural changes because this is easier and less costly, even if biological indicators are the better way to assess the effectiveness of CSE programmes.

CSE is a privileged means to create a shift in young people's minds to reach gender equality and enable them to empower themselves (Boonstra, 2011). Indeed, CSE programmes grounded on an empowerment-based approach, thus highlighting gender and power in their curricula, have shown noteworthy results. For instance, a three-year study conducted in junior secondary high schools in the Lagos State of Nigeria assessed the impact of the 'Family Life and HIV Education' curriculum delivered to young people. The curriculum covered subjects such as human sexual development and sexual health, skills for negotiating personal and intimate relationships, and gender-equitable attitudes. At the end of the study, young people presented greater knowledge of SRH, expression of gender-equitable attitudes, confidence about saying no to pressures to have sex and (among boys) a commitment not to pressure girls to engage in sex (Action Health Incorporated, 2010). Other studies in Nigeria and elsewhere showed how gender-sensitive programmes lead to the development of gender-equal and peaceful relationships (Madunagu, 2003; Verma et al., 2008).

Furthermore, there is increasing evidence that emphasizing gender and power in CSE programmes is more efficient in impacting positively on attitudinal and biological outcomes (i.e. decreasing rates of STDs and EUP). For instance, in recent literature, gender is referred to as 'a gateway to SRH outcomes' (Haberland, 2010; Middlestadt et al., 2012). Unfortunately, CSE and LSE programmes in the ESA region are still not emphasizing these issues enough, and a review of the literature on gender and CSE in South Africa has also shown that Life Orientation programmes can even reinforce gendered power relations because of persistent punitive, paternalistic approaches to young people's sexuality, among many other reasons (Shefer and Macleod, 2015).

CSE has the potential to be a catalyst for social change and to enhance non-violent relationships, based on respect between young people and control over their own lives and bodies. The Stepping Stones life skills programmes in South Africa and The Gambia are striking examples of effective sexuality education. In the two-year period after the intervention, boys and men shifted attitudes and were less engaged in violent behaviours: fewer were involved in incidents of intimate partner violence (Dunkle et al., 2006), rape (Jewkes et al., 2006) and transactional sex (Dunkle et al., 2007).

Strategies for scale-up

Scale-up of CSE in the ESA region

In view of the challenges and HIV and SRH-related issues faced by youth in the ESA region, it is critical that countries pursue efforts in the light of the ESA commitment to scale-up CSE. In 2016, only 10 in 21 countries of the region had coordination mechanisms, work plans and mobilized resources for implementation (UNESCO, UNFPA and UNAIDS, 2016).

UNESCO identifies the three following aspects to ensure an effective scale-up, notably based on evidence and successful strategies (Fonner et al., 2014; Haberland and Rogow, 2015):

- *The creation of an enabling environment for the implementation of CSE programmes,* with a conducive legal and policy environment, a strong leadership and a costed scale-up plan.
- *Decisions on the different technical considerations that will affect the scale-up,* such as the development and contents of a CSE curriculum framework, the choice of the CSE delivery model to use, the form of training that will be provided to the teachers and an effective M&E system.
- *Addressing factors that affect the delivery of CSE* through creating a conducive and safe physical and psychosocial environment in schools and communities with effective parental engagement and linkages to SRH services and out-of-school delivery.

The International Technical Guidance on Sexuality Education (UNESCO, 2018a) gives the following characteristics of effective CSE programs based on a review of various CSE programs from across the world:

Preparatory phase

1. Involve experts on human sexuality, behaviour change and related pedagogical theory.
2. Involve young people, parents/family members and other community stakeholders.
3. Assess the social SRH needs and behaviours of children and young people targeted by the programme, based on their evolving capacities.
4. Assess the resources (human, time and financial) available to develop and implement the curricula.

Content development

5 Focus on clear goals, outcomes and key learnings to determine the content, approach and activities.
6 Cover topics in a logical sequence.
7 Design activities that are context-oriented and promote critical thinking.
8 Address consent and life skills.
9 Provide scientifically accurate information about HIV and AIDS and other STIs, pregnancy prevention, early and unintended pregnancy and the effectiveness and availability of different methods of protection.
10 Address how biological experiences, gender and cultural norms affect the way children and young people experience and navigate their sexuality and their SRH in general.
11 Address specific risk and protective factors that affect particular sexual behaviours.
12 Address how to manage specific situations that might lead to HIV infection, other STIs, unwanted or unprotected sexual intercourse or violence.
13 Address individual attitudes and peer norms concerning condoms and the full range of contraceptives.
14 Provide information about what services are available to address the health needs of children and young people, especially their SRH needs.

Challenges for scaling up CSE in the ESA region

In understanding the gap between existing data on HIV knowledge levels and the persistently high rates of new HIV infections, it is necessary to examine in depth the quality of education as well as the domestic structures within which sexuality education is being housed. Many countries in the region face systemic challenges in delivering a quality education to all learners, including maths, literacy, science and other traditionally 'core' subjects. Sexuality education is subject to the same stresses as these other subjects: a high ratio of learners to teachers, weak programmes for teacher training and support, very limited teaching and learning resources and a persistence of traditional pedagogical approaches that prioritize a 'chalk and talk' approach over the active participation of learners (UNESCO, 2012; UNFPA, 2012). Hence, young people lack the favourable environment to cultivate critical thinking and the necessary skills to empower themselves and become confident citizens. This environment is however vital to achieve gender equality (Pettersson, 2014).

Teachers are at the core of catalytic actions in the scale-up of CSE. Governments and stakeholders need to emphasize the importance of the continuous training of teachers and to provide the adequate means to enable them to adapt to the requirements of teaching CSE. This includes the capacity to provide an interactive pedagogy, the confidence to talk about sexuality and the ability to create a healthy and respectful environment in the classroom. Then, major investments are needed in the provision of quality and sufficient teaching and learning materials for all schools.

The ESA region has seen relative success with reaching young people in the school system. However, achieving universal access to good-quality CSE will require specific strategies for reaching marginalized young people who are out of school. Evidence shows that the vulnerability of youth increases when they exit school upon completion or due to dropout (World Bank, 2015). In many countries, the dropout rate is especially high between primary and secondary levels, which is also often just at time of, or just after, sexual initiation (UNESCO, 2012). This means that even if CSE is scaled up nationally through formal education, a large number of young people will not access it (World Bank, 2015). For those who are in school, informal and non-formal sexuality education is important to reinforce and even go further than what is provided in the classroom. Thus, there is a need for an out-of-school CSE delivery strategy that uses the CSE curriculum or similar content used in schools to ensure continuity from school to out-of-school CSE provision (UNESCO, 2018b). This will be an important next step to reach young people living with disabilities or with HIV, those living in extreme poverty, those with higher HIV risk or teenage mothers. In the case of the latter, despite policies to the contrary, many schools in countries in the ESA region still adopt a punitive approach and exclude young mothers from school as soon as they get pregnant (UNESCO, UNFPA and UNAIDS, 2016).

Finally, cultural and religious conservatism often weakens expansion of CSE, and a major challenge resides in the overcoming of these resistances. In general, public discussions around sex and sexuality are highly sensitive, and parents as well as community leaders still fear that talking about sexuality will lead to earlier sexual debut or an increased number of sexual partners among young people (Barboza, 1993). The case of Nigeria is a remarkable example of how to address these issues through effective action. Stakeholders were reluctant to implement CSE, and policy-makers created early advisory and advocacy committees to facilitate the dialogue with and to inform key CSE stakeholders: community and religious leaders, school administrators and representatives of teacher unions and parents associations. Moreover, the model was adaptive to social and cultural characteristics of different federal states, and strategic changes of names of curriculum were made. For example, in the Sokoto State the name of the curriculum was changed from 'Family Life and HIV/AIDS Education' to 'School Health Education Program'. The scale-up had relative success, despite compromises and the fact that Islamic schools are still less likely to provide CSE than Christian schools (Huaynoca et al., 2013).

To deal with opposition, countries need to *build community support* by strategically choosing the issues to address, framing their work with care, having sensitive content vetted and actively reaching out to all stakeholders to explain what they were doing. A second key element is to *deal with backlash* by using supportive media persons as intermediaries, arranging for journalists to visit the schools and see for themselves what was going on, and organizing information-sharing discussion sessions.

Lessons learnt from implementing CSE programmes in the ESA region

1. Nationwide coverage of CSE is impossible without government leadership and ownership. For CSE expansion to be effective and sustainable, it must be integrated into existing systems and become part of the core business of a ministry of education. As such, this requires changes to policy, laws and budgets, which is impossible without high-level commitment and leadership. High-level leadership and ownership contribute to changing the environment in which CSE is offered and provide a mandate and justification to teachers and other implementers to provide CSE. They can also contribute to making the provision of CSE (and HIV-SRH services) acceptable to gatekeepers.
2. If CSE is to be effectively expanded, it requires integration of M&E into existing ministry systems. At the national level, tools such as the Annual School Census (ASC) and analysis by the Education Management Information System (EMIS) should include CSE components and, therefore, data collection forms and M&E training may need to be amended to reflect these additions. Such indicators, if introduced via the EMIS, can help countries track CSE delivery and enable policy and programmes to be adapted as needed.
3. To ensure full support for CSE, there is need to engage with key gatekeepers, at the state and community level, to garner their support in the creation of a conducive environment for CSE. Parents can play an important role in communicating with their children about sexuality, relationships and well-being. Studies have repeatedly shown that favourable parental attitudes influence children's attitudes. Parents and families play a key role in shaping attitudes, norms and values related to gender roles, sexuality and the status of adolescents and young people in the community (Svanemyr et al., 2015).
4. The respect of human rights needs to be a priority for countries which provide CSE to ensure an equal and safe access for all. This means, for instance, that countries should foreclose any punitive, criminalizing laws or policies regarding sexual orientation, consensual sex among minors or teenage pregnancy, and any other policy that would violate the basic human rights essential to CSE successful delivery.
5. Despite all countries in ESA now heading towards implementation of CSE, a number of ongoing challenges remain with some of the CSE curricula. The lack of appropriate attention to gender norms and roles

as well as power relations in CSE curricula represents a stark disconnect from the reality for most adolescent girls and young women. In addition, curricula are often missing essential content, especially around pregnancy prevention and gender.

6 Teacher training remains a weak point in most sexuality education programmes. Developing and updating training curricula and supporting teachers to examine their own values and biases remains a priority. The quality of CSE delivered to young people depends ultimately upon teachers' knowledge, confidence and skill to deliver the subject. Teachers must be adequately trained in the subject matter and in more participatory pedagogical approaches. Teachers frequently focused on knowledge rather than skills and used didactic methods rather than engaging pupils through participatory approaches. Increasingly, teacher-training programmes in the region are now focusing on examining personal attitudes and values to improve comfort and confidence as well as the content and teaching skills required.
7 While the ESA Commitment has increased inter-sectoral collaboration, more must be done to ensure that adolescents and young people receiving CSE have access to youth-friendly health services. Having the knowledge, attitudes and skills to make healthy decisions is insufficient without access to services and commodities. Too often, young people access services when it is too late, in part because of fear, discomfort, embarrassment and gatekeeper disapproval. The education sector has a role to play in improving linkages between schools and healthcare facilities, including through providing referrals.

Conclusion

Comprehensive sexuality education, if well implemented, has the potential to address many issues related to HIV and SHR faced by young people in the ESA region. ESA commitment has been a great boost to the CSE agenda in the ESA region and it can become a foundation for ensuring political engagement in different public health issues. Many ESA countries have embraced the concept of CSE and are supporting its implementation, which is vital to reduction of HIV rates in the region. However, most country policies and sociocultural environments are still not sufficiently capacitated to reach these goals, and the path will be long before a comprehensive, empowerment-based sexuality education can be provided to all young people in and out of school. Emphasizing gender is pivotal to this achievement, as evidence has shown, and further investigation needs to be undertaken to assess the interrelations between CSE, gender equality and human rights and their impact on the health and well-being of young people.

To achieve effective and widespread delivery, advocacy and information-building on CSE must be continuous, and the furthering of the scientific literature on CSE plays a major role here, as it is the base of any plausible advocacy. Future research is required to answer some unexplored questions, such as the factors affecting the successful transfer of knowledge and values within the classroom and why stubborn gaps remain between teachers' generally high knowledge levels on HIV/AIDS and low levels of student knowledge on HIV.

Another key area for assessment are the specific components to prioritize for ensuring effective CSE delivery, acknowledging that a comprehensive curriculum review is not always due to a lack of time and resources. Lastly, more inquiry is needed on how to reach the most vulnerable young people, especially marginalized young people outside of educational settings, and to ensure the quality and relevance of sexuality education to their lives and needs.

Appendix

Table A1.1 Positioning of CSE in the curriculum in selected ESA countries

Country	*Primary school (if integrated, please list the subjects)*	*Examinable (yes/no)*	*Secondary school (if integrated, please list the subjects)*	*Examinable (yes/no)*
Botswana	Infused into all the subjects	Yes except guidance and counselling	Infused into all subjects	Yes except guidance and counselling
Burundi	Integrated into carrier subjects: civics, biology and languages	Yes	Integrated into carrier subjects: civics, biology and languages (French, Kirundi and English)	Yes
Kenya	Integrated into the life skills curriculum, religious education, biology	No for life skills Core subjects are examinable	Integrated into the life skills curriculum, religious education, biology and other core subjects	No for life skills Core subjects are examinable
Lesotho	Integrated into personal, spiritual and social and scientific and technological learning areas in grades 4–6, stand-alone in grade 7	Not examinable but assessed	Taught as a stand-alone subject in secondary (grades 8 to 10)	Yes
Madagascar	Infused into all subjects	Dependent on subject	Infused into all subjects	Dependent on subject
Malawi	Integrated into life skills education with some elements in subjects such as social studies, primary science, home economics	Yes	Integrated into life skills education and some elements of CSE are integrated into other subjects such as social studies, biology, human ecology	Yes, it is examinable at senior secondary.
Mozambique	Integrated into Portuguese, social science, civic and moral education, and natural science	Yes	Integrated into Portuguese, history, geography, and natural science	Yes

(*Continued*)

Table A1.1 (Continued)

Country	*Primary school (if integrated, please list the subjects)*	*Examinable (yes/no)*	*Secondary school (if integrated, please list the subjects)*	*Examinable (yes/no)*
Namibia	Integrated into environmental studies, natural science and health education for grades 1–3 and life skills for grades 4–7	Environmental studies, natural science and health education are examinable Life skills subject is not examinable but it is *assessed*	Integrated into biology, life science and life skills	Biology and life science are examinable; however, life skills is not examinable but it is *assessed*
Rwanda	Integrated into science and elementary technology and social and religious studies	Yes	Integrated into biology and health sciences, general studies and communication skills, history and citizenship	Yes
South Africa	Integrated into life skills	Yes	Integrated into one subject: life orientation (grades 8–12)	Yes
South Sudan	Integrated into life skills and peace building education and biology, languages and extra-curricular activities	Yes CSE is integrated in examinable core subjects, though life skills is not examinable	Integrated into life skills and peace building education and other core subjects as well as extra-curricular activities	Yes
Eswatini	Integrated into health and physical education, languages, expressive arts, general studies	Yes	Integrated into life skills education, languages and science	Yes it is examinable in subjects where it is integrated
Tanzania	Integrated into science, personality development and sports, civic and moral education, science, science and technology	Yes	Biology and civics at lower secondary and general studies	Yes
Uganda	Integrated into English, science, social studies, religious education and geography	Yes	Integrated into life education (which includes physical education and sexuality education)	Yes
Zambia	Integrated into integrated science, social studies, home economics and religious education	Yes	Integrated into integrated science, biology, social studies, civic education, home economics and religious education	Yes
Zimbabwe	A mixture of stand-alone and integrated subjects	No	A mixture of stand-alone and integrated subjects	Yes

Source: UNESCO 2017.

References

Action Health Incorporated. 2010. *Foundation for a healthy adulthood: Lessons from school-based family life and HIV education curriculum implementation in Lagos state.* Lagos: Action Health Incorporated and Lagos State Ministry of Education.

AFIDEP and UNFPA. 2015. *Synthesis report on the demographic dividend in Africa.* Johannesburg: UNFPA East and Southern Africa Regional Office.

Amaugo, L.G., Papadopoulos, C., Ochieng, B.M. and Ali, N. 2014. The effectiveness of HIV/AIDS school-based sexual health education programmes in Nigeria: A systematic review. *Health Education Research,* 29(4), pp. 633–648. https://doi.org/10.1093/her/cyu002

Amo-Adjei, J. and Tuoyire, D. 2018. Timing of sexual debut among unmarried youth aged 15–24 years in sub-Saharan Africa. *Journal of Biosocial Science,* 50(2), pp. 161–177. doi:10.1017/S0021932017000098.

Barboza, Nathalie. 1993. *Breda series no. 2: Développement des programme et projets d'éducation en matière de population en Afrique francophone et lusophone* [*Breda series #2: The development of population education programmes and projects in francophone and Portuguese-speaking Africa*]. Dakar: UNESCO.

Boonstra, H.D. 2011. Advancing sexuality education in developing countries: Evidence and implications. *Guttmacher Policy Review,* 14(3).

Dunkle, K.L., Jewkes, R.K., Nduna, M., Jama, N., Levin, J., Sikweyiya, Y. and Koss, M.P. 2007. Transactional sex with casual and main partners among young South African men in the rural Eastern Cape: Prevalence, predictors, and associations with gender-based violence. *Social Science & Medicine,* 65, pp. 1235–1248. https://doi:10.1016/j.socscimed.2007.04.029.

Dunkle, K.L., Jewkes, R.K., Nduna, M., Levin, J., Jama, N., Khuzwayo, N., Koss, M.P. and Duvvury, N. 2006. Perpetration of partner violence and HIV risk behaviour among young men in the rural Eastern Cape, South Africa. *AIDS,* 20(16), pp. 2107–2114.

Fonner, V.A., Armstrong, K.S., Kennedy, C.E., O'Reilly, K.R. and Sweat, M.D. 2014. School based sex education and HIV prevention in low-and middle-income countries: A systematic review and meta-analysis. *PLoS One,* 9(3), p.e89692. doi:10.1371/journal.pone.0089692.

Guse, K., Levine, D., Martins, S., Lira, A., Gaarde, J., Westmorland, W. and Gilliam, M. 2012. Interventions using new digital media to improve adolescent sexual health: A systematic review. *Journal of Adolescent Health,* 51(6), pp. 535–543.

Haberland, N.A. 2010. *What happens when programs emphasize gender? A review of the evaluation research.* Presented at UNFPA global technical consultation on comprehensive sexuality education, Bogota, Colombia, November 30.

Haberland, N.A. 2015. The case for addressing gender and power in sexuality and HIV education: A comprehensive review of evaluation studies. *International Perspectives on Sexual and Reproductive Health,* 41(1), pp. 31–42.

Haberland, N.A. and Rogow, D. 2015. Sexuality education: Emerging trends in evidence and practice. *Journal of Adolescent Health,* 56(1), pp. S15–S21. https://doi.org/10.1016/j.jadohealth.2014.08.013

Huaynoca, S., Chandra-Mouli, V., Yaqub, N. and Denno, D.M. 2014. Scaling up comprehensive sexuality education in Nigeria: From national policy to nationwide application. *Sex Education,* 14(2), pp. 191–209. doi:10.1080/14681811.2013.856292.

Hindin, M.J., Kalamar, A.M., Thompson, T.A. and Upadhyay, U.D. 2016. Interventions to prevent unintended and repeat pregnancy among young people in low-and middle-income countries: A systematic review of the published and gray literature. *Journal of Adolescent Health*, 59(3), pp. S8–S15.

Jewkes, R., Dunkle, K., Koss, M.P., Levin, J.B., Nduna, M., Jama, N. and Sikweyiya, Y. 2006. Rape perpetration by young, rural South African men: Prevalence, patterns and risk factors. *Social Science & Medicine*, 63(11), pp. 2949–2961.

Madunagu, B., ed. 2003. *Training manual level 1: Adolescent sexuality, sexual and reproductive health and rights*. Calabar: Girls Power Initiative.

Maticka-Tyndale, E., Wildish, J. and Gichuru, M. 2010. Thirty-month quasi-experimental evaluation follow-up of a national primary school HIV intervention in Kenya. *Sex Education*, 10(2), pp. 113–130.

Mavedzenge, S. M. N., Doyle, A.M. and Ross, D.A. 2011. HIV prevention in young people in sub-Saharan Africa: A systematic review. *Journal of Adolescent Health*, 49(6), pp. 568–586.

Middlestadt, S.E., Pulerwitz, J., Acharya, K. et al. 2012. *Evidence for gender as a gateway factor to other behaviors: Ethiopia*. The Health Community Partnership's End of Project Meeting. www.jhuccp.org/legacy/pubs/HCP_endofproject/3Acharya.ppt. Accessed December 3, 2012.

Pettersson, T. 2014. *Basic values and civic education: A comparative analysis of adolescent orientations towards gender equality and good citizenship*. www.worldvaluessurvey.org/library/. Accessed August 11, 2014.

Ross, D.A., Changalucha, J., Obasi, A.I., Todd, J., Plummer, M.L., Cleophas-Mazige, B., Anemona, A., Everett, D., Weiss, H.A., Mabey, D.C. and Grosskurth, H. 2007. Biological and behavioural impact of an adolescent sexual health intervention in Tanzania: A community-randomized trial. *AIDS*, 21(14), pp. 1943–1955.

Shefer, T. and Macleod, C. 2015. Life orientation sexuality education in South Africa: Gendered norms, justice and transformation. *Perspectives in Education*, 33(2), pp. 1–10.

Svanemyr, J., Amin, A., Robles, O.J. and Greene, M.E. 2015. Creating an enabling environment for adolescent sexual and reproductive health: A framework and promising approaches. *Journal of Adolescent Health*, 56(1), pp. S7–S14.

Trenholm, Christopher, Devaney, Barbara, Fortson, Ken, Quay, Lisa, Wheeler, Justin and Clark, Melissa. 2007. *Impacts of four title V, section 510 abstinence education programs*. MATHEMATICA Policy Research. https://www.mathematica.org/our-publications-and-findings/publications/impacts-of-four-title-v-section-510-abstinence-education-programs.

UNAIDS and the African Union. 2015. *Empower young women and adolescent girls: Fast tracking the end of the AIDS epidemic in Africa*. Geneva: UNAIDS.

Underhill, K., Operario, D. and Montgomery, P. 2007. Systematic review of abstinence-plus HIV prevention programs in high-income countries. *PLoS Medicine*, 4(9), p.e275. https://doi.org/10.1371/journal.pmed.0040275

UNESCO. 2009. *International technical guidance on sexuality education: An evidence-informed approach for schools, teachers and health educators* (Volumes 1–2). Paris: UNESCO.

UNESCO. 2012. *Opportunities lost: The impact of grade repetition and early school leaving*. Global Education Digest 2012. Paris: UNESCO.

UNESCO. 2013. *Ministerial commitment on comprehensive sexuality education and sexual and reproductive health services for adolescents and young people in Eastern and Southern African (ESA)*. www.youngpeopletoday.org

UNESCO. 2017. *CSE scale-up in practice: Case studies from Eastern and Southern Africa.* Paris: UNESCO.

UNESCO. 2018a. *International technical guidance on sexuality education: An evidence-informed approach* (Revised Edition). Paris: UNESCO.

UNESCO. 2018b. *A civil society perspective: Fulfilling our promise to young people today: Progress review report on the implementation of the Eastern and Southern African ministerial commitment on comprehensive sexuality education and sexual and reproductive health services for adolescents and young people 2015–2017.* Paris: UNESCO.

UNESCO. 2018c. *Review of the evidence on sexuality education, report to inform the update of the UNESCO International Technical Guidance on Sexuality Education.* Developed by Paul Montgomery and Wendy Knerr. Oxford: Centre for Evidence-Based Intervention (CEBI), Department of Social Policy and Intervention, University of Oxford Press.

UNESCO, UNFPA and UNAIDS. 2016. *Fulfilling our promise to young people today: 2013–2015 progress review.* Durban: UNESCO, UNFPA and UNAIDS.

UNFPA. 2012. *Sexuality Education: A ten country review of school curricula in Eastern and Southern Africa.* New York, NY: UNFPA.

UNFPA. 2013. *Adolescent pregnancy: A review of the evidence.* New York: UNFPA.

UNICEF Evaluation Office. 2012. *Global evaluation of life skills education programmes.* Final Report. New York: UNICEF.

Verma, R., Pulerwitz, J., Mahendra, V.S., Khandekar, S., Singh, A.K., Das, S.S. and Barker, G. 2008. *Promoting gender equity as a strategy to reduce HIV risk and gender-based violence among young men in India.* Horizons Final Report. Washington, DC: Population Council.

World Bank Group. 2015. *Out-of-school youth in sub-Saharan Africa: A policy perspective,* Keiko Inoue, Emanuela di Gropello, Yesim Sayin Taylor, and James Gresham, editors. https://elibrary.worldbank.org/doi/10.1596/978-1-4648-0505-9_fm.

13 Using school-based early warning systems as a social and behavioral approach for HIV prevention among adolescent girls

A case study from Uganda

Julie DeSoto, Asha Belsan, Robert Wamala, Victor Ochaya, Rita Laura Lulua, Gloria Ekpo, Dennis Cherian and Shelby Benson

Introduction

A growing body of literature discusses social and behavioral approaches to HIV prevention. In a recent literature review of adolescent-focused HIV prevention research by Pettifor et al., (2018), the authors noted the need for combining HIV prevention strategies addressing individual, dyadic (peer/partner/parent), community (e.g. school environment), and societal-level risk and protective factors. In a systematic review of programs for HIV prevention among youth in sub-Saharan Africa, Harrison et al., (2010) concluded there should be emphasis on social risk factors for HIV, including gender, poverty, and alcohol, adding that future programs should work to change social norms and target structural factors contributing to HIV infection among adolescents. In 2008, Coates et al., called on the behavioral science community to better inform promising cognitive-behavioral, persuasive communications, and peer education approaches with theoretical frameworks. More recently, Govender et al., (2018) reviewed key challenges for mitigating HIV risk through sexual contact among young people in Eastern and Southern Africa (ESA), the region with the highest HIV burden. Overall, researchers and practitioners recommend that interventions focused on adolescents and young people should be developed using theoretical frameworks, contain multiple strategies, and comprehensively engage different levels of the ecosystem (schools, communities, individuals, families).

This chapter seeks to respond to these findings by outlining a school-based social and behavioral intervention used in Uganda. An overview of the model and its implementation is discussed, with emphasis on the importance of understanding enabling factors and barriers when adapting evidence-based HIV prevention approaches to specific contexts. To evaluate effectiveness of the project, the chapter presents findings from an external longitudinal study comparing intervention and control schools at two different times. These outcomes are further contextualized by standardized monitoring data collected by World Vision[1] and critical insights gathered from field implementers.

The model: strengthening school-community accountability for girls education

Previous research has identified attendance, behavior, and course performance (ABC predictors) as powerful indicators of secondary school dropout and completion rates. Evidence suggests that using an early warning system (EWS) to track these indicators is an effective approach for predicting and preventing secondary school dropout in the United States and elsewhere (Bruce et al., 2011; Heppen & Bowles Therriault, 2008; Neild, Balfanz & Herzog, 2007). This case study documents how the School-Community Accountability for Girls Education (SAGE) project in Uganda was designed and implemented to deliver a combination (ABC predictors plus EWS) school-based HIV prevention project for adolescent girls (AG). SAGE was a two-year PEPFAR-funded project (October 1, 2016–March 31, 2019). Its main goal was to reduce secondary school dropout and ultimately HIV infection among 38,750 AG aged 13–19 in 151 schools across ten districts of Uganda (Sembabule, Mubende, Oyam, Mukono, Gomba, Bukomansimbi, Lira, Rakai, Mityana, and Gulu). SAGE used an innovative EWS package to shift social norms and practices around girls' education, violence against children, reproductive health, and positive discipline. It provided a package of activities (detailed herein) to help girls stay in school and sought to reduce risks of early marriage, pregnancy, and gender-based violence (GBV) as mitigating factors against HIV acquisition. The SAGE model was developed using Urie Bronfenbrenner's ecological systems theory (Bronfenbrenner, 1979), in which different levels of the socioecological model were addressed during the life of the project (the individual, peers, families and schools at the microsystem, mass media, politics and community in the exosystem, and behavior change at the macrosystem). Figure 13.1 is adapted from Bronfenbrenner's (1979) conceptualization of the ecology of human development.

The different levels of the socioecological model were further contextualized for in-school adolescents in Uganda using Susan Sawyer's Life Course Perspective on adolescent health interventions. In this model, interventions considered that adolescents' health is affected by biological and social role changes accompanying puberty, which are shaped by social determinants affecting the uptake of health-related behaviors (Sawyer et al., 2012). Also used was the USAID Positive Youth Development (PYD) model (Figure 13.2), which organizes interventions around developing adolescents' assets,

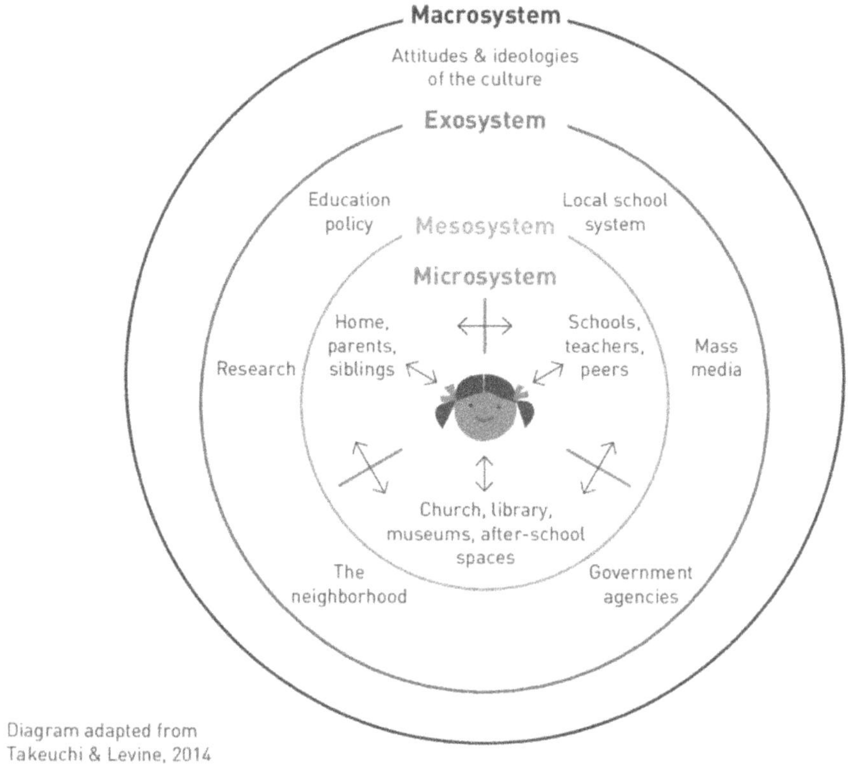

Figure 13.1 Adaption of Bronfenbrenner's ecological framework for human development

agency, and contribution to the project while supporting an enabling environment (USAID, 2019). Fredric H. Jones's Positive Discipline model was also incorporated, focusing on replacing corporal punishment in the classroom with teachers modeling appropriate behavior and building patterns of cooperation between students (Fred Jones Tools for Teaching, 2019).

SAGE theory of change and implementation framework

The SAGE theory of change posited that if adolescents at risk of secondary school dropout are detected through the EWS; an environment supporting reduced violence and positive gender norms is improved at home, in school, and in the community; and life skills interventions are accessible to girls, then adolescent girls will have the agency and social support necessary to stay in school, be violence-free, be HIV-free, and thrive.

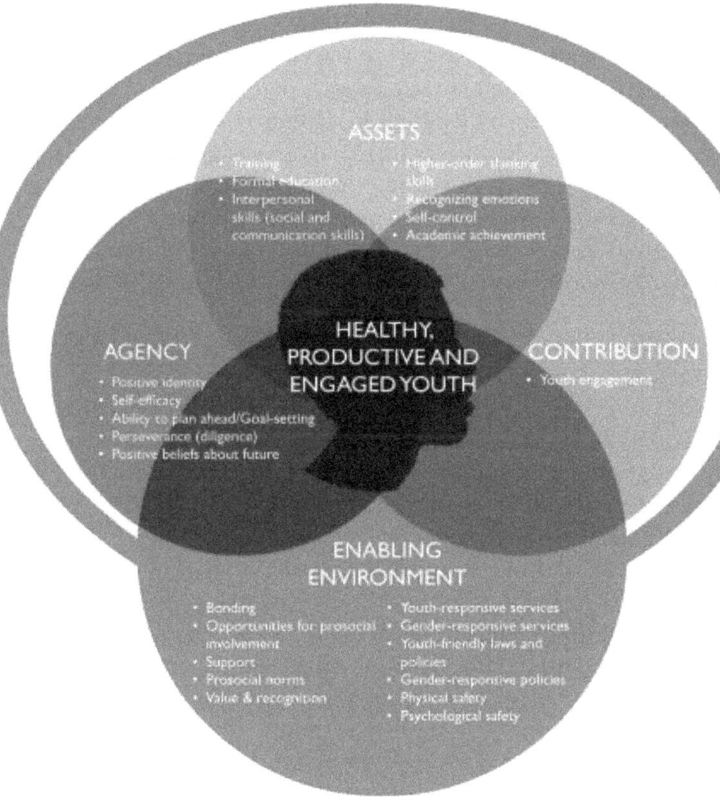

Figure 13.2 USAID Positive Youth Development (PYD) Framework

To respond to the theory of change, the project team developed the EWS package, a school-community monitoring and accountability mechanism helping girls stay in school by addressing all levels of the socioecological model. It involves adolescents, their schools, families, and communities in monitoring students' attendance and taking practical actions to support at-risk students to remain in school. Three key functions of the EWS package are to (1) predict dropout (using the register); (2) prevent dropout (creating an environment where girls are safe and encouraged to learn); and (3) return vulnerable girls to school (through home visits and mentoring) (visit www.worldvision.org/dreams for the full endline report).

The EWS package is an adolescent-led, adult-supported, and evidence-based monitoring and accountability mechanism. Building on guidelines and lessons learned from the five-year (September 27, 2010–September 29,

2015) USAID-funded Asia and Middle East Regional School Dropout Prevention Pilot (SDPP) Program in Cambodia, India, Tajikistan, and Timor-Leste, the SAGE EWS package identified critical vulnerabilities (e.g. economic status, death of one or more parents, parental attitudes towards early marriage) and risk factors (attendance patterns, behavior, and course performance) (SDPP Impact Evaluation, Creative Associates International, and Mathematica Policy Research, 2015). These triggered quick actions at the school and community to reduce dropout. World Vision adapted the model to the Uganda context (visit www.worldvision.org/dreams for the adapted manual) and added the adolescent-led peer educator (PE) innovation and action body structure known as the Stay in School Committee (SISC).

Using readily available school data and a project-designed register, schools track three predictors to identify and intervene with girls at risk of dropping out: attendance, behavior, and course performance (ABC). When a reduction in students' performance or attendance or a negative trend in classroom behavior occurs, teachers flag the girls for follow-up and refer them to the SISC (visit www.worldvision.org/dreamsfinal project report for flagging tool and metrics).

SAGE worked to improve student attendance norms by promoting adolescent leadership and community action to reduce dropout. PEs (adolescent girls in each grade chosen by peers by a vote) were trained in GBV reduction, sexual and reproductive health, HIV prevention, and safe school approaches. Once trained, these adult-supported PEs organized training for their peers according to a set plan. Teachers were trained on GBV reduction, positive discipline, and safe school practices. Communities received mass media and community-based dialogue interventions on girls' education, violence, HIV, and school attendance. Faith communities were trained using World Vision's Channels of Hope, a model that engages faith leaders in behavior change through messaging on relevant issues during faith-related gatherings.

The SISC is the main action and accountability body of the EWS package, where most decision-makers are AGs. Each school's SISC consists of 12 to 15 people: six AG PEs and one teacher, older girl, older boy, mother, father, faith leader, head teacher, and school administrator. Once a girl has been flagged, her case is referred to the SISC, which decides on next steps to ensure the girl is supported. The SISC serves as a school-community body tackling identified causes of absenteeism and monitoring and supporting girls to stay in school through the development and implementation of school-community action-oriented work plans. These work plans include home visits to the flagged girls, mobilizing support for school fees, and addressing safety and health issues as applicable.

Each SISC is held accountable for interventions on behalf of the most vulnerable girls. SISCs decide if a girl needs more support in school, what type of support, and if a home visit is needed. The types of support girls receive include PEs mentoring the girls one on one or in groups, teachers providing counseling and mentoring, fellow students organizing contributions of items the at-risk girls may lack (sanitary pads, money for meals, etc.), finding sponsors for school fees, training to make reusable sanitary pads, helping with notes and homework, and visiting homes to intervene around GBV, early marriage, or financial issues.

The selection and training of SISC members allows them to be effective advocates for AGs. Home visits are conducted by respected members of the community serving on the SISCs, trained on the issues that surround dropouts in this context. Visits usually consist of a meeting with the girl, her family member, and/or village elders. SISC members discuss the importance of girls' education and social issues. For example, the SISC may explain why early marriage is harmful and advocate for the girl to return to school. Often, a SISC member takes the girl back to the school the same day.

The project supported uptake of the EWS, fostered functionality of SISCs, empowered PEs, engaged communities, and helped ensure vulnerable AGs were linked to comprehensive sexual and reproductive health (SRH), HIV, and GBV services. To engage communities beyond the SISC, World Vision trains faith leaders in GBV issues using the Channels of Hope for Gender curriculum (refer to the final project report at www.worldvision.org/dreams for an in-depth description of each project activity).

Data (SAGE baseline and endline)

Previous research indicates school attendance serves as a protective factor against the acquisition of HIV (Stoner et al., 2017). Thus the main objective of this study was to explore the impact of the EWS package in reducing school dropout and increasing school retention among AGs ages 15–19 (as measured by dropouts averted and girls returned to school). The longitudinal study was conducted by Dr. Robert Wamala and his research team based at Makerere University. It gathered data using cross-sectional baseline and endline surveys between 2016 and 2019. The evaluation was meant to demonstrate the extent to which the AG-led EWS helps reduce secondary school dropout among girls. Cross-sectional baseline and endline surveys were conducted for SAGE in 2016 and 2019, respectively. The baseline and endline were conducted in ten intervention districts matched with three comparison (control) districts: Apac, Kayunga and Masaka. In each of these 13 districts, five public secondary schools were randomly selected to serve as supervision areas (SA) for the monitoring of the project performance. Pooled cross-sectional sample surveys conducted at baseline and endline of the project assessed the impact of the project. The quantitative data component of the baseline study was based on a lot quality assurance sampling (LQAS) of AGs and a multi-stage cluster sample of caregivers as described in the subsequent sections.

Survey sampling design

School-based surveys of in-school AGs and community-based surveys of caregivers were conducted. The control and intervention districts were socio-demographically similar. The following sections provide a detailed explanation of the design for each of the topical areas.

Stated study assumptions

1 Percentage of AGs with access to HIV prevention interventions; assumed to be 50% in the target districts.
2 Retention of AGs in Senior 4 in target schools was 34% (MoESTS, EMIS, 2013).
3 Percentage of the AGs with comprehensive knowledge about HIV prevention, care, and treatment; assumed to be 50%.
4 Percentage of parents or caregivers actively involved in strategies aimed at reducing HIV acquisition among AGs and in improving retention of their daughters at school; assumed to be 50%.

Of 151 schools where the program was implemented, this study was conducted in five intervention schools and five control schools in each selected district. In total, there were 1310 participants, 950 participants from intervention schools and 360 from control schools. In the intervention districts, an LQAS sample was selected from each of the randomly selected schools. In each school, a list of AGs aged 15–19, organized by class (Senior 1 to Senior 6), was generated by teachers. A systematic random sample of 19 girls was taken from the list. The endline survey was based on a random sample of schools, not necessarily those visited at baseline. Since there are only three districts in the control arm, a LQAS of 24 AGs was sampled from each of the selected schools. Overall, 15 schools and 360 AGs were selected from control districts. This increase in sample size from the control schools was motivated by the fact that LQAS samples across the intervention schools were to be pooled and compared with results from a pooled LQAS sample across control schools. This comparison assured a minimum detectable effect size of 10% (with 80% power and 95% certainty) due to SAGE interventions. Effect size is related to each of the indicators found in the Tables 13.3, 13.4, and 13.5 with consideration of the study's stated assumptions.

This study's data analysis was done using STATA 13.0 at two stages. First, a descriptive summary of participant characteristics was provided through frequency distributions and summary statistics, where applicable. A similar approach was adopted in describing adolescents based on key indicators. Second, differentials in the four key assumptions above between the control and intervention areas were investigated using the Pearson chi-square test. The test was used to assess differences in distribution of participants

Table 13.1 Description for sampling procedure of adolescent girls per district (baseline and endline)

Group	*# schools*	*Sample size per school*	*# districts*	*# AG participating in baseline*	*# AG participating in endline*
Intervention	5	19	10	950	950
Control	5	24	3	360	360
TOTAL # AG sample size in control + intervention					1310

Note: The schools were adopted as the supervision areas in each district.

Table 13.2 Description for sampling procedure of caretakers per district (baseline and endline)

Group	*# villages*	*Sample size per village*	*# districts*	*# parent/caregiver participating in baseline*	*# parent/caregiver participating in endline*
Intervention	2	21	10	420	420
Control	4	21	3	252	252
TOTAL # parent/caregiver sample size in control + intervention					672

between the control and treatment group. No significant difference in distribution of participants at baseline was found with regards to age, class, religion and living arrangements. The difference-in-difference (DID) analysis shows differentials in project indicators between baseline and endline. DID analysis was based on linear regressions. For each indicator, difference scores were computed between control and treatment at the baseline and then at endline to enable comparisons. These findings are presented in the section "Key Findings of the Pre and Post Surveys".

Limitations

One of the key limitations of the study is the lack of adjustment for confounders. The study used a simple DID analysis based on the assumption that there would not have been a diffusion of the intervention to the control group (i.e. no contamination). The limitation of the study is that it did not test for parallel trend assumption. The DID model makes a counterfactual assumption (parallel trend assumption) that a treatment group would grow at the same rate as a control group if there were no intervention. Another limitation was that there were different sets of participants from the baseline to the endline study. Care was taken to ensure distances between intervention and control schools, decreasing the likelihood of DREAMS programming influencing control schools. Although statistically representative, the survey study examined only a small portion of the total

Table 13.3 Outcome 1: secondary schools strengthened to support adolescent girl retention activities

Section A: Project monitoring data as of March 2019

Indicators	*Project monitoring data 2016*	*Project monitoring data 2019*
Proportion (%) of girls retained in school for life of project	88.5%	99.7%

Section B: Baseline and endline survey data (2016 to 2019; 2.5 years)

Indicators	*Baseline value*			*Endline value*				
	Treat.	*Cont.*	*Diff.*	*Treat.*	*Cont.*	*Diff.*	*Diff. in diff. value*	*p-value*
Proportion (%) of girls 15–19 who report staying/going to school during their menstrual cycle	94.5%	95.9%	–1.4%	97.1%	97.9%	–0.8%	0.6%	0.783
% of AGs absent from school for at least a month in a term during the past 12 months	12.7%	8.8%	3.9%	10.2%	11.1%	–0.9%	–4.8%	0.105
% of AGs enrolled in school during the previous school year prior to the survey	80.7%	81.7%	–1.0%	88.7%	87.4%	1.3%	2.3%	0.539
% of AGs reporting feeling safe and protected in their communities	75.8%	77.7%	–1.9%	82.3%	85.8%	–3.5%	–1.6%	0.686
% of AGs who feel safe and protected while traveling to/from school	68.6%	71.0%	–2.4%	75.2%	73.1%	2.1%	4.5%	0.323

Note: Assessment is made using single difference-in-difference analysis, where proportions are estimated using linear regression; *** $p < 0.01$; ** $p < 0.05$; * $p < 0.1$.

Table 13.4 Outcome 2: HIV prevention activities for adolescents strengthened

Indicators	*Baseline value*			*Endline value*			*Results*	
	Treat.	*Cont.*	*Diff.*	*Treat.*	*Cont.*	*Diff.*	*Diff. in diff. value*	*p-value*
% of AG who correctly reject major misconceptions about HIV transmission	63.2%	61.3%	1.9%	68.8%	75.1%	–6.3%	–8.2%	0.084*
% of AG having comprehensive knowledge about HIV prevention	48.3%	48.8%	–0.5%	49.2%	59.1%	–9.9%	–9.4%	0.066*
% of AG who have taken an HIV test in past 12 months prior to the survey	85.2%	79.3%	5.9%	91.2%	74.5%	16.7%	10.8%	0.030**
% of AG who have taken an HIV test and have been told their results	92.5%	94.4%	–1.9%	96.3%	97.1%	–0.8%	1.1%	0.673
% of AG who have had sexual intercourse	15.6%	9.6%	6.0%	8.0%	9.2%	–1.2%	–7.2%	0.017***
% of AG (15–19) who have had sexual intercourse before the age of 15	33.4%	19.7%	13.7%	26.0%	21.8%	4.2%	–9.5%	0.474

Note: Assessment is made using single difference-in-difference analysis, where proportions are estimated using linear regression; *** $p < 0.01$; ** $p < 0.05$; * $p < 0.1$.

Table 13.5 Outcome 3: increased engagement of all staff, adolescents, parents, and key community stakeholders in discussions on GBV prevention, referrals, care, and treatment

Indicators	*Baseline value*			*Endline value*			*Results*	
	Treat.	*Cont.*	*Diff.*	*Treat.*	*Cont.*	*Diff.*	*Diff. in diff. value*	*p-value*
School-related sexual and gender-based violence								
% of AG who experienced SRGBV (any) in the last 12 months	77.4%	79.9%	–2.5%	65.6%	73.6%	–8.0%	–5.5%	0.197
% of AG who have experienced SRGBV (any) in the last six months	69.5%	69.2%	0.3%	56.4%	63.1%	–6.7%	–7.0%	0.148
Bullying and other forms of non-sexual violence								
% of AG who experienced any form of bullying in past six months prior to the survey	69.1%	74.0%	–4.9%	56.9%	60.1%	–3.2%	1.7%	0.712
% of AG who experienced any form of bullying in past 12 months prior to the survey	72.9%	79.9%	–7.0%	60.7%	63.4%	–2.7%	4.3%	0.340
Corporal punishment								
% of AG experiencing any form of corporal punishment in past six months prior to the survey	77.6%	69.2%	8.4%	64.1%	73.2%	–9.1%	–17.5%	0.000***
% of AG experiencing any form of corporal punishment in past 12 months prior to the survey.	82.7%	80.3%	2.4%	70.9%	76.6%	–5.7%	–8.1%	0.045**

Note: Assessment is made using single difference-in-difference analysis, where proportions are estimated using linear regression; *** $p < 0.01$; ** $p < 0.05$; * $p < 0.1$.

project scope. To address this, the authors further contextualize these findings in later sections of this chapter.

Household/community-based survey of caregivers

In each intervention district, a random sample of two villages was selected. In each selected village, 21 eligible households were sampled through village segmentation. An eligible household was one with at least one in-school AG aged 15–19; only one adult was interviewed in each household. A simple random sample of four villages was also taken in the control districts. In each selected village, 21 eligible households were sampled through village segmentation. The procedure for selecting school-based AGs and community-based caregivers in each of the districts is summarized in Tables 13.1 and 13.2.

In total, 672 completed surveys of parents or caregivers were obtained from the control and intervention areas. This demonstrates a 100% interview completion rate at baseline and endline. Interviews and surveys occurred in schools and communities for both AGs and caregivers, respectively. When an adolescent or caregiver could not be contacted, a replacement was allocated to achieve the required sample size. The figure represents an interview completion rate of 98.5%; this achievement is adequate to provide findings from the selected schools.

Key findings of the pre and post surveys

Table 13.3 indicates that while there were slight improvements across indicators at endline, the intervention showed no significant effects. This is probably due to the limited length of the intervention. Two indicators that showed notable change are AGs who felt safe and protected while traveling to school (4.5% increase) and AGs who felt safe and protected in their communities (1.6% decrease). This seems to demonstrate that school efforts to increase safety were effective, while community interventions were not. This may also demonstrate increased AG awareness of safety issues in their communities as a result of the project's sensitization efforts.

Indicators around HIV prevention and transmission in Table 13.4 show no significant impact ($p < 0.05$). This could be because school retention was the focus, and not enough emphasis was placed on HIV knowledge. However, we see a significant positive effect in the number of AG who took an HIV test (10.8% increase), which is known to be a protective factor against HIV infection. Similarly, we see a significant positive change in AGs who had sexual intercourse and age of sexual debut (with a reduction of 7.2% ever having sex and 9.5% fewer having sex before the age of 15).

Indicators for outcome 3 in Table 13.5 show significant impact. AG who experienced school-related gender-based violence (SRGBV) significantly decreased at 6 and 12 months by 7% and 5.5%, respectively ($p < 0.05$).

Table 13.6 Outcome 4: Gender norms and school participation

Indicators	*Baseline value*			*Endline value*			*Results*	
	Treat.	*Cont.*	*Diff.*	*Treat.*	*Cont.*	*Diff.*	*Diff. in diff. % value*	*p-value*
Gender norms and school participation								
% of AG who disagree with at least three harmful norms and attitudes that violate the rights of AG	46.2%	50.0%	-3.8%	38.6%	49.6%	-11.0%	-7.2%	0.161

Note: Assessment is made using single difference-in-difference analysis, where proportions are estimated using linear regression; *** $p < 0.01$; ** $p < 0.05$; * $p < 0.1$.

This demonstrates a correlation between the length of the project and the reduction of SRGBV experienced by AG. Similarly, bullying decreased by 4.3%. Perhaps most significantly, rates of corporal punishment decreased at 6 and 12 months by 17.5% and 8.1%, respectively, the gains increasing during the project's presence in schools.

Table 13.6 shows a decrease of 7.2% of AGs who disagree with at least three harmful norms and attitudes that violate their rights. This suggests that the normative change interventions attempting to influence attitudes about AG education were successful.

Contextualizing project outcomes

While the externally commissioned study yields important information about the overall project outcomes, SAGE coordinators also collected two other sources of data to contextualize these results. First, SAGE conducted sustained and systematic monitoring data, tracking participants in all intervention schools. SAGE produced monitoring data that corroborated results from the study (higher improvements in school retention at the end of the project). Of the 44,351 AGs supported by the project, 99.7% were retained in school. Of those, 2352 were flagged for SISC action and 95% remained in school after additional support came from SISC members, PEs, and school administration. Through SAGE, 339 girls (14% of those flagged at risk) who had already dropped out or were in the process of leaving received home visits to their parents/caregivers by adult members of a SISC. Of these at-risk girls, only 132 (5.6% of those flagged at risk) dropped out, and 17 of them (13% of dropouts) returned to school. In addition, 31,730 AGs have been mentored by community role models, 5285 have received life-skills training, and 8433 have learned how to make reusable sanitary pads. Also,

23,539 have received HIV testing services through the project, and 509 have been extensively trained and empowered to serve as PEs on the SISC.

Second, SAGE coordinators engaged in longitudinal and sustained qualitative data gathering.

Qualitative methods were employed to collect data from different stakeholders, including focus group discussions (FGD) and key informant interviews (KII). Participants were chosen from ten selected schools and surrounding communities in five intervention districts (Lira, Oyam, Mukono, Mubende, & Mityana) using convenience sampling. Respondent confidentiality was protected by masking traits of individuals or groups that could make them identifiable. A total of 13 KIIs were conducted with teachers, parents, government officials, school administrators, and other key informants using a structured interview guide. Then, 12 FGDs were conducted using a FGD checklist with 6–13 AG or parents in each group. A total of 81 adolescent girls 13–19 years old enrolled in secondary school and 48 parents/caregivers of AG (23 female; 25 male) participated in these FGDs.

These methods were deemed appropriate for collecting both in-depth and community information on knowledge, attitudes, and practices in addition to expert knowledge on the subject matter under assessment: HIV infections among adolescents and secondary school girl child dropout. The qualitative data was used to contextualize the quantitative findings from World Vision's university research partner. The information was also used to explore whether other sociocultural attributes influenced secondary school dropout rates for girls. Responses from the transcribed notes of the interviewer/moderator were assigned codes and labels that were used during data analysis. All data collected were analyzed based on content and selected topics as stated in the terms of reference. This provided the content and thematic analysis for the study (World Vision, 2019). While not the focus of the chapter, these qualitative data raised important insights about the project that were not considered in the externally conducted study.

Challenges

Notable challenges faced during implementation were the lack of conditional cash transfers for school fees, high levels of GBV in the community and schools, and exclusion of boys as direct beneficiaries. These challenges were difficult to overcome due to the project's short length of time for the intervention, as building stakeholder buy-in, piloting, and scaling a project in 151 schools, and being able to work with the AGs only while school was in session did not allow enough time for significant social norms change. Once implementation began, it became clear that many AGs dropped out of school because they lacked financial resources for school fees. This remained a challenge throughout the intervention. While the project team expected GBV to be an issue, the baseline results showed that more than

70% of AGs had experienced SRGBV, which called for a major course correction in programming. Financial and other resources were diverted to extensive GBV-reduction training for teachers, school administrators, and community dialogues. Efforts to shift perceptions on violence against children was one of the biggest challenges that SAGE faced. SAGE enforced policies by training teachers on the risks of corporal punishment and the benefits of using positive discipline in the classroom. This showed notable incremental positive change in social norms around corporal punishment and violence against children (e.g. a decrease of 17.5% in corporal punishment over 2.5 years). This incremental shift encouraged other project approaches, such as the AG-led EWS and peer-to-peer support structures, that enabled PEs to advocate for at-risk girls and for the SISC to act to retain them in school.

More broadly, there remains a disconnect between policy and practice concerning use of school attendance rosters. Most SAGE schools had not regularly taken roll in the classrooms even though government guidelines include this mandate. Teachers often do not understand the economic and social drivers or implications of school dropout, particularly for girls. Similarly, although gender equality is championed at the national level, it is not prioritized in homes and communities in much of Uganda. For example, the SAGE baseline study showed that only 54% of AGs strongly agree with the statement, "Girls and boys have equal opportunity to go to school", and only 56% of parents and caregivers strongly agreed with the statement, "In our community, we believe girls should be educated as much as boys".

Finally, in Uganda, it is uncommon to directly engage adolescents in the implementation of projects. The SAGE project worked within traditional family, gender, and leadership norms to sensitize participating schools and communities on the importance of AG leadership of the project. For instance, maintaining a six-girl majority in the SISC where AGs were decision-makers and equal contributors in a group of adults was unconventional yet instrumental in reaching the target population with the project interventions.

Recommendations and future approaches

Four key recommendations drawn from the projects are (1) school-based projects addressing dropout should include conditional cash transfers for AGs who lack resources for school fees, (2) social and behavioral interventions for AGs should include both interventions for violence reduction and HIV prevention, (3) these social and behavioral approaches should engage AGs and adolescent boys simultaneously, and (4) ample time should be allotted in projects working to change negative social norms around violence, education, and health. Qualitative data showed that most AGs in the project who were at risk of dropping out, or did drop out, were facing an inability to pay for school fees or basic scholastic requirements (World

Vision, 2019). Dropping out meant they had a higher likelihood of engaging in risky sexual behaviors, including relationships with older men who were more likely to transmit HIV (World Vision, 2019; Pettifor et al., 2013). Girls cited lack of school fees as the catalyst that forced them into high-risk situations like sexually exploitative acts, brewing local alcohol, or early marriages. The exclusion of boys and young men from activities is a concern that should be addressed with urgency. This issue is especially salient in contexts where GBV and sexual and reproductive health are strongly associated with HIV prevalence in AGs. Our findings show that boys can be supported to be advocates against perpetrators of violence; boys can also protect themselves from HIV and AIDS, which in turn protects their sexual partners.

At a systems level, engaging with national and local government leaders is recommended to address the gap between national dialogue, policies, and practice. SAGE spent considerable time building awareness of the project among national and district government officials and engaging staff at health clinics and stakeholders in communities and schools. Without these important relationships in place, implementation would have been less effective.

We recommend that adolescents are kept at the core of programmatic strategies. AGs were consulted at each stage of design and implementation and seen as thought leaders. SAGE sought to give PEs an opportunity to grow through life-skills programming, including leadership, communication, sexual and reproductive health, HIV prevention and treatment, and menstrual hygiene management training. In turn, AGs led other aspects of the project, such as mentorship, designing health messages for their peers, and conducting trainings for fellow students. Adolescents must be empowered to take a central role in their health, trust healthcare providers, feel a sense of confidentiality, and be able to access services at convenient times. Although health clinics were engaged and sensitized to serve adolescents, there was not an adequate comprehensive support network, and a gap remains with referrals. Schools should collaborate with health facilities to provide spaces for adolescents to receive relevant health information, responses to their questions, and links to health services. Promisingly, AGs have embraced HIV testing services (HTS) and most now know their status (see Table 13.4).

Further research should seek to better understand why girls drop out of school. Teachers reported that out of 501 AGs who dropped out, 36% (132) had been flagged by the EWS as being at risk. Of those who were not flagged, teachers reported that 24% dropped out due to lack of school fees, 18% dropped out due to pregnancy, 10% changed schools, and 6% got married. AGs who dropped out and who were not flagged by the EWS dropped out for reasons that in-school tracking of ABC predictors may not catch, such as school fees, pregnancy, and changing schools.

SAGE demonstrated the feasibility of implementing a social and behavioral approach to adolescent health promotion that employs a multi-sectoral and combination approach. School-based interventions are recommended because young people do not often visit health clinics and are generally assumed to be healthy (WHO, 2010). These interventions also have the potential to reduce stigma by normalizing HIV testing and counseling and creating an environment where adolescents can support one another to be tested, adhere to medication, and feel connected to their peers. There is great potential in programming that cross-cuts education, gender, and health sectors.

Conclusion

The adolescent-led EWS is a potentially effective tool to identify AGs at risk of dropping out of school and may be successful when scaled up elsewhere (including in primary schools) to reduce HIV-related vulnerabilities. In the three total sets of data (externally conducted survey, monitoring data, and qualitative), the project recommends there is much to be optimistic about with the EWS package.

The project monitoring and qualitative data suggests that the EWS package can effectively predict school dropout. The retention rate for the AG beneficiaries in the 151 schools was 99.7%, compared with a national rate of <70% for girls. This is a remarkable achievement, given that the project did not rely on cash transfers but rather on a combination approach of socio-behavioral interventions bridging the school, home, and community environments of AGs and supporting them to stay in school. The project monitoring and qualitative data indicates that the SAGE model is also highly effective at returning girls to school. Nearly all the girls (95%) identified by the EWS as being at high risk of dropping out were retained in school, including the 17 girls who had already dropped out and returned to school following the SISC intervention. Monitoring data and qualitative results also implied that tracking all three ABC predictors is important to flag all at-risk AGs in different school contexts. While coursework performance had the highest individual predictive value of the ABC predictors (75.4%), 37% of cases were identified by two or three indicators, which suggested that all three have value. The qualitative data suggests that ABC predictors alone are not enough but must be used with a combination package of socio-behavioral approaches for schools and communities to reduce dropout.

Given the complexity of the EWS package, it is important to consider which of the components have the highest prevention value. Increased confidence and empowerment of AGs played a central role in the EWS. Further research should examine programming that increases the number of AGs trained. Positive discipline training encouraged teachers to refrain from corporal punishment. In schools where this was strongly adopted, the qualitative data showed improved teacher-student relationships. Further assessment should look at whether student performance and attendance increased in classrooms where teachers practiced positive discipline. Finally, qualitative data showed that the model was more successful in schools where the head teacher and focal teacher were supportive and engaged and fulfilled their project-specific roles.

The SAGE model appears to be sustainable. Activities were built on already existing resources (people who advocate for girl child education, ministry activities, existing school programs, etc.). Qualitative data indicated that the transition of the EWS implementation to government and school officials should be completed on a school-by-school basis. This will help plan for low-cost continuation of activities, such as linking schools with manufacturers of reusable menstrual pad materials, redesigning the EWS register so it is more affordable to produce, and encouraging the Ministry of Health to include school HTS in their budgets. The SAGE model can be replicated in other contexts outside Uganda. We recommend additional implementation studies in other contexts.

Note

1 World Vision is a Christian humanitarian organization dedicated to working with children, families, and their communities worldwide to reach their full potential by tackling the causes of poverty and injustice.

References

Bronfenbrenner, U. (1979). *The ecology of human development.* Cambridge, MA: Harvard University Press.

Bruce, M., Bridgeland, J. M., Fox, J. H., and Balfanz, R. (2011). *On track for success: The use of early warning indicator and intervention systems to build a grad nation.* Baltimore, MD: Johns Hopkins University, School of Education, Everyone Graduates Center. Available at: http://eric.ed.gov/?id=ED526421.

Coates, T. J., Richter, L., and Caceres, C. (2008). Behavioural strategies to reduce HIV transmission: How to make them work better. *Lancet, 372*(9639), 669–684. doi:10.1016/S0140-6736(08)60886-7.

Creative Associates International, and Mathematica Policy Research. (2015). *Findings from the four country school dropout prevention pilot program impact evaluation.* Available at: http://schooldropoutprevention.com/wp-content/uploads/2016/03/Summary_Findings_Report_English_FINAL.pdf [Accessed 21 July 2019].

Fred Jones Tools for Teaching. *Overview.* Available at: www.fredjones.com/overview [Accessed 7 July 2019].

Govender, K., Masebo, W., Nyamaruze, P., Cowden, R. G., Schunter, B. T., and Bains, A. (2018). HIV prevention in adolescents and young people in the eastern and southern African region: A review of key challenges impeding actions for an effective response. *The Open AIDS Journal, 12,* 53–67. doi:10.2174/1874613601812010053. Available at: https://www.ncbi.nlm.nih.gov/pmc/articles/PMC6062910/

Harrison, A., Newell, M. L., Imrie, J., and Hoddinott, G. (2010). HIV prevention for South African youth: Which interventions work? A systematic review of current evidence. *BMC Public Health, 10,* 102. doi:10.1186/1471-2458-10-102.

Heppen, J.B., and Bowles Therriault, S. (2008). *Developing early warning systems.* Washington, DC: National High School Center, American Research Institutes.

Ministry of Education and Sports Uganda, and Education Information Management System. (2014). *Education and sports sector fact sheet 2002–2015.* Available at: http://education.go.ug/data/dcat/2/Data-and-Statistics.html [Accessed 20 April 2018].

Neild, R.C., Balfanz, R., and Herzog, L. (2007). An early warning system. *Educational Leadership, 65,* 28–33.

Pettifor, A., Bekker, L.G., Hosek, S., DiClemente, R., Rosenberg, M., Bull, S.S., Allison, S., Delany-Moretlwe, S., Kapogiannis, B.G., and Cowan, F. (2013). Preventing HIV among young People: Research priorities for the future. *Journal of Acquired Immune Deficiency Syndromes, 63*(2), S155–S160. doi:10.1097/QAI.0b013e31829871fb.

Pettifor, A., Stoner, M., Pike, C., and Bekker, L. G. (2018). Adolescent lives matter: Preventing HIV in adolescents. *Current Opinion in HIV and AIDS, 13*(3), 265–273. doi:10.1097/COH.0000000000000453. Available at: https://www.ncbi.nlm.nih.gov/pmc/articles/PMC5902132/

Sawyer, S., Afifi, R.A., Bearinger, L.H., Blakemore, S.J., Dick, B., Ezeh, A.C., and Patton, G.C. (2012). Adolescence: A foundation for future health. *Lancet, 379*(9826), 1630–1640. doi:10.1016/S0140-6736(12)60072-5.

Stoner, M. C. D., Pettifor, A., Edwards, J.K., Aiello, A.E., Halpern, C.T., Julien, A., Selin, A., Twine, R., Hughes, J.P., Wang, J., Agyei, Y., Gomez-Olive, F.X., Wagner, R.G., Macphail, C., and Kahn, K. (2017). The effect of school attendance and school dropout on incident HIV and HSV-2 among young women in rural South Africa enrolled in HPTN 068. *AIDS (London, England), 31*(15), 2127–2134. doi:10.1097/qad.0000000000001584.

USAID. (2019). *Positive youth development (PYD) framework.* Available at: www.youthpower.org/positive-youth-development-pyd-framework [Accessed 2 July 2019].

World Health Organization. (2010). *Social determinants of health and well-being among young people: Health behaviour in school-aged children (HBSC) study.* Available at: www.euro.who.int/__data/assets/pdf_file/0003/163857/Social-determinants-of-health-and-well-being-among-young-people.pdf [Accessed 20 April 2018].

World Vision. (2019). *DREAMS: Determined, resilient, empowered, AIDS-free, mentored and safe women.* Available at www.worldvision.org/dreams [Accessed 7 July 2019].

Conclusion

Kaymarlin Govender and Nana K. Poku

The writers of this book have come together to provide critical insights on HIV interventions in terms of 'what works', why they work and the limitations in our knowledge to curb the sexual transmission of HIV among young people across Eastern and Southern Africa (ESA). While the UNAIDS-prescribed prevention targets for 2020 are likely to be missed (UNAIDS, 2020), the writers of the volume are driven by the collective purpose to move swiftly towards ending the HIV pandemic as a public health threat by 2030, if not before.

As we have noted in preceding chapters, across the region, efforts to mitigate the risk for the acquisition of HIV among young people have produced mixed results. This is mostly due to the HIV pandemic being characterised by its heterogeneous and dynamic nature, the slow progress in reducing the number of new HIV infections and the many factors that are linked with the sexual transmission of HIV (see Chapter 1). For several years, adolescent girls and young women (AGYW) have been the 'face' of ongoing acquisition of HIV in the region; young men have been reluctant to seek HIV services with AIDS-related deaths increasing; there are also rising rates of new HIV infections among young key populations (YKP) with widespread prejudice, stigma, sexual exploitation and human rights violations limiting their access to HIV and sexual and reproductive health (SRH) services.

While new HIV infections are stabilising in some of the hardest-hit countries, the rate of new infections is still far too high and the future cost of maintaining an ever-expanding pool of people reliant on daily treatment for survival is unsustainable. Financial resources to support the increasing number of people on antiretroviral treatment (ART) have taken away the investments for intensifying prevention efforts in the region's youthful population. In addition, the span (and costs) of the Sustainable Development Goals (SDGs) have shown that HIV/AIDS is not the only global priority and it now has to share the stage with the growing burden of non-communicable diseases, re-emerging infections and new public health threats such as the coronavirus disease 19 (COVID-19) pandemic.

Speeding up the reduction of new HIV infections and securing and protecting the sexual and reproductive health of young people becomes even more of an imperative to avoid these looming future challenges. In the sections below, we draw on some key insights on 'what works' in preventing the sexual transmission of HIV, discuss gaps in knowledge on the implementation of interventions and present some possibilities for sector wide HIV prevention programming going forward.

What works in addressing psychosocial, behavioural and structural drivers of HIV risk

There is currently a wide range of tools that work for the primary prevention of HIV for different sub-populations, e.g. condoms, voluntary medical male circumcision, oral pre-exposure prophylaxis (PrEP), clean needles as well as risk reduction information and the promotion of specific behaviours, such as regular HIV testing, information sharing between partners about HIV serostatus and the use of HIV viral load monitoring before making decisions about sex and drug-using activities (Hargreaves et al., 2020).

Even so, the effectiveness of these prevention tools among young people in ESA have been limited primarily by the interplay between individual, interpersonal, social and structural factors (Govender et al., 2019a). Interventions to especially address psychosocial, behavioural and structural drivers of HIV risk have not been emphasised in resource allocations and policy dialogues in ESA. Reasons include gaps in knowledge on how to improve women's use of HIV prevention tools, obstacles to challenging prevailing stigmas (stigmas associated with being HIV positive and or having expressions of different gender or sexual orientation) that are associated with poor uptake of prevention services and the difficulties associated with attempting to change cultural norms of masculinity (e.g. inconsistent condom use, multiple sexual partners, low HIV testing behaviours) that ultimately contribute to the spread of HIV. Furthermore, HIV prevention programming is hampered by complexities involved in combining these different types of interventions in certain contexts to substantively reduce new HIV infections. Programming is also impeded by the failure to address human rights, gender and other equity barriers in accessing services. In this section, we draw on some key points made by writers in this book regarding evidence on what works in primarily reducing the sexual transmission of HIV.

Gafos and colleagues, in their review of a decade of evidence (see Chapter 7), discussed the benefits of social and structural interventions that address education, poverty and gender equality to mitigate HIV vulnerability among young people in ESA. The case for increasing educational enrolment is strong, with evidence suggesting that each additional year of schooling reduces the risk of HIV (Barnighausen et al., 2007), particularly for young women. Similarly, school attendance and educational attainment can impact on future socio-economic status, self-esteem, social networks and exposure to HIV prevention education (Jukes et al., 2008). Youth poverty can also be a motivator for engaging in risky sex, as has been emphasised in the results of a recent phylogenetic study showing age disparate sexual partnerships between younger women and older men in a HIV hyper-endemic area of South Africa (De Oliveira et al., 2017). Emerging evidence on the benefits of interventions to alleviate youth poverty has increased the urgency of implementing the UNAIDS fast-track target to strengthen national and child social protection polices (UNAIDS, 2018).

As regards gender-based violence (GBV), research shows that intimate partner violence (IPV) – physical, sexual and psychological – increases susceptibility to HIV among young women (Durevall and Lindskog, 2015; Jewkes et al., 2010). Even though violence among AGYW is seen as a problem that will take generations to change, several GBV interventions have shown that it is possible to reduce GBV incidence and improve HIV risk outcomes (refer to Chapter 7).

More generally, while the evidence for psychosocial and structural interventions for affecting HIV risk pathways is encouraging, there are still significant gaps in our knowledge. We are not clear on exactly how to implement structural interventions in an effective manner in specific settings. Further, mechanisms through which structural interventions operate to mitigate HIV risk and acquisition are not necessarily straightforward or have sustained effects. For instance, in the case of cash transfers interventions to improve school attendance, success is dependent on the nature (conditional or unconditional cash transfers), scope (type of youth that are reached or not reached) and duration of the intervention, including specification of HIV and related outcomes. The significance of context is also aptly demonstrated in the HPTN068 study, which showed that providing equivalent cash transfers in settings with prevailing high levels of social protection (e.g. existing child support grant to poor households, free schooling and school feeding programmes) may not be beneficial to HIV outcomes. Such interventions will have better effects where there is low social protection coverage or low school attendance (Pettifor et al., 2016). Further, incentives to keep girls in schools (as measured only through school attendance) excludes girls who have dropped out of school, those who are pregnant from poor homes (noting that there a few countries in ESA region which have policies that encourage girls to re-enter school after birth of their children, see Chapter 12), leaving them vulnerable to exploitative sexual relationships.

While efforts to shift gender norms and reduce GBV show some promise, outcomes have not been convincing, partly due to the design weaknesses in GBV interventions (lack of standardised measures for gender norms, short-term duration of interventions and failure to directly measure clinical or biological outcomes (pregnancy, HIV incidence). Even so, the entrenched and prevailing gender dynamics that dominate women's lives are a huge challenge for HIV prevention efforts. The recent findings of the ECHO multi-country study in South Africa, Kenya, Eswatini and Zambia is a poignant illustration (Evidence for Contraceptive Options and HIV

Outcomes (ECHO) Trial Consortium, 2019). While the study showed no links between use of birth control methods and HIV infection, it sketches a grim picture of our fight against HIV, where young women continue to bear the brunt of the epidemic. Despite individualised HIV prevention packages provided to all participants during the study, HIV incidence was alarmingly high (infection rate of almost 4%). Even when HIV prevention commodities like condoms were available, condom use was low, reflecting the struggles heterosexual women have to go through in convincing their sexual partners to use condoms.

Female-centred approaches are key to HIV prevention and better sexual health among young people. This can only be realised if their male sexual partners are seen as part of the solution and not just the problem. Mantell and colleagues (see Chapter 9) assert that patriarchal norms (physical strength, sexual domination over women, independence and emotional bluntness) that govern men's behaviours also drive poor health outcomes in men; these norms are developed and institutionalised as boys' transition into adulthood. Men's use of violence within relationships, sexual infidelity and heavy alcohol use have been associated independently with GBV and HIV infection (Jewkes et al., 2014). Shifting hegemonic masculine norms in GBV interventions targeted at young men have produced mixed results (see reviews on interventions targeted at young men in Chapters 7 and 9). For example, young men who completed the GBV Stepping Stones intervention in South Africa (Jewkes et al., 2008) showed lower incidence of herpes infection (HSV-2) and related sexual and alcohol use behaviours, while the Regai Dzive Shiri (Zimbabwe) (Cowan et al., 2010) and the Fataki campaign (Kaufman et al., 2013) showed no effects for shifting gender norms in young men. A more recent full trial of the Stepping Stones and Creating Futures intervention did however show a reduction of men's self-reported perpetration of intimate partner violence, however a similar finding was not present for young women in the study (Gibbs et al., 2020).

Shifting gender/sexual norms for young people is complicated; there is no magic bullet. Gittings and colleagues (see Chapter 10), in their research with young men at risk for HIV, suggest that interventions also should consider the dynamics of engagement (demographic and personal qualities of facilitators, participants, researchers, and programme workers) and contextual mediators (socio-economic, cultural and geographical) that work to influence gender norms. Social change is not linear, rather it is refracted through fluctuating life circumstances of participants, their sexual relationships and the communities in which they live in that ultimately shape HIV risk. Interventions that rely on gender transformative principles through employing critical thinking and learning activities in process-type engagements with participants are more likely to see shifts in social norms. These authors also raise an ethical issue: what does it mean to be working with young men for HIV prevention in settings where women and girls are more biologically and socially vulnerable to HIV infection, especially if such work is seen to compete for the same resources? Interventions with men therefore also needs to be able to articulate how its methods and objectives are aligned with broader feminist principles of inquiry (see, Govender, 2012).

Freedman and colleagues (see Chapter 8) assert that in certain settings, structural factors are more likely to drive inequities in health outcomes for young people. Members of young key populations face, what they term, 'compounded vulnerabilities' since they share a number of specific barriers and challenges concerning their sexual and reproductive health that is linked to legal, social and political structures, which undermine their ability to access healthcare. Social, health and human rights struggles related to citizenship is thus reflected in HIV and SRH outcomes. The authors go on to argue that the paucity of research with young key populations and the neglect in using a more expansive social determinants of health framework (Solar and Irwin, 2010) makes it difficult to decipher and affect pathways linked to better sexual and reproductive health.

Siloed approaches to HIV programming based on rigid categories of social identity and sexual or drug use practices, without the recognition that such practices are in constant flux among young people, are additional barriers to preventing HIV. It therefore seems that a predominantly HIV-dominated intervention response with little attention paid to young people's holistic reproductive health, (including access to contraception, the problem of unintended pregnancy or unsafe abortion) obscures that systemic links between both. This is because SRH challenges bare inextricably linked with HIV prevention efforts (e.g. elimination of mother-to-child transmission of HIV or safer conception strategies). Moving forward requires, first and foremost, addressing the substantial evidence gap surrounding the diverse nature of young people's lives, as well as addressing head-on the prevailing and seemingly intransigent levels of stigma, discrimination and exclusion that drives HIV risk and access to SRH services for these groups. It also entails moving beyond the locality of specific interventions and working more broadly to strengthen HIV and SRH-related rights of young key populations in law, programming and policy (see Levy et al.,'s 2019 review of successful programmes targeting gender inequality and restrictive gender norms).

While biomedical interventions combined with social protection programmes can reduce new HIV infections among young people, it is also important to support those already living with HIV to lead healthy lives, through viral suppression and engaging in safer sex and planned parenthood. Young people living with HIV (YPLHIV) are not a homogenous group. Social vulnerabilities may stem from geographical location (rural, urban), orphanhood (maternal, paternal, dual), length of illness and mode of HIV acquisition (perinatal infection vs behaviourally infected). We are aware of chronic vulnerabilities suffered by children who were perinatally infected with HIV, however recent research also shows that horizontally HIV-infected children are also prone to having poor clinic experiences, lack of ART adherence and multiple psychological challenges (Sherr et al., 2018). The recent findings of the HPTN 084 trial on the effectiveness of a long-acting antiretroviral (ARV) injection now significantly increases options for HIV positive women who struggle to take the daily tablet (WHO, 2020). Zungu and colleagues (Chapter 11) further assert that social support grants, travel vouchers to get to facilities and school lunch programmes are essential to improving adherence in low-resource settings. They also point out that the 'care' element of these combination interventions needs more emphasis. Psychosocial support and care at home and clinics has been strongly associated with reduced unprotected sex, especially among AGYW living with HIV (Toska et al., 2017). An emergent concern is how to strengthen community systems to support ART adherence, enabling beneficiaries' access to livelihood opportunities and health services (Busza et al., 2014). Developing capabilities among people living with HIV to realise their aspirations (completing school, finding employment, managing parenthood) needs to be emphasised in future programming.

The evidence, in sum, suggests that interventions, in combination, that tackle upstream drivers of HIV and SRH risk (gender inequalities, poverty, education, repressive social norms and policies, intersectional stigma) have the potential to interrupt multiple pathways of vulnerability, thereby enabling young people to remain HIV negative and also preventing continued transmission of HIV among YPLHIV. As such, no single casual pathway can be drawn from a single social or structural driver to a set of practices or behaviours; rather, a range of potential outcomes may arise. Making inferences about correlations between drivers of HIV risk and HIV burden, therefore, involves identifying 'sociologically plausible' pathways drawn from extant social sciences literature and epidemiological data (Auerbach, Parkhurst and Caceres, 2011).

A key resource for developing relevant HIV prevention interventions is knowledge and experiences *in situ,* together with knowledge about how young people navigate and are made vulnerable by structural challenges in specific contexts. This approach will help explain why adolescent girls (15-19 years) acquire HIV much earlier in some countries in the region (e.g. South Africa and Kenya, see chapter 1). Cowden and colleagues (in Chapter 2), in elucidating pathways of HIV risk use a psychosocial and development approach to show that transitions from childhood to young adulthood is associated with potentially disruptive role transitions (especially with the onset of puberty) and social and economic inequalities often amplify risk for HIV. These authors also emphasise how people can develop capabilities (resiliency) through drawing on a range of resources (both individual and social) to buffer these environmental insults (Ungar, 2004). The developmental processes associated with life course transitions are not necessarily linear (Sameroff, 2009) and devoid of context. These ideas resonates with the 'slow research' agenda that has been gaining ground recently (Adams et al., 2014), where in-depth understandings of context and locally constructed experiences of sexual risk and health can also be relevant to HIV prevention (see earlier work on AIDS-competent communities and health enabling environments (Campbell et al., 2009).

Based on the above, prevention interventions with young people needs to consider not only 'what prevention interventions work' but under 'what circumstances' and 'who is the target population' of interest. The importance of recognising the heterogeneity of a single population and the need for differentiated HIV prevention approaches is evidenced in the HIV prevention cascade perspective. The 'prevention cascade' is useful because it provides a guide to the design and monitoring of HIV prevention programmes through a multi-pronged approach that includes demand-side interventions, supply-side interventions and adherence interventions (Hargreaves et al., 2016; 2020). Therefore, interventions that are well conceptualised, with intersectoral partnerships and finely attuned to local realities of young people are more likely to be effective in preventing HIV (see Chapter 13, where DeSoto and colleagues discuss their lessons learnt from a community-based HIV program to reduce school drop-out among adolescent girls).

Conversely, questions also remain about the scalability and relevance of HIV interventions within the rapidly evolving and sector-wide approaches to health programming. The many health and development priorities facing nations in the ESA region, in the light of dwindling resources, mean that opportunities for synergies outside the HIV sector is now urgent and necessary. In the following section, we put forward some considerations for future HIV prevention programming.

Evolving the prevention response: synergies, co-investments and contextual enablers

The Sustainable Development Goal (SDG) 3, healthy lives and well-being and pandemic preparedness, presents some opportunities and challenges for a more inclusive approach to HIV/AIDS programming, given that limited global resources for HIV programming are being spent on HIV prevention (Resch, Ryckman and Hecht, 2015). The value of a synergetic type approach is that when opportunities exist to address one set of issues; this can lead to multiple development outcomes (Isbell et al., 2016).

As indicated previously, there is now overwhelming evidence in ESA for an interlinked set of structural drivers leading jointly to poor HIV and SRH outcomes (e.g. unwanted pregnancies, poor access to contraception among AGYW as a result of gender inequalities and poverty is linked with higher concentrations of HIV infection).

There is also evidence for a range of structural HIV interventions to mitigate poverty, poor education and GBV that can achieve multiple downstream impacts: keeping girls in school, improving future livelihoods and improving HIV and sexual health outcomes.

At national levels, HIV programming in ESA has been historically premised on government and development assistance for health (DAH) funding being very rigid, vertical and disease-specific (Sundewall and Forsberg, 2020), with non-HIV sectors and funders not willing to consider the spillover effects of their policies and programmes on HIV, or vice versa. Notwithstanding these institutional challenges, the shift towards holistic healthcare under the banner of Universal Health Coverage (UHC) (Political Declaration of the High-level Meeting on Universal Health Coverage, 23 September 2019) has spurned the need for delivering a basic package of health services (across different sectors and different SDG targets) (also refer to: The global financing facility framework for women, children and adolescents: Roadmap for advancing gender equality, 2020). Investing across a broad set of HIV and SRH interventions to address the most common health needs of the population is being typically defined in a country's essential health-care package, with such a package becoming increasingly central to how resources, including DAH should be allocated (Sundewall and Forsberg 2020).

Cost-effectiveness data has also shown that pooling of resources across sectors through a co-financing mechanism can jointly improve HIV and related health outcomes (Remme et al., 2014). Conceptual shifts towards integrated approaches (HIV and SRH) to health delivery have already occurred; for example the Southern Africa Development Community (SADC) implemented the Minimum Standards for the Integration of HIV and Sexual and Reproductive Health (Southern African Development Community, 2015); (also note the Eastern and Southern Africa (EAC) Ministerial Commitment to Comprehensive Sexuality Education, 2013).

Even so, there are many challenges to implementing multi-sectoral health programming in low-resource settings which include: different prioritization processes, predominance of single-modality economic models, poor domestic resource mobilisation and institutional barriers to adopting co-financing models (limited financial autonomy of government and non-government budget holders, potential loss of budget control and threats to current institutional arrangements) (Remme and Mcguire, 2018). In addition, funding for health is scattered across government ministries and external donors, which complicates resource allocation for essential health benefits packages, with lost opportunities for HIV prevention also being incurred. More feasibility work is required to assess the practicalities of operationalizing the co-financing approach in governmental planning and budgeting. In addition, there is a need to support in-country technical capacity to improve local capability and ownership in recording and analyzing data, and to support health planning and budget allocation exercises as well as increasing reliance on domestic funding (Remme et al., 2014).

Apart from operational challenges related to delivery of health packages (which include HIV and SRH services), there are ongoing dialogues with between government and stakeholders on the key elements of these health benefits packages. While HIV basic services are covered, key SRH services are sometimes not included because of political, religious, legal and moral concerns (e.g. safe abortion services, interventions for MSM communities, people who sell sex and people who inject drugs) (refer to Prioritising Essential Packages of Health in Six countries in Sub Saharan Africa report, 2019). The point is aptly made by Machawira and colleagues (see Chapter 12) that even with EAC Commitments to Comprehensive Sexuality Education, most country policies and sociocultural environments are still not conducive to reaching the goals of empowerment-based sexuality education for young people.

So how should we ensure sector-wide participation in prioritization processes for health service packages? Inclusivity and transparency are indeed challenges, and civil society needs to hold governments and other health providers more accountable. There are examples where advocacy by gender activists for inclusion of specific health services has worked (e.g. inclusion of cervical cancer services as part of an essential health package in Eswatini; National Cancer Prevention and Control Strategy, 2019). Activating multiple constituencies to obtain more accurate and timely in-country data on HIV, SRH and other health indicators to inform decision-making is important. The All In approach for optimizing HIV data on adolescents in ESA countries, through engaging players across the health and development sectors, is a multi-sectoral strategy which has shown some promise (see Armstrong and colleagues, Chapter 4).

At a regional level, African intergovernmental bodies have elaborated a wide array of policy documents that address the health and well-being of young people, many of them connected to HIV and SRH programming. Even so, many of these frameworks are top down, with insufficient emphasis on building national ownership, coupled with faltering political will and lack of consultation and accountability to constituents (Gabelnick and colleagues, see Chapter 3). Advocacy for regional HIV and SRH programming is not new, especially given the links between HIV and migration in a rapidly growing youthful population in sub-Saharan Africa (Iliffe, 2006). There are some good examples of cross-border health initiatives that cater for health needs of mobile and remote populations (e.g. North Star Alliance Roadside Wellness Clinics along trucking routes in ESA; Govender et al., 2019b), but enabling foreign migrants to access HIV and SRH services in 'receiver' countries is a growing challenge (Gupta et al., 2012) with some arguing for the establishment of regional health passports as an option for improving regional health and security (Šehović, see Chapter 6).

While country efforts towards UHC are being formalised, we should however not lose important research, policy and programming opportunities to strengthen investments in programming for particularly young and marginalised groups (AGYW, YPWSS, MSM, LGBTI communities). Our experience on investing in reducing new HIV infections among AGYW through evidence based and multi-sectoral programming (e.g. PEPFAR-funded DREAMS HIV prevention programming; Global Fund programming to reduce human rights barriers to accessing HIV and SRH services, see Chapter 3) has provided some key lessons on implementation, it also raises some general issues for future programming. How can we collectively capitalise on these opportunities and use them as avenues to engage with young people themselves on the multiple issues affecting their lives? Why is embracing diversity among young people is key to effective HIV/and SRH research and programming? How would the prioritisation of young people increase prospects for more inclusive and ethically sound research, policy and programming?

Misalignments with international and regional human rights laws and commitments compromises young people's fundamental health rights because of insufficient guidance on how to navigate the legal-ethical complexities associated with capacity to consent for research on HIV and access to SRH services (UNFPA, 2017). Behaviours deemed illegal (under-age consensual sex, same-sex behaviour, sex work) could mean the systematic exclusion of vulnerable participants who are potential beneficiaries of such research and interventions. Given these imperfect legal frameworks that exist in many countries in ESA, Strode and Slack (see Chapter 5) assert that we should be more transparent on how we make decisions regarding the nature and extent of issues entailed in consenting and participation processes. Adolescents should also understand the personal implications of consent to research, the extent of privacy clauses and requirements of mandatory reporting. Adopting approaches to adolescent participation in HIV and SRH research needs to be thoughtful, well-grounded in relevant ethics principles (The United Nations General Assembly, 1989) and guided by their *primary* role to protect research participants rather than to adopt the role of law enforcement. In-country, research ethics committees (RECs) are key institutions who play a role in determining whether adolescent protocols are 'ethically acceptable' and sometimes will have to make uncomfortable decisions to enable balanced, nuanced, well-justified ethical approaches.

In sum, if we are to capitalise on emerging synergies in policy and programming for HIV and related health outcomes, we then need to address multiple contextual enablers. These include more granular-level data on HIV and SRH drivers to improve programme efficiencies and better decision-making; strong political will with inclusiveness in decision-making; intergovernmental mechanisms to facilitate programming and accountability; strong monitoring and evaluation frameworks; cost effective analysis with local expertise for implementation.

At a wide-ranging level, there is also a need to capacitate civil society to push for investments in social and human rights programming to reduce forms of stigma, shift harmful social norms and promote social inclusion of its sexually and gender diverse minorities. More support is required for public interest litigation, training and advocacy to advance sexual and human rights of young people and instigate reform of national laws that do not comply with international human rights law (Southern African Litigation Centre 2017). It is encouraging to note the current and ongoing advocacy work for law and policy reform (UNFPA, 2017). The recent landmark decision by the high court of Botswana (on June 11, 2019) decriminalizing same-sex sexual contact (Collison, 2019) has been as a result of long-term public activism and support by human rights organizations. There could be many sexual and reproductive health gains for all if more societies on the continent could honor, celebrate and protect the innate diversity of human sexuality. The immediate likelihood of a broader and similarly inspired wave of change across the region looks uncertain, but Botswana has shown that it is possible.

The evidence for social and structural interventions in reducing new infections among young people has shown that progress is indeed possible (see also reviews by Harrison et al., 2015; Govender et al., 2018), however as we have outlined thus far, there are indeed many challenges in getting the difference sectors to work together, achieve health and development synergies, promote the full inclusion of its diverse citizenry, improve efficiencies in programming and benefit from joint outcomes.

The SDG framework offers new hope to realise our ultimate goal in getting to zero new HIV infections through integrated HIV and SRH programming (under UHC) and opportunities to deliver multiple impacts at scale. While there is a need for integrated services, optimal paths will differ between settings, populations and services. In the strive for UHC, there is a genuine risk of wholesale relinquishment of the exceptionalism approach to HIV (Bekker et al., 2018) AIDS exceptionalism has brought an array of human, financial and technical skills to fighting the HIV epidemic. It has also ensured global commitment to producing systemic, incremental interventions and also to engaging diverse communities in far reaching ways. As global attention shifts towards achieving the SDG 3 goal of universal health coverage, there needs to be a rigorous appraisal of the risks and benefits of mainstreaming the HIV and SRH response into national health systems. Ending the HIV epidemic for young people requires more resources, global commitment to addressing related health issues, and more emphasis on people-centred systems.

References

Adams, D.A., Jajosky, R.A., Ajani, U., Kriseman, J., Sharp, P., Onweh, D.H., Schley, A.W., Anderson, W.J., Grigoryan, A., Aranas, A.E. and Wodajo, M.S. 2014. *Summary of notifiable diseases – United States, 2012.* https://europepmc.org/article/med/27736829.

Auerbach, J.D., Parkhurst, J.O. and Caceres, C.F. 2011. Addressing social drivers of HIV/AIDS for the long-term response: Conceptual and methodological considerations. *Global Public Health,* 6(Suppl 3), S293–S309.

Barnighausen, T., Hosegood, V., Timaeus, I.M. and Newell, M.L. 2007. The socioeconomic determinants of HIV incidence: Evidence from a longitudinal, population-based study in rural South Africa. *AIDS,* 21(Suppl 7), S29–S38.

Bekker, L.G., Alleyne, G., Baral., S, Cepeda, J., Daskalakis, D., Dowdy, D., . . . Beyrer, C. 2018. Advancing global health and strengthening the HIV response in the era of the sustainable development goals: The International AIDS Society-Lancet Commission. *Lancet (London, England),* 392(10144), 312–358. doi:10.1016/S0140-6736(18)31070-5.

Busza, J., Besana, G.V., Mapunda, P. and Oliveras, E. 2014. Meeting the needs of adolescents living with HIV through home based care: Lessons learned from Tanzania. *Children and Youth Services Review,* 45, 137–142, February.

Campbell, C., Nair, Y., Maimane, S. and Gibbs, A. 2009. Strengthening community responses to AIDS: Possibilities and challenges. In P. Rohleder, L. Swartz and S. Kalichman (Eds.), *HIV/AIDS in South Africa 25 years on* (pp. 221–235). London: Springer Verlag.

Collison, C. 2019. Botswana decriminalises homosexuality in historic judgment. *Mail and Guardian,* 11 June. https://mg.co.za/article/2019-06-11-botswana-high-court-ruling-a-victory-for-countrys-queer-communities [Accessed 22 July 2019].

Cowan, F. M., Pascoe, S. J., Langhaug, L. F., Mavhu, W., Chidiya, S., Jaffar, S., Mbizvo, M. T., Stephenson, J. M., Johnson, A. M., Power, R. M., Woelk, G., Hayes, R. J. and Regai Dzive Shiri Trial, T. 2010. The Regai Dzive Shiri project: Results of a randomized trial of an HIV prevention intervention for youth. *AIDS,* 24, 2541–2552.

De Oliveira, T., Kharsany, A., Gräf, T., Cawood, C., Khanyile, D., Grobler, A., Puren, A., Madurai, S., Baxter, C., Karim, Q. and Karim, S. 2017. Transmission networks and risk of HIV infection in KwaZulu-Natal, South Africa: A community-wide phylogenetic study. *Lancet HIV,* 4, e41–e50.

Durevall, D. and Lindskog, A. 2015. Intimate partner violence and HIV in ten sub-Saharan African countries: What do the demographic and health surveys tell us? *Lancet Glob Health,* 3, e34–e43; Cross-sectional study. *PLoS One,* 6, e24256.

Eastern and Southern Africa (ESA). 2013. *Ministerial Commitment Meeting and Affirmation Ceremony.* Report [pdf]. www.youngpeopletoday.org/wp-content/uploads/2018/06/2013-ESA-Commitment-Report_Feb.pdf.

Evidence for Contraceptive Options and HIV Outcomes (ECHO) Trial Consortium. 2019. HIV incidence among women using intramuscular depot medroxyprogesterone acetate, a copper intrauterine device, or a levonorgestrel implant for contraception: A randomised, multicentre, open-label trial. *Lancet (London, England),* 394(10195), 303–313. doi:10.1016/S0140-6736(19)31288-7.

Gibbs, A., Dunkle, K., Ramsoomar, L., Willan, S., Jama Shai, N., Chatterji, S., Naved, R. and Jewkes, R. 2020. New learnings on drivers of men's physical and/or sexual violence against their female partners, and women's experiences of this, and the implications for prevention interventions. *Global health action,* 13(1), 1739845. doi: 10.1080/16549716.2020.1739845.

Global Financing facility: Roadmap for advancing gender equality. 2020. https://www.globalfinancingfacility.org/sites/gff_new/files/documents/GFF-Roadmap-for-Advancing-Gender-Equality_EN.pdf

Govender, K. 2012. Researching young masculinities: Theorizing processes of identification in the research setting. *International Proceedings of Economics Development & Research,* 31, 234–238.

Govender, K., Masebo, W., Nyamaruze, P., Cowden, R. G., Schunter, B. T. and Bains, A. 2018. HIV prevention in adolescents and young people in the Eastern and Southern African region: A review of key challenges impeding actions for an effective response. *The Open AIDS Journal,* 12, 53–67. doi:10.2174/1874613601812010053.

Govender, K., Cowden, R. G., Oppong Asante, K., George, G. and Reardon, C. 2019a. Sexual risk behavior: A multi-system model of risk and protective factors in South African adolescents. *Prevention Science.* Advance online publication. doi:10.1007/s11121-019-01015-3.

Govender, K., Beckett, S., Masebo, W., Braga, C., Zambezi, P., Manhique, M., . . . Durevall, D. 2019b. Effects of a Short Message Service (SMS) Intervention on Reduction of HIV Risk Behaviours and Improving HIV Testing Rates Among Populations located near Roadside Wellness Clinics: A Cluster Randomised Controlled Trial in South Africa, Zimbabwe and Mozambique. *AIDS and Behavior,* 23(11), 3119–3128.

Gupta, R. K., Jordan, M. R., Sultan, B. J. et al. 2012. Global Trends in antiretroviral resistance in treatment-naive individuals with HIV after rollout of antiretroviral treatment in resource settings: A global collaborative study and meta regression analysis. *Lancet*, 380, 1250–1258.

Hargreaves, J. R., Delany-Moretlwe, S., Hallett, T. B., Jonson, S., Kapiga, S., Bhattacharjee, P., Dollabetta, G. and Garnett, G. P. 2016. The HIV prevention cascade: Integrating theories of epidemiological, behavioural, and social science into programme design and monitoring, London school of hygiene and tropical medicine, London. *Lancet HIV*, 3, e318–e22. doi:10.1016/S2352-3018(16)30063-7.

Hargreaves, JR., Davey, C., Auerbach, J., Blanchard, J., Bond, V., Bonell, C., Burgess, R., Busza, J., Colbourn, T., Cowan, F., Doyle, A., Hakim, J., Hensen, B., Hosseinipour, M., Lin, L., Johnson, S., Masuka, N., Mavhu, W., Mugurungi, O., . . . Yekeye, R. 2020. Three lessons for the COVID-19 response from pandemic HIV. *The Lancet HIV*, 7(5). doi:10.1016/S2352-3018(20)30110-7.

Harrison, A., Colvin, C.J., Kuo, C., Swartz, A. and Lurie, M. 2015. Sustained high HIV incidence in young women in Southern Africa: Social, behavioral, and structural factors and emerging intervention approaches. *Current HIV/AIDS Reports*, 12(2), 207–215. doi:10.1007/s11904-015-0261-0.

Iliffe, J. 2006. *The African AIDS epidemic: A history*. Oxford: James Currey.

Isbell, M. T., Kilonzo, N., Mugurungi, O. and Bekker, L.-G. 2016. We neglect primary HIV prevention at our peril. The Lancet HIV, 3(7).

Jewkes, R., Nduna, M., Levin, J., Jama, N., Dunkle, K., Puren, A. and Duvvury, N. 2008. Impact of stepping stones on incidence of HIV and HSV-2 and sexual behaviour in rural South Africa: Cluster randomised controlled trial. *British Medical Journal*, 337, a506.

Jewkes, R. K., Dunkle, K., Nduna, M. and Shai, N. 2010. Intimate partner violence, relationship power inequity, and incidence of HIV infection in young women in South Africa: A cohort study. *Lancet*, 376, 41–48.

Jewkes, R., Gibbs, A., Jama-Shai, N., Willan, S., Misselhorn, A., Mushinga, M., Washington, L., Mbatha, N. and Sikweyiya, Y. 2014. Stepping stones and creating futures intervention: Shortened interrupted time series evaluation of a behavioural and structural health promotion and violence prevention intervention for young people in informal settlements in Durban, South Africa. *BMC Public Health*, 14.

Jukes, M., Simmons, S. and Bundy, D. 2008. Education and vulnerability: The role of schools in protecting young women and girls from HIV in Southern Africa. *AIDS*, 22(Suppl 4), S41–S56.

Kaufman, M. R., Mooney, A., Kamala, B., Modarres, N., Karam, R. and Ng'wanansabi, D. 2013. Effects of the Fataki campaign: Addressing cross-generational sex in Tanzania by mobilizing communities to intervene. *AIDS Behaviour*, 17, 2053–2062.

Levy, J.K., Darmstadt, G.L., Ashby, C., Quandt, M., Halsey, E., Nagar, A., and Greene, M.E. 2019. Characteristics of successful programmes targeting gender inequality and restrictive gender norms for the health and wellbeing of children, adolescents, and young adults: a systematic review *Lancet Glob Health*, 8: e225–36.

National Cancer Prevention and Control Strategy. 2019. *Report* [pdf]. Ministry of Health Kingdom of Eswatini. www.iccpportal.org/system/files/plans/ESwatini%20NCCP%202019.pdf [Accessed 22 July 2019].

Pettifor, A., Macphail, C., Hughes, J. P., Selin, A., Wang, J., Gomez-Olive, F. X., Eshleman, S. H., Wagner, R. G., Mabuza, W., Khoza, N., Suchindran, C., Mokoena, I., Twine, R., Andrew, P., Townley, E., Laeyendecker, O., Agyei, Y., Tollman, S. and Kahn, K. 2016. The effect of a conditional cash transfer on HIV incidence in young women in rural South Africa (HPTN 068): A phase 3, randomised controlled trial. *Lancet Global Health*, 4, e978–e988.

Prioritizing Essential Packages of Health Services in Six countries in Sub-Saharan Africa. 2019. *Partnership for Maternal, Newborn & Child Health.* https://www.who.int/pmnch/media/news/2019/Full-report.pdf [Accessed 15 Sep. 2020].

Political Declaration of the High-level Meeting on Universal Health Coverage "Universal health coverage: moving together to build a healthier world" 23 September 2019. https://www.who.int/news-room/events/detail/2019/09/23/default-calendar/un-high-level-meeting-on-universal-health-coverage

Remme, M. and Mcguire, F. 2018. *STRIVE technical brief: Development synergies and co-financing.* London: STRIVE.

Remme, M., Vassall, A., Lutz, B., Luna, J. and Watts, C. 2014. Financing structural interventions: Going beyond HIV-only value for money assessments. *AIDS*, 28(3), 425–434.

Resch, S., Ryckman, T. and Hecht, R. 2015. Funding AIDS programmes in the era of shared responsibility: An analysis of domestic spending in 12 low-income and middle-income countries. *Lancet Global Health*, 3(1), e52–61.

Sameroff, A. 2009. The transactional model. In A. Sameroff (Ed.), *The transactional model of development: How children and contexts shape each other* (pp. 3–21). Washington, DC: American Psychological Association.

Sherr, L., Cluver, L. D., Toska, E. and He, E. 2018. Differing psychological vulnerabilities among behaviourally and perinatally HIV infected adolescents in South Africa - Implications for targeted health service provision. *AIDS Care*, 30(Suppl 2), 92–101. doi:10.1080/09540121.2018.1476664.

Solar, O. and Irwin, A. 2010. *A conceptual framework for action on the social determinants of health* (76 p.). Geneva: WHO World Health Organization. http://www.who.int/social_determinants/publications/9789241500852/en/

Southern Africa Development Community (SADC). 2015. *Minimum standards for the integration of HIV and sexual and reproductive health in the SADC region* [pdf]. http://menengage.org/wp-content/uploads/2016/09/Minimum-Standards-for-Integration-of-HIV-and-SRH-in-SADC-Region.pdf.

Southern Africa Litigation Centre. 2017. *Human rights of key populations in Southern Africa Southern Africa litigation centre.* www.southernafricalitigationcentre.org/annual-reports-and-newsletters/ [Accessed 22 July 2019].

Sundewall, J. and Forsberg B. C. 2020. Understanding health spending for SDG 3. *The Lancet*, ISSN: 0140-6736.

The United Nations General Assembly. 1989. *Convention on the rights of the child: Adopted and opened for signature, ratification and accession by general assembly resolution 44/25 of 20 November 1989.* https://ec.europa.eu/anti-trafficking/sites/antitrafficking/files/un_convention_on_the_rights_of_the_child_1.pdf.

Toska, E., Pantelic, M., Meinck, F., Keck, K., Haghighat, R. and Cluver, L., 2017. Sex in the shadow of HIV: A systematic review of prevalence, risk factors, and interventions to reduce sexual risk-taking among HIV-positive adolescents and youth in sub-Saharan Africa. *PLoS One*, 12(6), p.e0178106. https://doi.org/10.1371/journal.pone.0178106

UNAIDS. 2018. *Social protection: A fast-track commitment to end AIDS. Guidance for policy-makers, and people living with, at risk of or affected by HIV.* Geneva: UNAIDS.

UNAIDS. 2020. Fast-track: Ending the AIDS epidemic by 2030. https://reliefweb.int/report/world/fast-track-ending-aids-epidemic-2030-0

UNFPA. 2017. *Harmonizing the legal environment for adolescent sexual and reproductive health and rights: A review of 23 countries in East and Southern Africa.* Johannesburg: UNFPA.

Ungar, M. 2004. A constructionist discourse on resilience: Multiple contexts, multiple realities among at-risk children and youth. *Youth & Society*, 35(3), 341–365. doi:10.1177/0044118X03257030.

WHO. 2020. Trial results reveal that long-acting injectable cabotegravir as PrEP is highly effective in preventing HIV acquisition in women. https://www.who.int/news/item/09-11-2020-trial-results-reveal-that-long-acting-injectable-cabotegravir-as-prep-is-highly-effective-in-preventing-hiv-acquisition-in-women

Index

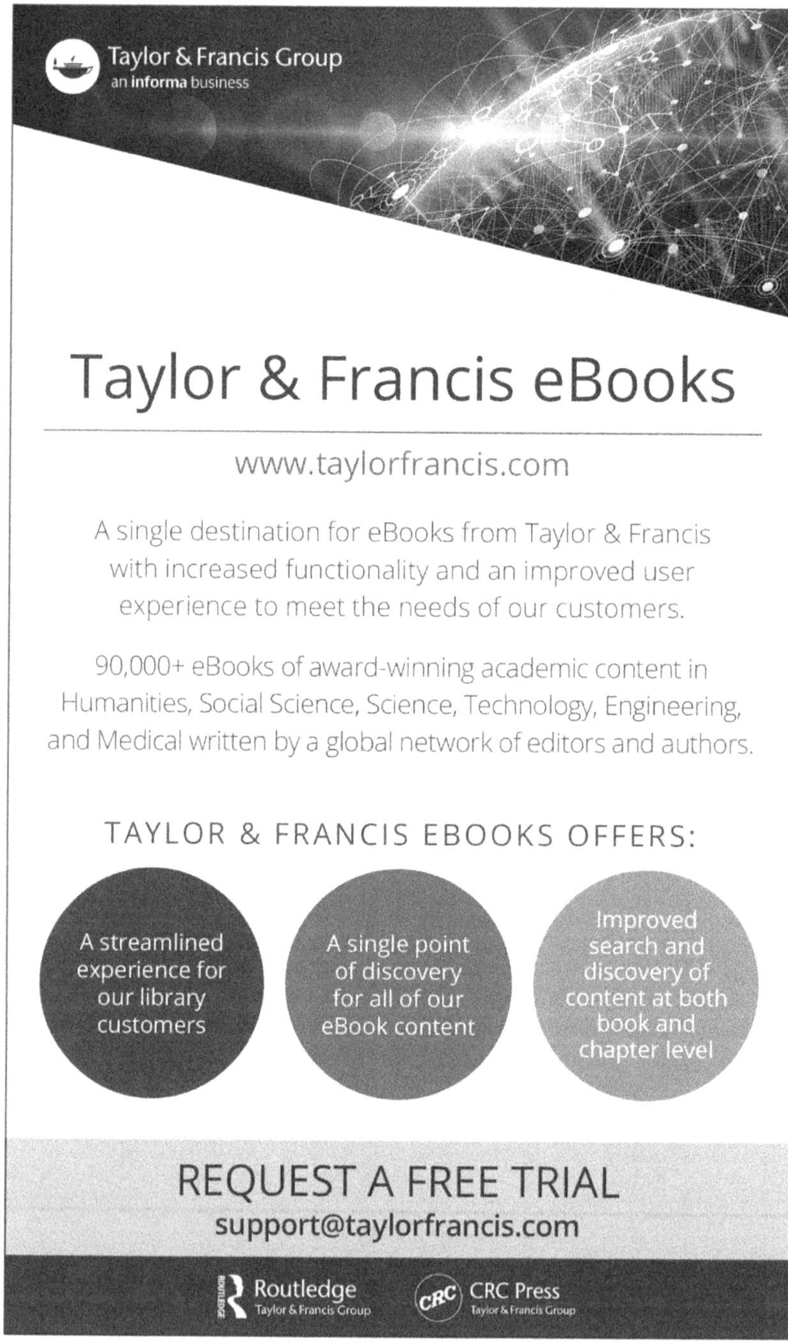
Taylor & Francis Group
an informa business
Taylor & Francis eBooks
www.taylorfrancis.com
A single destination for eBooks from Taylor & Francis with increased functionality and an improved user experience to meet the needs of our customers.
90,000+ eBooks of award-winning academic content in Humanities, Social Science, Science, Technology, Engineering, and Medical written by a global network of editors and authors.
TAYLOR & FRANCIS EBOOKS OFFERS:
A streamlined experience for our library customers
A single point of discovery for all of our eBook content
Improved search and discovery of content at both book and chapter level
REQUEST A FREE TRIAL
support@taylorfrancis.com
Routledge
Taylor & Francis Group
CRC Press
Taylor & Francis Group